Total Hip Replacement: Techniques and Complications

Total Hip Replacement: Techniques and Complications

Edited by Fisher Lloyd

STATES
ACADEMIC PRESS
www.statesacademicpress.com

States Academic Press,
109 South 5th Street,
Brooklyn, NY 11249, USA

Visit us on the World Wide Web at:
www.statesacademicpress.com

ISBN: 978-1-63989-526-7

Cataloging-in-Publication Data

Total hip replacement : techniques and complications / edited by Fisher Lloyd.
p. cm.
Includes bibliographical references and index.
ISBN 978-1-63989-526-7
1. Total hip replacement. 2. Hip joint--Surgery. 3. Total hip replacement--Complications. I. Lloyd, Fisher.
RD549 .T68 2022
617.581 059 2--dc23

Table of Contents

Preface

This book was inspired by the evolution of our times; to answer the curiosity of inquisitive minds. Many developments have occurred across the globe in the recent past which has transformed the progress in the field.

Total hip replacement is a surgical procedure which is used to treat fracture, arthritis or other conditions which restrict the movement of the hip joint. The surgery involves removing and replacing the damaged cartilage and bone with prosthetic components. The hip joint implants are composed of two parts, a ball portion and a socket portion. These two components can be either press fit or cemented into place. The technique for the surgery is chosen on the basis of the strength and quality of the bone. A combination of the two with a non-cemented socket and a cemented stem can also be used. From theories to research to practical applications, case studies related to all contemporary topics of relevance to total hip replacement have been included in this book. It elucidates new techniques and their applications in a multidisciplinary manner. The book is appropriate for students seeking detailed information in this area as well as for experts.

This book was developed from a mere concept to drafts to chapters and finally compiled together as a complete text to benefit the readers across all nations. To ensure the quality of the content we instilled two significant steps in our procedure. The first was to appoint an editorial team that would verify the data and statistics provided in the book and also select the most appropriate and valuable contributions from the plentiful contributions we received from authors worldwide. The next step was to appoint an expert of the topic as the Editor-in-Chief, who would head the project and finally make the necessary amendments and modifications to make the text reader-friendly. I was then commissioned to examine all the material to present the topics in the most comprehensible and productive format.

I would like to take this opportunity to thank all the contributing authors who were supportive enough to contribute their time and knowledge to this project. I also wish to convey my regards to my family who have been extremely supportive during the entire project.

Editor

1

Failure Mechanisms in Hip Resurfacing Arthroplasty

Hiran Wimal Amarasekera

Abstract

Hip resurfacing arthroplasty has been a popular alternative for total hip replacement in young active patients since the early 1990s.

Early results have been promising and a large number of arthroplasties were performed in the United Kingdom, North America, and Western Europe during the last decade. However, due to a series of complications, such as pseudo-tumours, femoral neck fractures avascular necrosis and aseptic loosening, the long-term results were poor and failure rate has been high.

This chapter attempts to identify the different biological and biomechanical mechanisms that may contribute to these failures. It also discusses some considerations to be noted when designing resurfacing implants in the future.

This is a research study based on the author's primary research work carried out with retrieval specimens taken from failed hip arthroplasties.

Keywords: Hip Resurfacing, pseudo-tumours, retrieval specimens, metal-on-metal designs, surgical approaches, avascular necrosis, aseptic lymphocyte-dominated vasculitis-associated lesions (ALVAL)

1. Introduction

1.1. History

The concept of hip resurfacing arthroplasty or surface replacement of the hip was originally introduced by John Charnley in the 1950s [1] but had to abandon the idea due to high wear rate [2]. Since then, many surgeons, such as *Wagner et al* [3], have been using hip resurfacing arthroplasty as an alternative to total hip replacements (THR). [4, 5]

Due to high wear rate and metal plastic debris giving rise to a number of complications, this procedure did not gain popularity among orthopaedic surgeons until the early 1990s.

1.2. Modern hip resurfacing

In the early 1990s, there was resurgence in hip resurfacing arthroplasties when *McMinn et al.* introduced metal-on-metal-resurfacing. [6] Instead of metal-on-plastic, the design was changed to metal-on-metal. Since then, there has been a rapid increase in hip resurfacing throughout the world mainly in Europe, the United Kingdom [7], and North America peaking in late the 90s and the early part of this decade. [8]

The main reasons for this popularity among surgeons were the advantages of hip resurfacing as compared to the conventional hip replacements such as minimal bone loss, less dislocation rates, and easier conversion to a revision. Due to these factors resurfacing was introduced mainly as an alternative to THR in young active adults. [9] Modern hip resurfacing also addressed the problems associated with previous designs. The new design was built using better materials (metal-on-metal), modified surgical techniques including new surgical approaches, and better instrumentation for implant positioning. [10]

1.2.1. Indications for modern hip resurfacing

Indications were broad-based, but the ideal candidate is described as young, active adult males in their late forties to early sixties [9] with good bone stock having primary or secondary osteoarthritis.

Hip resurfacings have been done in young females [11], including patients with dysplasia and avascular necrosis (AVN) of the femoral head. [12]

1.2.2. Complications of hip resurfacing

There are many complications associated with hip resurfacing some are common for any orthopaedic procedure such as infection, nerve palsy, deep vein thrombosis, and dislocation. Even though the complications are similar the complication rates differ between hip resurfacing and total hip arthroplasty.

These complications can be classified in many ways:

1. Based on common and specific: Common to all hip arthroplasties and specific to hip resurfacing
2. Based on timing: Early and late
3. Based mainly on site of failure; femoral or acetabular components: Femoral, acetabular, both, or none

Common complications to all hip arthroplasty procedures include bleeding, nerve damage, deep vein thrombosis, malpositioning of implants, and dislocations. Out of these, dislocation is relatively rare in hip resurfacing compared to THR due to the larger size head in the femoral component. However, the large head increase the surface area and can lead to high wear rates leading to eventual failure. Malpositioning is a contributory factor for the high wear rates. [13]

The complications that are more specific to hip resurfacing arthroplasty can be further divided into early and late complications.

The early complications are usually seen within the first weeks to the early years. These are loosening of implants, femoral neck fractures, femoral head notching [14] and AVN. [15]

The late complications are set of complications recognized recently, following the long-term outcome of patients. [16] Among these are osteolysis, pseudo-tumours, bone resorption, ALVAL, loosening of components, high metal ion levels in blood, and tissue metallosis. These complications can eventually lead to failure of the hip resurfacing implant. [17, 18]

2. Causes of failure/complications in hip resurfacing

1. AVN of the femoral head
2. Loosening of implants
3. Femoral neck fractures
4. Impingement
5. High metal ion levels in blood
6. Metallosis
7. Pseudo-tumours formation
8. ALVAL
9. Resorbtion of head

2.1. Pathogenesis of early complications

It is widely believed that early complications such as AVN, femoral neck fractures, and loosening of implants, are mainly associated with the decrease in the blood flow to the femoral head. Understanding the basic mechanisms of failure in each complication will help us to prevent these at present and design better implants in the future.

2.1.1. Reducing blood flow to the femoral head possibly leading to AVN and implant failure

This has been mainly attributed to the posterior surgical approach that reduces the femoral head blood flow by damaging the branches of the medial circumflex femoral artery. Unlike in THR where the femoral head and neck is removed in resurfacing the neck and part of the head is preserved, the blood flow to this area appear to play a crucial role in the long-term outcome. This is the main reason why many surgeons have challenged the posterior approach. Alternatively many surgical approaches have been tried. Many studies have attempted to demonstrate this by comparing the blood flow between posterior and other approaches [19 - 22].

Ganz et al has described trochanteric flip approach as an alternative surgical approach to the posterior approach to be used during hip resurfacing to preserve the blood flow. [23]

Even though many studies show a clear drop in blood flow intra-operatively during posterior approach, post-operatively some studies fail to establish a clinical significance and a direct link to this fall as a cause of AVN; other studies show this as a transient drop that recovers during the post-operative period [24]. Some have argued that AVN is not caused by the procedure. [25] Some have even used hip resurfacing as a treatment option for patients having established AVN and Perthes disease. [12, 26, 27, 28]

Due to these reasons, many studies have been conducted comparing different surgical approaches when hip resurfacing is performed. This has also led to many different surgical approaches being tried by many surgeons in the past decade. [29] The posterior, poster-lateral [30], direct lateral, Ganz trochanteric flip [31], direct anterior [32], and antero-lateral [33] approaches. [34] Some complications of resurfacings shown in Fig 1A-1C.

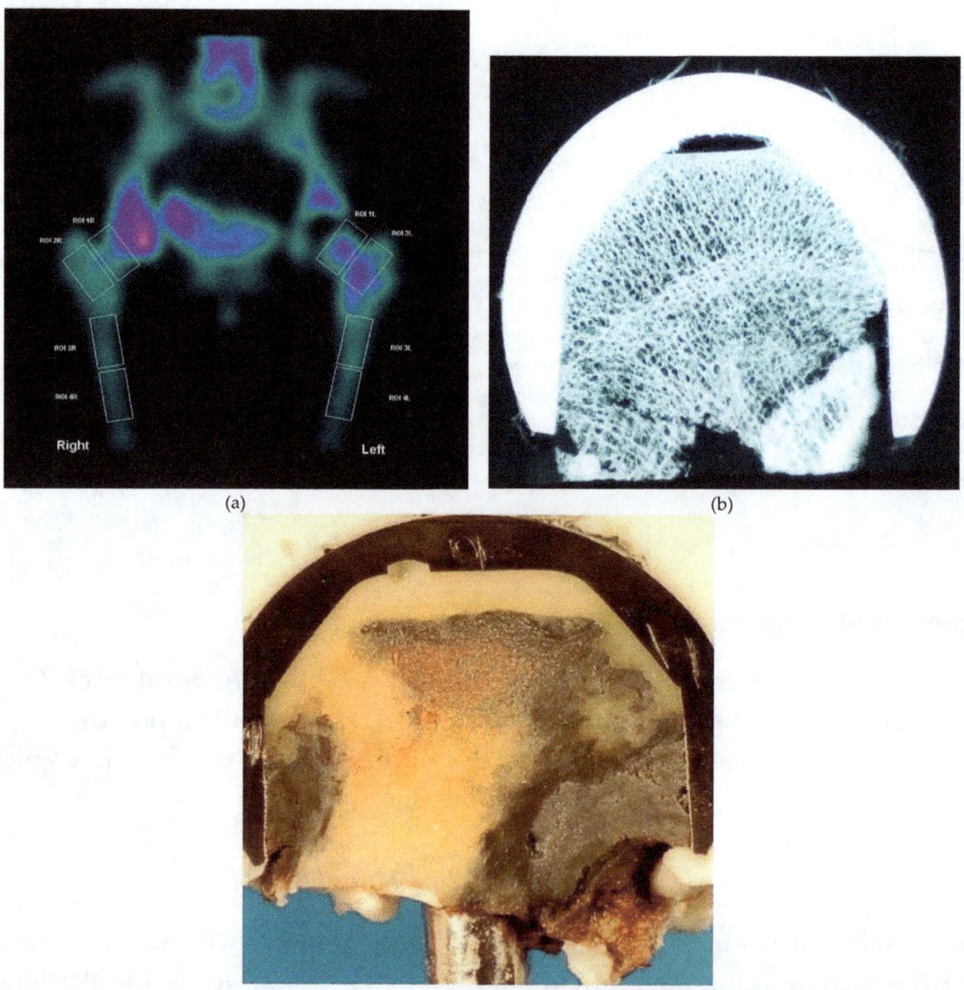

Figure 1. (a). Single cut section of a Single Positron emission Computed Tomography (SPECT) image. The most likely areas to develop AVN and fractures are ROI L (L: Operated, R: Normal). (b). Mocroradiograph shows bone thinning under the metal implant with a fracture at the lower margin. (c). The cut section of a retrieval head with metallosis and early pseudo-tumour formation

2.1.2. Femoral neck fractures following hip resurfacing

Femoral neck fractures is a common and specific complication of hip resurfacing (Fig. 1B and 2). There are many factors attributed to this including AVN, poor patient selection (patients with osteoporosis such as older age groups, post menopausal female patients), and poor implant positioning that may cause notching. [15] Some also believe that notching may affect the blood flow. [14] Proper patient selection and careful surgical technique is important to minimise neck fractures. [35 - 37]

The ideal patient for hip resurfacing is the young active adult male. [38] Hip resurfacing in post-menopausal females is not recommended. Hip resurfacing in younger females is a debatable issue among many surgeons as revision rates and femoral neck fractures appear to be higher in females than in males. [39] Bone density and good bone stock appear as an important feature to prevent complications. [40] Obesity is another risk factor for neck fractures. [35]

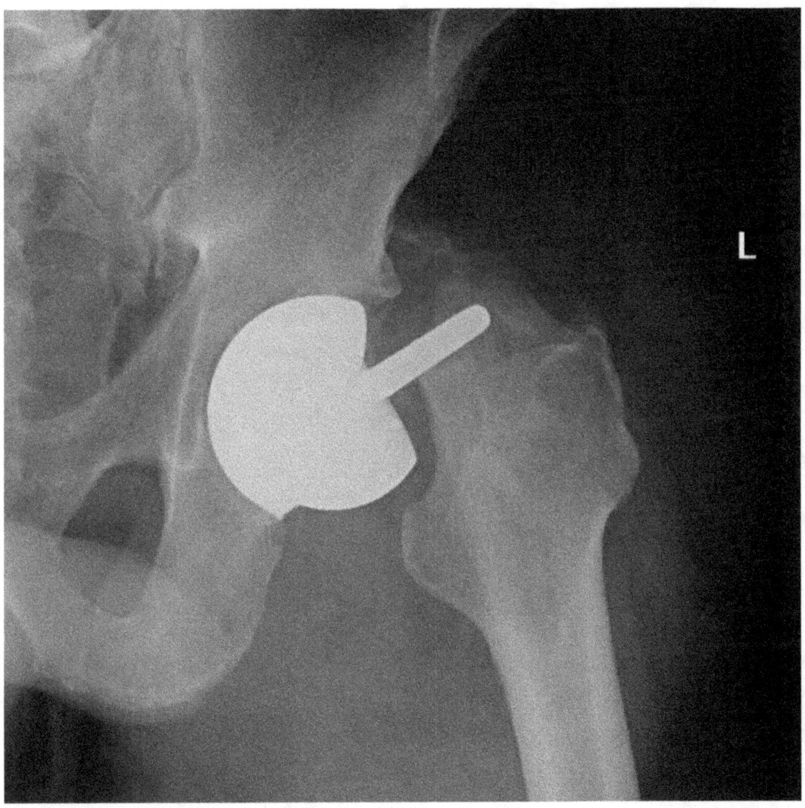

Figure 2. X-ray of a femoral neck fracture following hip resurfacing arthroplasty

2.1.3. Loosening of components

Loosening of components is another cause for early and late failure of resurfacing, mainly acetabular failure, in young adults. [41] Loosening can be further divided to acetabular, femoral or both. Loosening of components can be due to many reasons. Poor positioning, poor cementing, poor surgical technique, and infection can all cause loosening. Even though cementing of both components are common, some prefer cementing the femoral head with un-cemented acetabular component, while some do not use cement at all. [42, 43] Initial failure rates for cemented acetabular component were high and led to the re-introduction of the cementless components. [44] If cement is used, the cementing technique becomes a key factor in improving long and short-term results. [45] Another complication associated with cementing is the possibility of thermal necrosis (Fig. 3) that can lead to loosening and this needs to be minimised for better outcomes. [46]

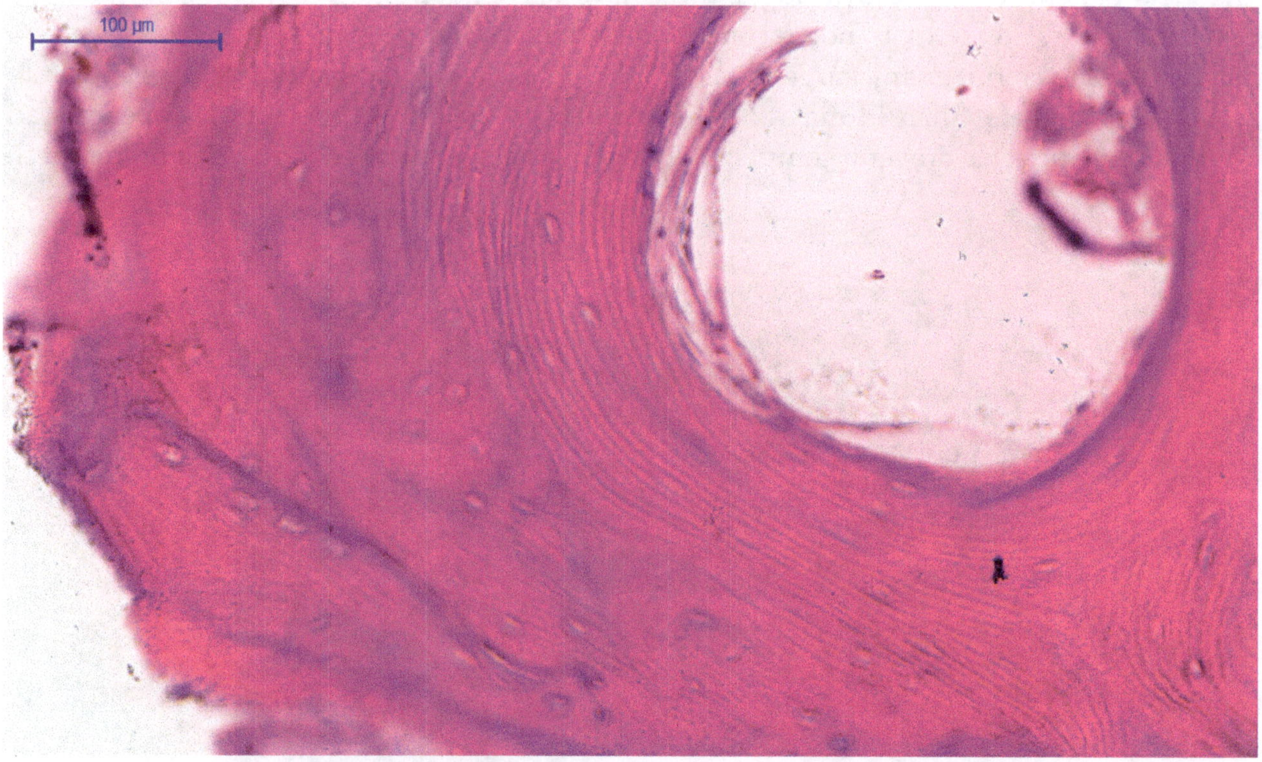

Figure 3. Features of necrosis at the margin of cemented implant with empty lacunae, most likely due to thermal necrosis (Cement metal interface) (H & E 20X)

2.2. Pathogenesis and possible mechanisms of failure in late complications

Most late complications that lead to eventual failure of the implants seem to be associated with high wear rates leading to increased metal ion released to soft tissues and blood leading to the following changes:

1. High metal ions in the blood
2. Metal sensitivity
3. Metallosis in tissues
4. ALVAL
5. Development of pseudo tumours (Fig. 4)

6. Osteolysis

7. Bone resorption

Pseudo-tumours have been reported [47] following resurfacing arthroplasty (Fig. 1C and 4). In a Canadian study of around 3,400 hips, pseudo-tumours were reported in four, giving a prevalence of 0.10%. [48].

The commonest hypothesis suggested for pseudo-tumour formation is the release of metal ions due to the increased surface area and malpositioning of implants. [49] This triggers a delayed Type IV hypersensitivity reaction leading to osteolysis and ALVAL presenting as pseudo tumours. [50 - 53]

Acetabular component malpositioning appear to cause more ALVAL formation due to high wear. [50, 54, 55] Blood metal ion levels, mainly Cobalt and chromium (Co and Cr), have been found to be high following resurfacing arthroplasty but the link between high blood ion levels and the formation of pseudo-tumours is not well established. [56] Some studies suggest the presence of asymptomatic pseudo-tumours with high blood ion levels among patients after resurfacing arthroplasty (RA). [57]

Blood metal ion levels may be high following both THR and RA, as many studies suggest [58 - 61], but the local effect on the hip may differ between the two.

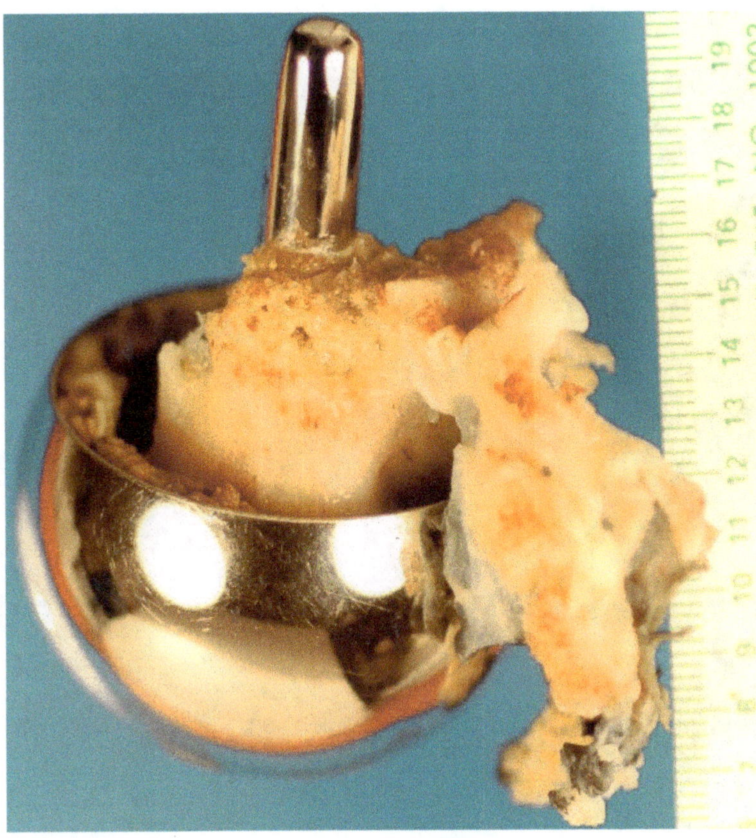

Figure 4. Retrieved head with extensive resorption of head osteolysis and growth of a pseudo-tumour

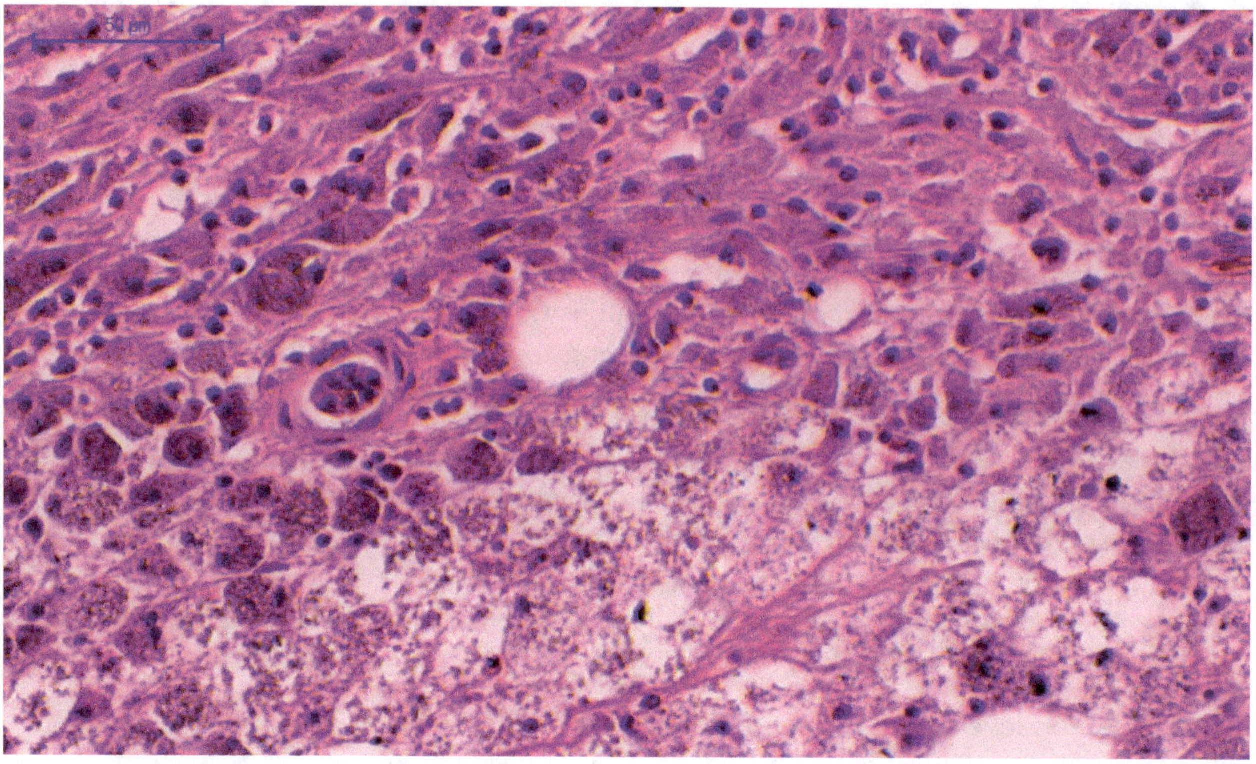

Figure 5. Large number of lymphocytic infiltration with metal particles engulfed macrophages forming multinucleated foreign body Giant cells (H & E 40X)

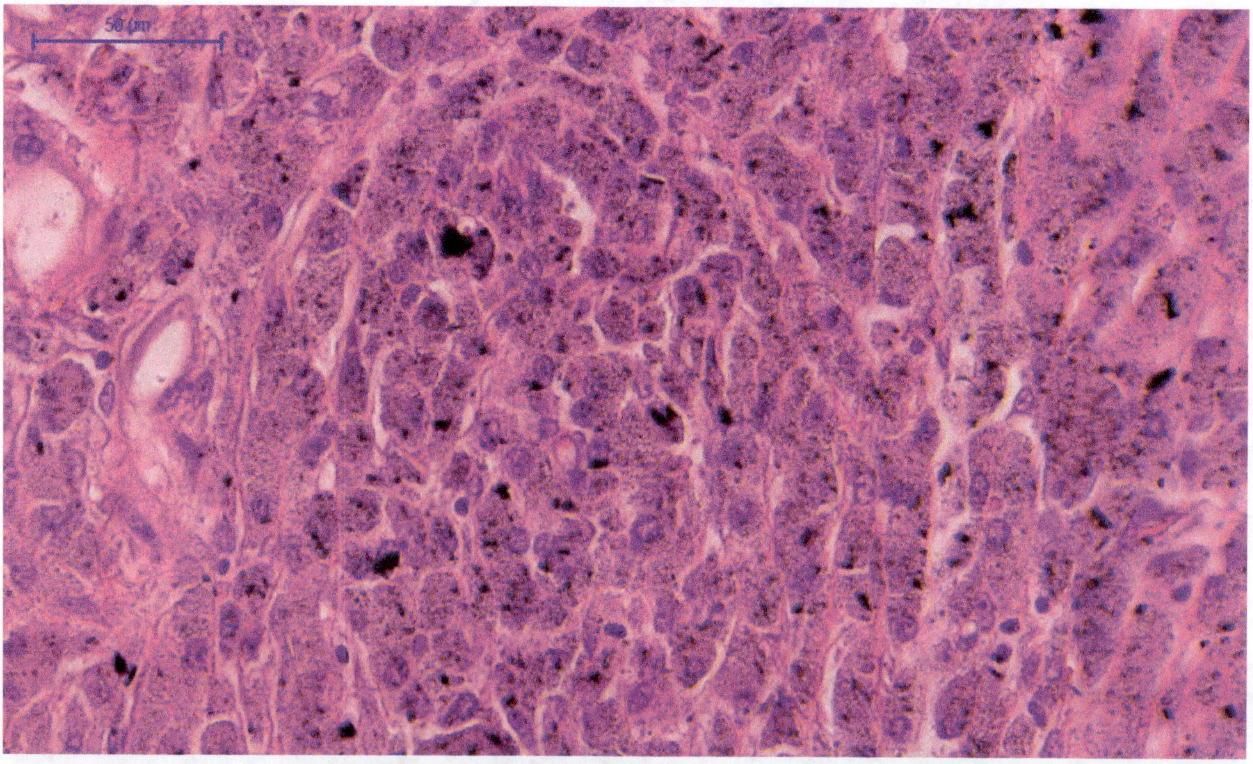

Figure 6. Large number of metal particles (black) seen in bone tissue from a retrieved femoral head (H & E 40X)

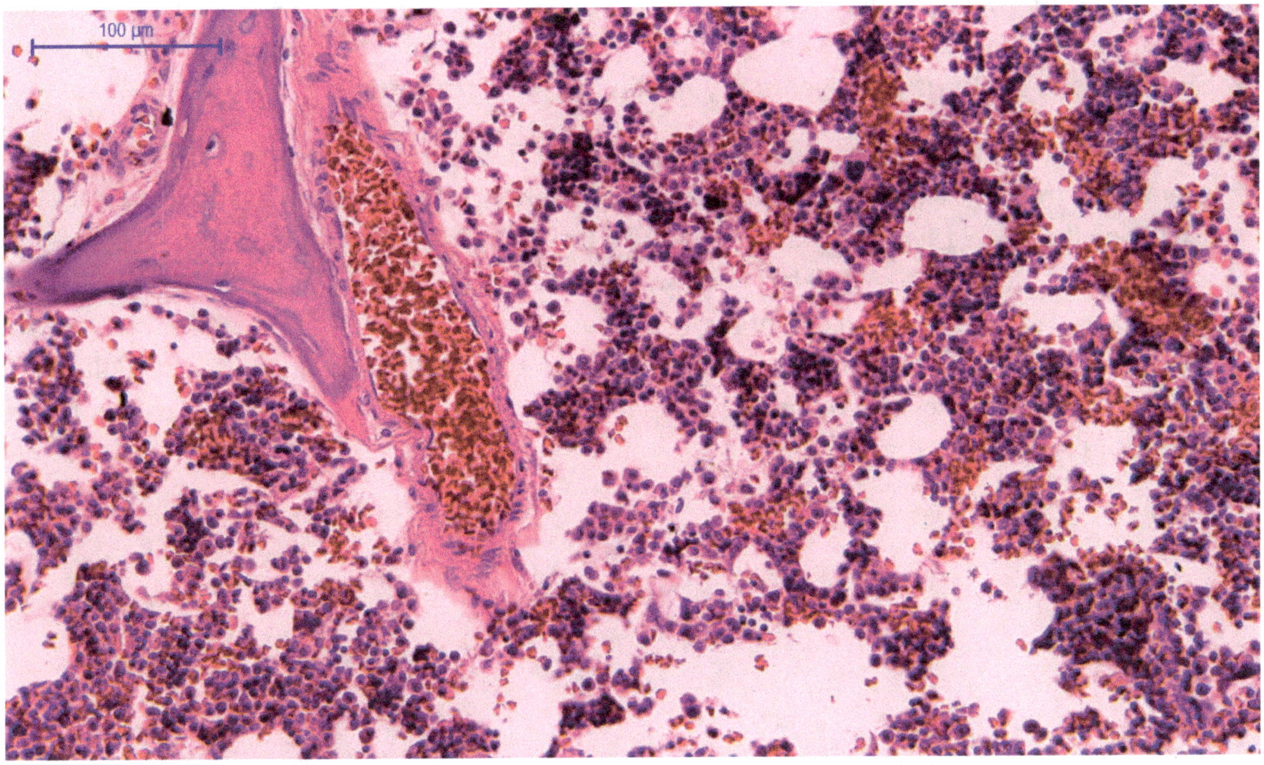

Figure 7. Highly vascular bone in osteolysis and pseudo-tumour formation showing a blood vessel, aggregation of lymphocytes inflammatory cells, and live bone characterised by nucleated lacunae (H & E 20X)

Pseudo-tumours appear to be highly vascular with blood vessels red blood cells, lymphocytes macrophages, and inflammatory cells with live bone until osteolysis occurs. (Figs. 1C, 5–7)

Common cause for aseptic failure of acetabular component is most likely due to osteolysis triggered by the metal particles. [62]

3. Hypothesis of late failure in hip resurfacing

After considering multiple factors that seem to contribute to the eventual failure of the resurfacing implant, I have recognized two possible pathways that may lead to the failure of the implant in the late stages. These are:

3.1. Uncoordinated osteoblast-osteoclast activity

This process seems to be similar to the process seen in fracture healing. However, compared to fracture healing, which occurs in a well-coordinated systematic stepwise manner, here it happens haphazardly. In osteoblastic activity, new bone formation and signs of healing is seen in one part of the bone; simultaneously, osteolysis bone breakdown and remodelling with osteoclastic activity is seen in the other end. Bone remodelling is a process that is essential in the healing of a bone where a fine balance exists between osteoclastic activity and osteoblastic activity. When this fine balance is broken, uncontrolled osteoclastic activity can cause destruction on a large volume of the femoral head leading to complete osteolysis and bone resorption. This is an uncoordinated process and as long as the initial stimuli that triggered remains, the process seems to continue and eventually leading to bone resorption.

This can present as loosening, pain, malpositioning, and femoral neck fractures. Over activity of osteoclasts initially lead to focal areas of destruction (Fig. 10) that eventually leads to osteolysis of the whole femoral head (Fig. 13). However, in patients where osteoclasts and osteoblast act in a normal coordinated way, well-formed new bone growth can occur resulting in a well-fixed and stable metal/cement bone interface (Fig. 12). The factors that cause increased uncontrolled osteoclasts activity are not clearly understood. This is an area that will need further research. In this series, we found both patterns in patients. A hypothesis of the probable pathway is given below (Fig. 8).

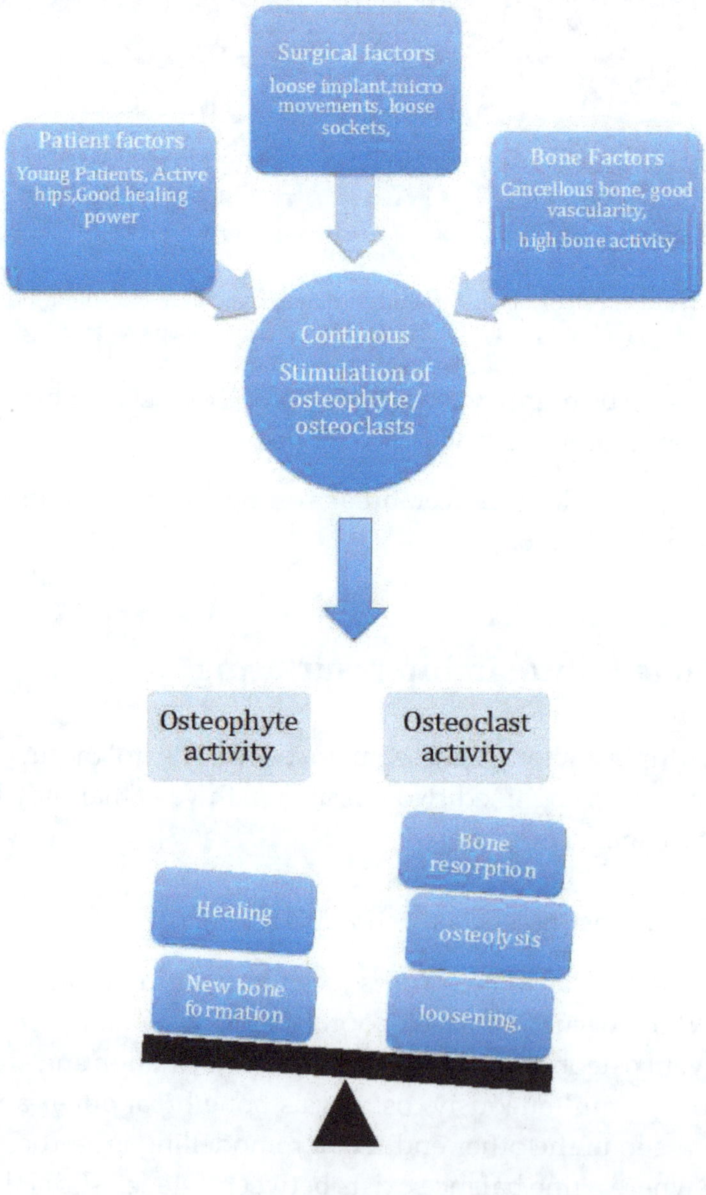

Figure 8. Multiple factors leading to increased bone activity

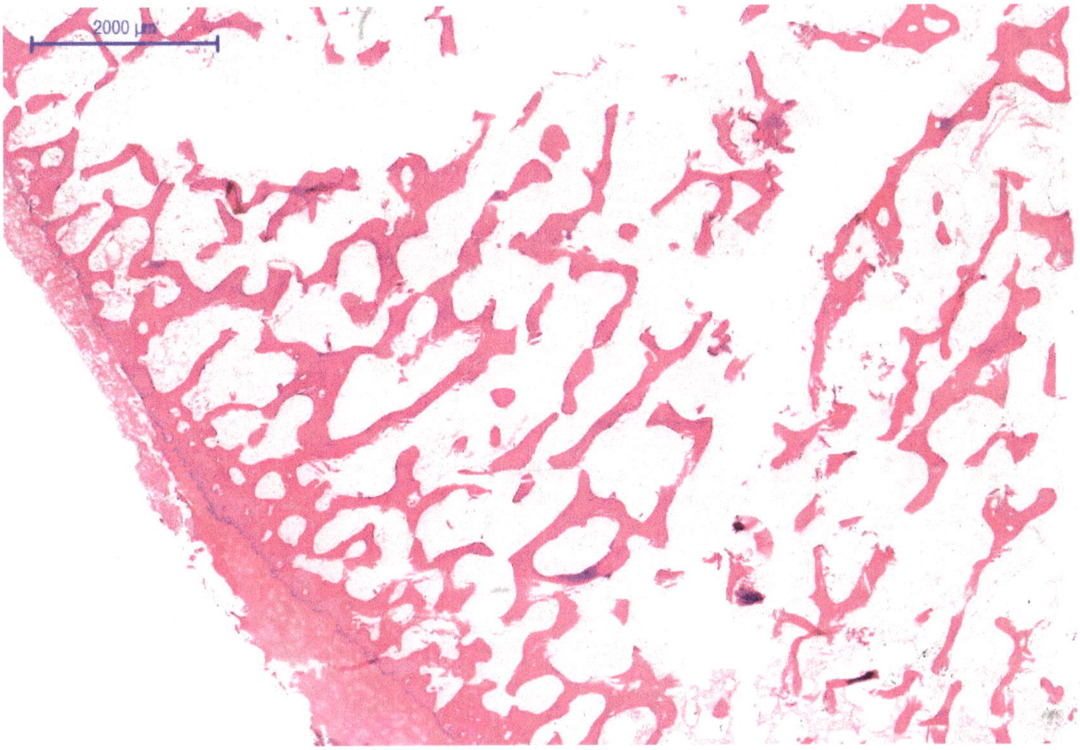

Figure 9. New bone formation from the outer margin while bone remodelling and resorption is shown from a more central area (above). (H & E P 8 ant slice 1X)

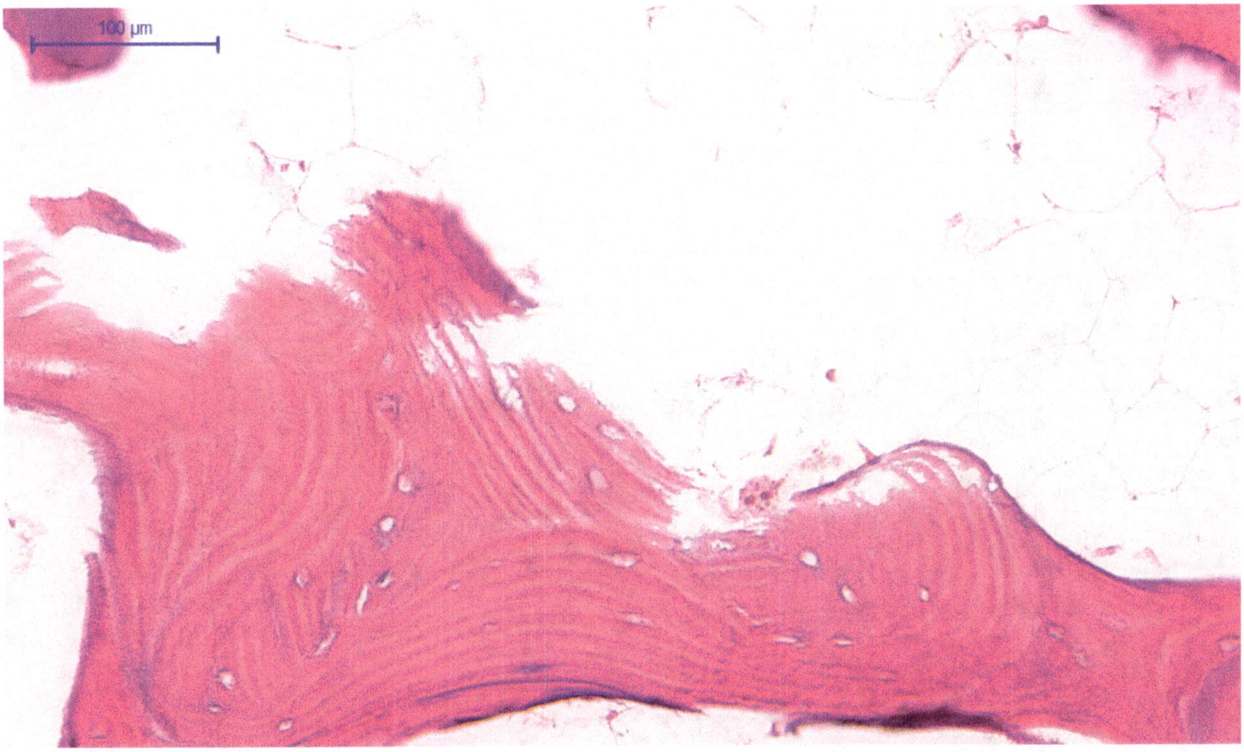

Figure 10. Slide of the central area showing osteoclastic activity with serrated bone margins with an osteoclast causing bone resorption. (H & E 20X)

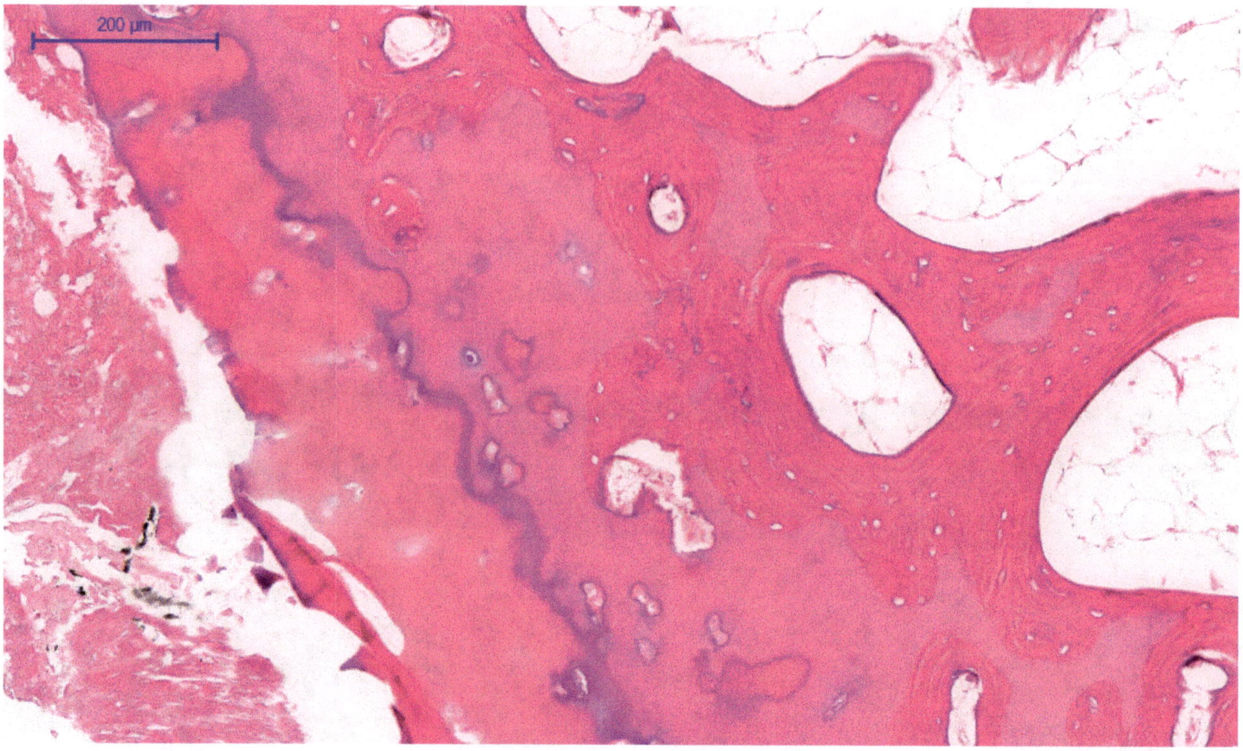

Figure 11. Same slide margin of the bone showing new bone formation (H & E 10X)

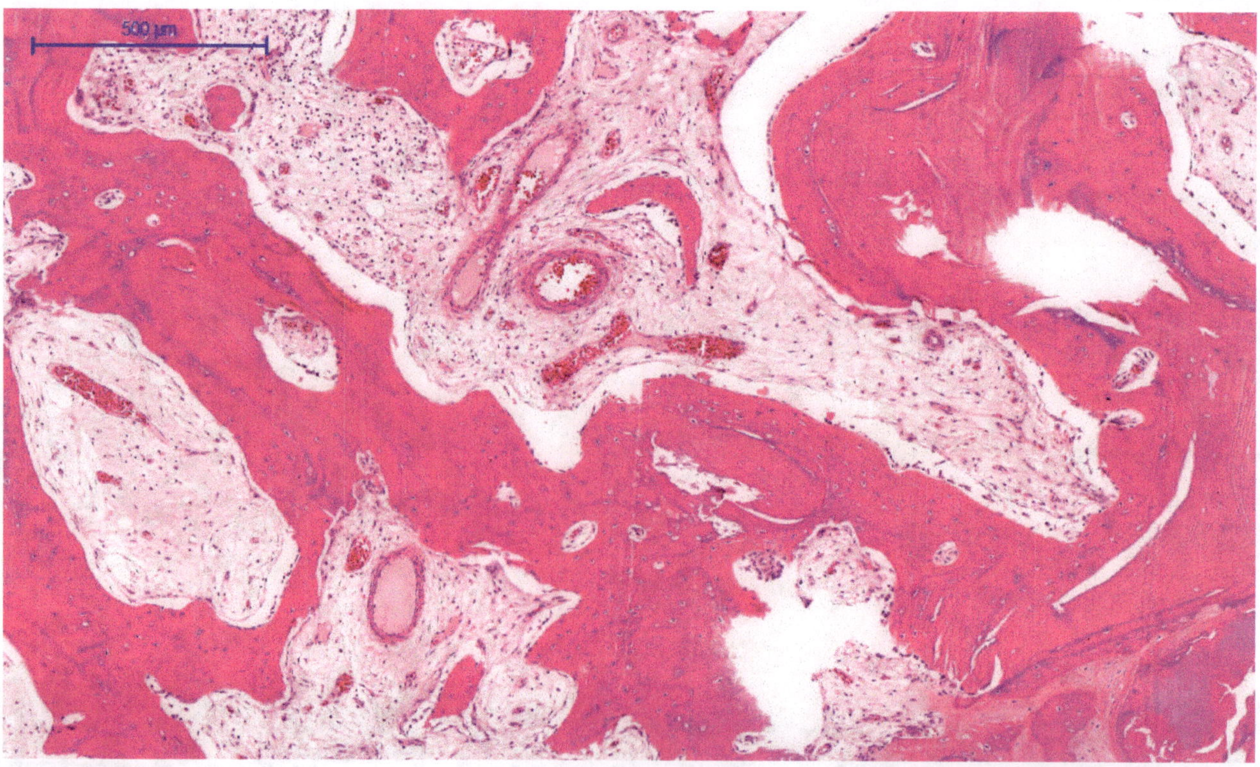

Figure 12. The posterior slice of the same patient (P8) with highly active bone with multiple blood vessels, new bone formation osteoblastic activity, live nucleated lacunae with minimal osteoclasts and bone resorption. (H & E P8 post slice 5x)

In contrast, patients showing loosening, gross osteolysis, bone resorption, show high osteoclastic activity with absence of osteoblastic features or new bone formation.

However, we also noted that both groups show good vascularity with active bones with good blood supply.

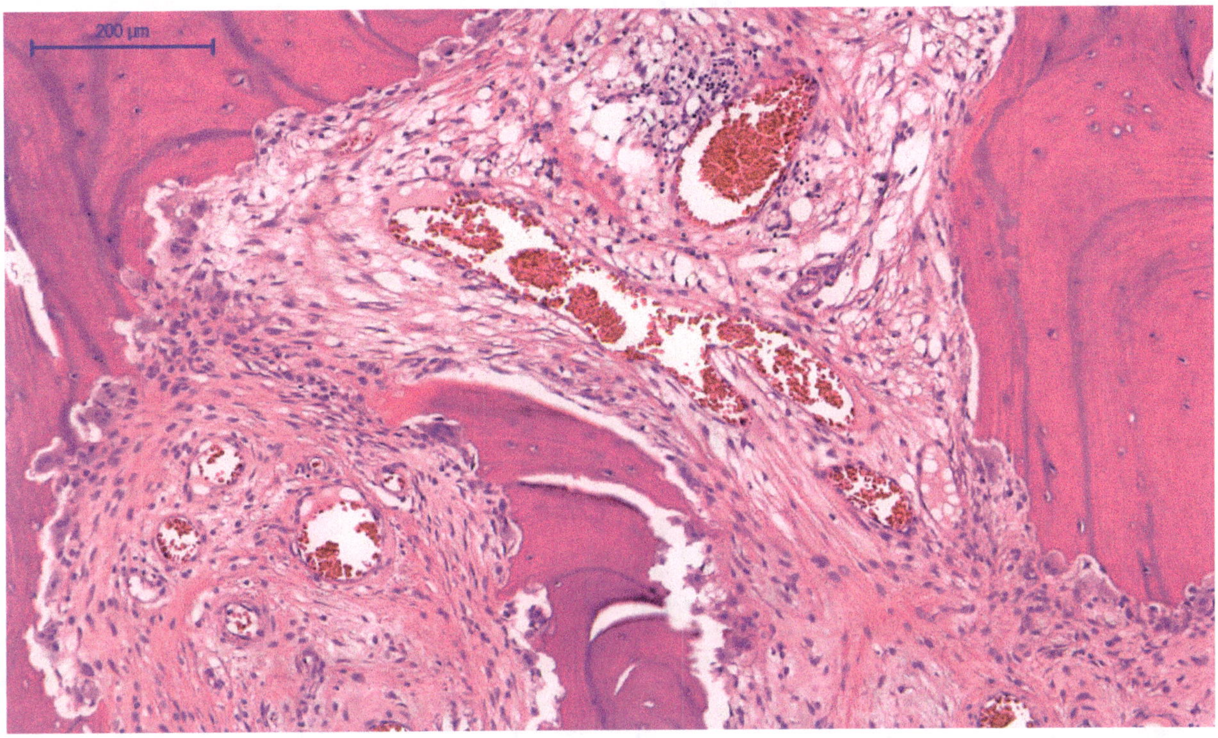

Figure 13. High osteoclastic activity leading to osteolysis along the bone showing serrated bone margin. Note the blood vessels showing good vascularity. (H & E 10x)

3.2. Immune response to foreign bodies leading to delayed hypersensitivity

This mechanism is more established as a number of studies has looked into metal ion release, osteolysis, pseudo-tumour formation, and ALVAL formation.

Metal ions have been implicated as triggering a foreign body type reaction leading to a delayed Type IV hypersensitivity. This has been attributed as a final common pathway leading to osteolysis bone destruction and failure. [51, 52, 57, 60] This may be a cause for unexplained groin pain seen in most of these [63] (Fig 13).

It is also worth mentioning that foreign body granulomas or pseudo-tumours per se may not lead to osteolysis. They can remain asymptomatic. [57, 47] However with time, as they grow in the bone and the under surface of the implant, they can act as a space occupying lesion separating the bone from the metal leading to loosening and malpositioning.

Secondly, they can also trigger immunological reactions that lead to osteolysis and femoral head resorption. As there is no direct evidence for this, this is another area that warrants further investigations and research.

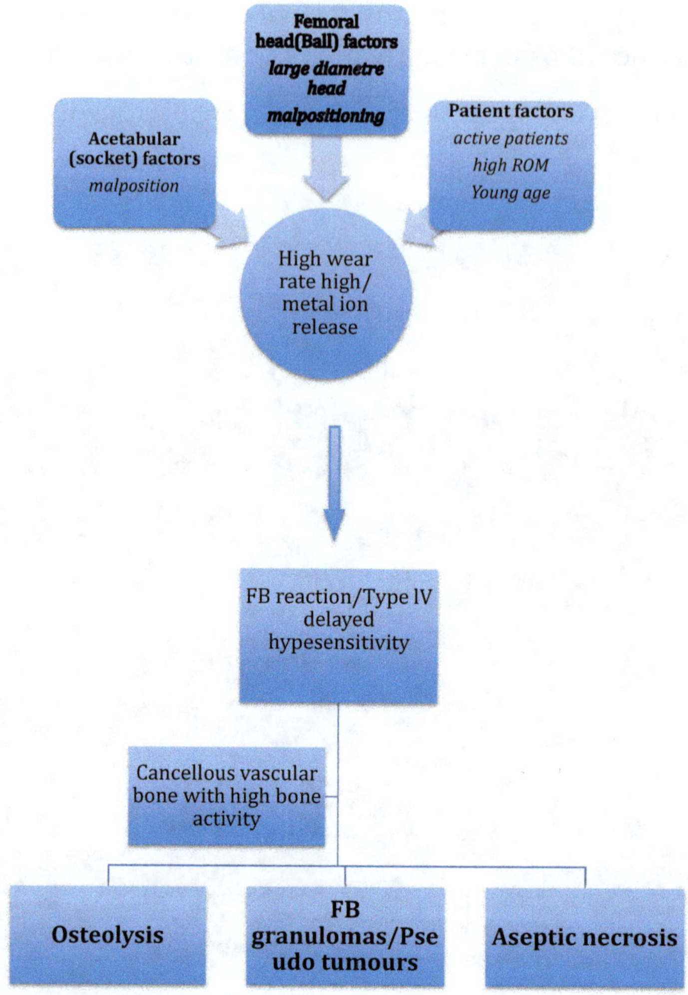

Figure 14. Mechanisms that may lead to immune response seen following hip resurfacing arthroplasty

4. Conclusions

There are many areas where new studies can be done to improve our understanding of the causes and mechanisms of failure of modern metal-on-metal hip arthroplasty.

As we have demonstrated, the causes for failure seem to be multifactorial (Fig. 14) partly due to the mechanisms that are well understood and partly due to mechanisms that at present are ill understood such as persistent groin pain and influence on metal ions.

We might have to rethink the design, taking into account that these biological factors such as femoral head and head neck are developmentally, functionally, structurally, and histologically different bones from the cortical bone. The interaction between metal and bone or cement and bone is different between the two bone types. Secondly, fixing the implant into the most mobile portion (ball of the hip joint) seem to act as a stimulation to trigger many biological responses and inflammatory reactions and immune reactions leading to new bone formation (osteoblastic response) or osteolysis (osteoclastic response).

Micro movement, caused by the loosening and release of high metal particles, made worse by a large diameter head in an environment of high bone activity with good vascularity and healing, in the femoral head seems to trigger ill-understood immune response that is osteo-clastic in nature. As the fixation of the femoral component is totally dependant in this area of bone, any microscopic osteolysis can lead to loosening leading to further osteolysis and leading to a vicious cycle (Fig. 15). One option is to break this vicious cycle by having at least a part of the fixation in a less active cortical bone.

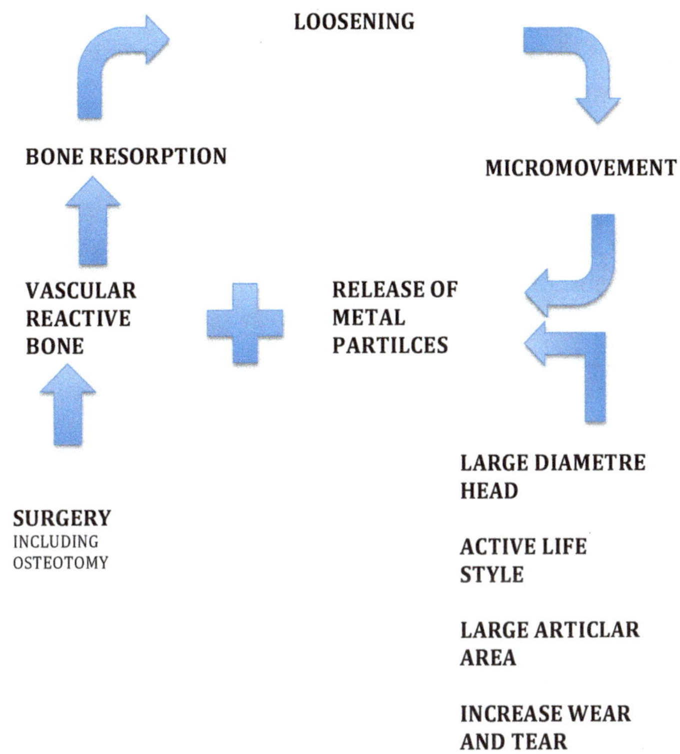

Figure 15. Vicious cycle leading to loosening

The exact relationship between the vascularity of the femoral head and the outcome of resurfacing arthroplasty is not well-established. On one hand, it is argued that vascularity is an essential element for the healing of the resurfaced femoral head to obtain a well-fixed component at the metal bone interface.

However, in spite of good vascularity, cementing can cause thermal necrosis (Fig. 3) at the cement bone interface; but all these implants do not seem to fail. "Does thermal necrosis result in failure of resurfacing arthroplasty?" is a research question that is worth exploring.

Secondly, a good vascular supply can act as a double-edged sword as it enhances bone activity, and with that can stimulate osteoclastic and immune responses (Fig. 13).

These cast doubts whether the trochanteric flip approach is necessarily a good thing as the bone activity in this approach is much higher than other approaches due to the additional osteotomy.

Thirdly, in patients who had AVN caused by non-surgical causes resurfacing arthroplasty [26, 64, 65] or partial resurfacing [66] has been used as a mode of treatment. Therefore, it is worth studying the long-term outcomes in this group in order for us to understand the relationship between vascularity and hip resurfacing.

This retrieval analysis did not demonstrate any relationship between the development of AVN and surgical approach.

One key drawback in finding the exact relationship between vascularity of the bone and AVN is the inability to work out the "critical ischemia" for bone tissue (minimal blood flow needed to keep the bone alive). Experiments that may help us to determine the "critical ischemia" of the femoral head will help us answer this question. [22]

Another limitation is difficulty in finding the bone activity in the femoral head covered by the metal implants. Even though SPECT [67, 68] and Positron Emission Tomography (PET) [69] have been used to study vascularity attenuation caused by the metal implants, they cause difficulty in interpreting the results accurately. [24, 70]

Patient No/Approach Non Posterior (NP) Posterior P	**Last follow up since THR (M)**	**Persistent Problems (Y/N)**
1 NP	42	Y (Groin Pain)
2 NP	26	N
3 NP	23	Y (Groin Pain)
4 NP	23	Y (Groin Pain)
5 NP	13	N
6 NP	Loss for follow up	
7 P	28	Died (? CAUSE) Infection
8 P	33	Y (Groin Pain)
9 P	25	Y (Groin Pain)
10 P	30	N
11 P	3.5	Y (Groin Pain)
12 P	21	N

Table 1. Follow up of revision surgery for failed hip resurfacing arthroplasty (note groin pain seem to be persistent even after revision in both groups).

According to this study, patients who had a revision for unexplained groin pain had groin pain even years after conversion to a THR (Table 1). The patients who had only a revision of acetabular component had to be revised within a mean duration of 14.5 months (10-16) to a THR due to persistent problems. These lead us to believe either the damage led to the development of the groin pain that may be irreversible or initial factors that triggered the groin pain persists even after the conversion to a total hip replacement. Therefore, we need to rethink whether THR is the first and the only option in treating patients with persistent unexplained groin pain.

In conclusion, we believe that the failure of hip resurfacing is due to multiple factors, eventually leading to common pathological pathways leading to failure.

The significance of the contribution of each factor to the final pathways is not clear.

The fact that femoral component is fixed in the most mobile area of the joint in a relatively active patient, continuously moving the hip impacting on a relatively weak cancellous bone that constantly attempts to heal, while a large diameter head releasing high levels of metal ions leading to immunological response appear to be a recipe for disaster that finally leads to the failure of metal-on-metal hip resurfacing arthroplasty.

Acknowledgements

Special Thanks to Prof. Pat Campbell, Joint Replacement Centre University of California Los Angeles (UCLA), USA; Prof. Damian Griffin Warwick Orthopaedics, University of Warwick Medical School, University Hospitals of Coventry and Warwickshire, United Kingdom; Dr. Nick Parsons Warwick Orthopaedics, University of Warwick Medical School, University Hospitals of Coventry and Warwickshire, United Kingdom.

Author details

Hiran Wimal Amarasekera[1,2*]

Address all correspondence to: hiruwan@hotmail.com

1 Neville Fernando Teaching Hospital and South Asian Institute of Medicine, Colombo , Sri Lanka

2 Warwick Orthopaedics, University of Warwick,Coventry, United Kingdom

References

[1] Charnley J. Using Teflon in arthroplasty of the hip-joint. The Journal of bone and joint surgery American volume 1966;48(4):819.

[2] McMinn D, Daniel J. History and modern concepts in surface replacement. Proc Inst Mech Eng H 2006;220(2):239-51.

[3] Wagner H. Surface replacement arthroplasty of the hip. Clinical orthopaedics and related research 1978(134):102-30.

[4] Head WC. Wagner surface replacement arthroplasty of the hip. Analysis of fourteen failures in forty-one hips. The Journal of bone and joint surgery American volume 1981;63(3):420-7.

[5] Grujic H, Olerud S, Soreff J. Wagner resurfacing hip arthroplasty: preliminary results. Acta Orthop Scand 1982;53(5):785-9.

[6] McMinn D, Treacy R, Lin K, et al. Metal on metal surface replacement of the hip. Experience of the McMinn prothesis. Clinical orthopaedics and related research 1996(329 Suppl):S89-98.

[7] National joint registry England and Wales, 2004.

[8] Prime MS, Palmer J, Khan WS. The National Joint Registry of England and Wales. Orthopedics 2011;34(2):107-10.

[9] McMinn DJ, Daniel J, Ziaee H, et al. Indications and results of hip resurfacing. International orthopaedics 2011;35(2):231-7.

[10] Rechl H, Pilge H, Rudert M. [Development of hip resurfacing]. Der Orthopade 2008;37(7):626-33.

[11] Gross TP, Liu F. Prevalence of dysplasia as the source of worse outcome in young female patients after hip resurfacing arthroplasty. International orthopaedics 2012;36(1):27-34.

[12] Bose VC, Baruah BD. Resurfacing arthroplasty of the hip for avascular necrosis of the femoral head: a minimum follow-up of four years. The Journal of bone and joint surgery British volume 2010;92(7):922-8.

[13] Underwood RJ, Zografos A, Sayles RS, et al. Edge loading in metal-on-metal hips: low clearance is a new risk factor. Proc Inst Mech Eng H 2012;226(3):217-26.

[14] Beaule PE, Campbell PA, Hoke R, et al. Notching of the femoral neck during resurfacing arthroplasty of the hip: a vascular study. The Journal of bone and joint surgery British volume 2006;88(1):35-9.

[15] Kohan L, Field CJ, Kerr DR. Early complications of hip resurfacing. The Journal of arthroplasty 2012;27(6):997-1002.

[16] Amstutz HC, Le Duff MJ. Eleven years of experience with metal-on-metal hybrid hip resurfacing: a review of 1000 conserve plus. The Journal of arthroplasty 2008;23(6 Suppl 1):36-43.

[17] Morlock MM, Bishop N, Stahmer F, et al. [Reasons for failure of hip resurfacing implants. A failure analysis based on 250 revision specimens]. Der Orthopade 2008;37(7):695-703.

[18] Morlock MM, Bishop N, Zustin J, et al. Modes of implant failure after hip resurfacing: morphological and wear analysis of 267 retrieval specimens. The Journal of bone and joint surgery American volume 2008;90 Suppl 3:89-95.

[19] Amarasekera H, Costa M, Prakash U, et al. FEMORAL BLOOD FLOW DURING HIP RESURFACING: A COMPARISON OF TWO APPROACHES USING LASER DOPPLER FLOW MEASUREMENT. Journal of Bone & Joint Surgery, British Volume 2012;94-B(SUPP III):148.

[20] Beaule PE, Campbell P, Shim P. Femoral head blood flow during hip resurfacing. Clinical orthopaedics and related research 2007;456:148-52.

[21] Griffiths DE, Acton K, Hull JB. Hip resurfacing with preservation of femoral head blood supply. Surgeon 2008;6(2):115-9.

[22] Amarasekera HW, Costa ML, Foguet P, et al. The blood flow to the femoral head/neck junction during resurfacing arthroplasty: A COMPARISON OF TWO APPROACHES USING LASER DOPPLER FLOWMETRY. The Journal of bone and joint surgery British volume 2008;90(4):442-5.

[23] Ganz R, Gill TJ, Gautier E, et al. Surgical dislocation of the adult hip: A TECHNIQUE WITH FULL ACCESS TO THE FEMORAL HEAD AND ACETABULUM WITHOUT THE RISK OF AVASCULAR NECROSIS. The Journal of bone and joint surgery British volume 2001;83-B(8):1119-24.

[24] Amarasekera H, Roberts P, Costa M, et al. Scintigraphic assessment of bone status at one year following hip resurfacing: comparison of two surgical approaches using SPECT-CT scan. Bone and Joint Research 2012;1(1):86-92.

[25] Campbell P, Mirra J, Amstutz HC. Viability of femoral heads treated with resurfacing arthroplasty. The Journal of arthroplasty 2000;15(1):120-2.

[26] Boyd HS, Ulrich SD, Seyler TM, et al. Resurfacing for Perthes disease: an alternative to standard hip arthroplasty. Clinical orthopaedics and related research 2007;465:80-5.

[27] Grecula MJ. Resurfacing arthroplasty in osteonecrosis of the hip. Orthop Clin North Am 2005;36(2):231-42, x.

[28] Schmalzried TP. Total resurfacing for osteonecrosis of the hip. Clinical orthopaedics and related research 2004(429):151-6.

[29] Gerdesmeyer L, Gollwitzer H, Bader R, et al. [Surgical approaches in hip resurfacing]. Der Orthopade 2008;37(7):650-8.

[30] McBryde CW, Revell MP, Thomas AM, et al. The influence of surgical approach on outcome in Birmingham hip resurfacing. Clinical orthopaedics and related research 2008;466(4):920-6.

[31] Beaule PE, Shim P, Banga K. Clinical experience of Ganz surgical dislocation approach for metal-on-metal hip resurfacing. The Journal of arthroplasty 2009;24(6 Suppl):127-31.

[32] Kreuzer S, Leffers K, Kumar S. Direct anterior approach for hip resurfacing: surgical technique and complications. Clinical orthopaedics and related research 2011;469(6): 1574-81.

[33] Jacobs MA, Goytia RN, Bhargava T. Hip resurfacing through an anterolateral approach. Surgical description and early review. The Journal of bone and joint surgery American volume 2008;90 Suppl 3:38-44.

[34] H A. Surgical approaches to the hip joint and its clinical implications in adult hip arthroplasty. In: Knove P, ed. Arthroplasty. 1 ed. Croatia: INTECH, 2013:3-19.

[35] Marker DR, Seyler TM, Jinnah RH, et al. Femoral neck fractures after metal-on-metal total hip resurfacing: a prospective cohort study. The Journal of arthroplasty 2007;22(7 Suppl 3):66-71.

[36] Amanatullah DF, Cheung Y, Di Cesare PE. Hip resurfacing arthroplasty: a review of the evidence for surgical technique, outcome, and complications. Orthop Clin North Am 2010;41(2):263-72.

[37] Amstutz HC, Takamura KM, Le Duff MJ. The effect of patient selection and surgical technique on the results of Conserve(R) Plus hip resurfacing--3.5- to 14-year follow-up. Orthop Clin North Am 2011;42(2):133-42, vii.

[38] Della Valle CJ, Nunley RM, Barrack RL. When is the right time to resurface? Orthopedics 2008;31(12 Suppl 2).

[39] Jameson SS, Langton DJ, Natu S, et al. The influence of age and sex on early clinical results after hip resurfacing: an independent center analysis. The Journal of arthroplasty 2008;23(6 Suppl 1):50-5.

[40] Bitsch RG, Jager S, Lurssen M, et al. Influence of bone density on the cement fixation of femoral hip resurfacing components. Journal of orthopaedic research : official publication of the Orthopaedic Research Society 2010;28(8):986-91.

[41] Kim PR, Beaule PE, Laflamme GY, et al. Causes of early failure in a multicenter clinical trial of hip resurfacing. The Journal of arthroplasty 2008;23(6 Suppl 1):44-9.

[42] Hull P, Baxter JA, Lewis C, et al. Metal-on-metal hip resurfacing with uncemented fixation of the femoral component. A minimum 2 year follow up. Hip international : the journal of clinical and experimental research on hip pathology and therapy 2011.

[43] Ritter MA, Lutgring JD, Berend ME, et al. Failure mechanisms of total hip resurfacing: implications for the present. Clinical orthopaedics and related research 2006;453:110-4.

[44] Beaule PE, Le Duff M, Campbell P, et al. Metal-on-metal surface arthroplasty with a cemented femoral component: a 7-10 year follow-up study. The Journal of arthroplasty 2004;19(8 Suppl 3):17-22.

[45] Campbell P, Takamura K, Lundergan W, et al. Cement technique changes improved hip resurfacing longevity - implant retrieval findings. Bulletin of the NYU hospital for joint diseases 2009;67(2):146-53.

[46] Gill HS, Campbell PA, Murray DW, et al. Reduction of the potential for thermal damage during hip resurfacing. The Journal of bone and joint surgery British volume 2007;89(1):16-20.

[47] Malviya A, Holland JP. Pseudotumours associated with metal-on-metal hip resurfacing: 10-year Newcastle experience. Acta Orthop Belg 2009;75(4):477-83.

[48] A survey on the prevalence of pseudotumors with metal-on-metal hip resurfacing in Canadian academic centers. The Journal of bone and joint surgery American volume 2011;93 Suppl 2:118-21.

[49] Brooks P. Component malposition in hip resurfacing. Orthopedics 2010;33(9):646.

[50] Delaunay C, Petit I, Learmonth ID, et al. Metal-on-metal bearings total hip arthroplasty: the cobalt and chromium ions release concern. Orthop Traumatol Surg Res 2010;96(8):894-904.

[51] Akbar M, Brewer JM, Grant MH. Effect of chromium and cobalt ions on primary human lymphocytes in vitro. J Immunotoxicol 2011;8(2):140-9.

[52] Kwon YM, Thomas P, Summer B, et al. Lymphocyte proliferation responses in patients with pseudotumors following metal-on-metal hip resurfacing arthroplasty. Journal of orthopaedic research : official publication of the Orthopaedic Research Society 2010;28(4):444-50.

[53] Mahendra G, Pandit H, Kliskey K, et al. Necrotic and inflammatory changes in metal-on-metal resurfacing hip arthroplasties. Acta Orthop 2009;80(6):653-9.

[54] Hart AJ, Skinner JA, Henckel J, et al. Insufficient Acetabular Version Increases Blood Metal Ion Levels after Metal-on-metal Hip Resurfacing. Clinical orthopaedics and related research 2011;469(9):2590-7.

[55] Mai MC, Milbrandt JC, Hulsen J, et al. Acetabular cup malalignment after total hip resurfacing arthroplasty: a case for elective revision? Orthopedics 2009;32(11):853.

[56] Kim PR, Beaule PE, Dunbar M, et al. Cobalt and chromium levels in blood and urine following hip resurfacing arthroplasty with the Conserve Plus implant. The Journal of bone and joint surgery American volume 2011;93 Suppl 2:107-17.

[57] Kwon YM, Ostlere SJ, McLardy-Smith P, et al. "Asymptomatic" pseudotumors after metal-on-metal hip resurfacing arthroplasty: prevalence and metal ion study. The Journal of arthroplasty 2011;26(4):511-8.

[58] Antoniou J, Zukor DJ, Mwale F, et al. Metal ion levels in the blood of patients after hip resurfacing: a comparison between twenty-eight and thirty-six-millimeter-head metal-on-metal prostheses. The Journal of bone and joint surgery American volume 2008;90 Suppl 3:142-8.

[59] Beaule PE, Kim PR, Hamdi A, et al. A prospective metal ion study of large-head metal-on-metal bearing: a matched-pair analysis of hip resurfacing versus total hip replacement. Orthop Clin North Am 2011;42(2):251-7, ix.

[60] Moroni A, Savarino L, Hoque M, et al. Do ion levels in hip resurfacing differ from metal-on-metal THA at midterm? Clinical orthopaedics and related research 2011;469(1):180-7.

[61] Matthies A, Underwood R, Cann P, et al. Retrieval analysis of 240 metal-on-metal hip components, comparing modular total hip replacement with hip resurfacing. The Journal of bone and joint surgery British volume 2011;93(3):307-14.

[62] Buechel FF, Drucker D, Jasty M, et al. Osteolysis around uncemented acetabular components of cobalt-chrome surface replacement hip arthroplasty. Clinical orthopaedics and related research 1994(298):202-11.

[63] Campbell P, Shimmin A, Walter L, et al. Metal sensitivity as a cause of groin pain in metal-on-metal hip resurfacing. The Journal of arthroplasty 2008;23(7):1080-5.

[64] Larson AN, McIntosh AL, Trousdale RT, et al. Avascular necrosis most common indication for hip arthroplasty in patients with slipped capital femoral epiphysis. J Pediatr Orthop 2010;30(8):767-73.

[65] Drescher W, Pufe T, Smeets R, et al. [Avascular necrosis of the hip - diagnosis and treatment]. Z Orthop Unfall 2011;149(2):231-40; quiz 41-2.

[66] Siguier T, Siguier M, Judet T, et al. Partial resurfacing arthroplasty of the femoral head in avascular necrosis. Methods, indications, and results. Clinical orthopaedics and related research 2001(386):85-92.

[67] McMahon SJ, Young D, Ballok Z, et al. Vascularity of the femoral head after Birmingham hip resurfacing. A technetium Tc 99m bone scan/single photon emission computed tomography study. The Journal of arthroplasty 2006;21(4):514-21.

[68] Leunig M, Ganz R. Vascularity of the femoral head after Birmingham hip resurfacing. A technetium Tc 99m bone scan/single photon emission computed tomography study. The Journal of arthroplasty 2007;22(5):784-5; author reply 85-6.

[69] Forrest N, Welch A, Murray AD, et al. Femoral head viability after Birmingham resurfacing hip arthroplasty: assessment with use of [18F] fluoride positron emission

tomography. The Journal of bone and joint surgery American volume 2006;88 Suppl 3:84-9.

[70] Amarasekera HW, Costa ML, Parsons N, et al. SPECT/CT bone imaging after hip resurfacing arthroplasty: is it feasible to use CT attenuation correction in the presence of metal implants? Nuclear medicine communications 2011;32(4):289-97.

2

Arthroplasty for Proximal Femur Fracture

Mark Curtin, Eoghan Pomeroy and James Broderick

Abstract

With an increasing global incidence of hip fractures, designing appropriate treatment strategies for hip fractures is fundamentally important to healthcare professionals, policymakers, and payers of healthcare services. We will evaluate the role of total hip replacement (THR) in the setting of trauma for the acute treatment of hip fractures. In this chapter, we will compare hemiarthroplasty and total hip replacement in the acute setting while also examining the role of arthroplasty in the setting of failed internal fixation, as well as in pathologic fractures. We will describe the pearls and pitfalls of surgical technique in these scenarios, highlighted with case examples.

Keywords: arthroplasty, trauma, hemiarthroplasty, THR, salvage

1. Introduction

The incidence of the neck of femur fracture is increasing alongside the increasing proportion of elderly patients with multiple comorbidities in our population statistics [1]. It is currently estimated that more than 80,000 hip fractures are treated each year in the United Kingdom—the great majority of these fractures require some form of surgical treatment, as nonoperative management is associated with high morbidity and complication rates [2–5]. Deciding on the most appropriate intervention is often challenging; factors such as fracture location and configuration, bone stock, physiological age, mobility, comorbidity, and implant selection are only some of the considerations in such cases. Optimal care for these patients requires multidisciplinary intervention across a broad range of services including surgery, anaesthesia, physiotherapy, geriatrics, and rehabilitative medicine.

Fractures are broadly categorised as intracapsular or extracapsular and can be classified as stable or unstable. In general, extracapsular fractures are treated by reduction and osteosynthesis, as are selected intracapsular fractures. Displaced intracapsular fractures are conventionally treated by hemiarthroplasty, but total hip replacement [THR] has a role either as a primary intervention in the younger more active patient or as a salvage procedure for failed osteosynthesis or hemiarthroplasty. Well-recognised goals of operative treatment include immediate pain relief, a rapid return to ambulation, an accelerated period of rehabilitation, and maintenance of independent living. Arthroplasty is generally considered to be a highly effective treatment for many painful hip conditions. By definition total hip replacement requires prosthetic replacement of the femoral and acetabular joint surfaces. All implants require an interface for skeletal fixation which can be achieved using bone cement or by biological fixation. In addition the implant must be able to accommodate an articular surface to provide a low-friction, physiological range of motion. Identifying the most appropriate treatment strategy for hip fractures avoids secondary hospital admissions, costly and often complicated reoperations, loss of independence, and physical disability. Designing optimal treatment strategies for hip fractures is fundamentally important to healthcare professionals, policymakers, and payers of healthcare services.

Stable fractures can be treated by osteosynthesis with predictable and favourable results [6, 7]. Conversely, surgical fixation of unstable fracture patterns remains challenging due to deficient bone stock and osteoporosis [8, 9]. In the past, fixed nail-plate devices used for the fixation of these fractures had high rates of cut-out and fracture displacement. Sliding hip screws have become the predominant method of fixation of these fractures with reduced rates of cut-out and fracture displacement compared with fixed nail-plate devices [10–14]. Cephalomedullary fixation has also demonstrated reduced cut-out rates in osteoporotic bone and is the preferred method of fixation for unstable intertrochanteric fractures [15, 16].

Complications of internal fixation are well documented including perforation of the femoral head, excessive sliding with secondary shortening, plate pull-out, and plate breakage [17, 18]. In cases where fixation is tenuous, a period of restricted mobilisation is suggested [19] during which morbidities such as pressure sores, respiratory tract infections, atelectasis, and deep vein thrombosis may develop. Despite considerable advances in internal fixation methods, the failure rate of the sliding hip screw is 6.8–9.8%, while the failure rate of cephalomedullary nails ranges from 7.1 to 12.5% in unstable fractures [20–22].

While internal fixation is widely viewed as the preferred treatment for young patients and elderly patients with stable fractures, there is still no standard treatment for active patients above 70 years of age [23, 24]. A suggested treatment algorithm can be seen in **Chart 1**. While hemiarthroplasty is expeditious and permits early mobilisation, in certain cases revision to a THR is required due to painful acetabular erosion or protrusion [25]. Radiographic studies have demonstrated that most of the motion in hemiarthroplasties occurs at the interface of the bipolar component and the acetabulum, not between the femoral head and the bipolar component. The significance of acetabular erosion and groin pain after a hemiarthroplasty is a topic of debate among the orthopaedic community. Many studies contributing to the pool of knowledge on the topic use outdated implants. Added to this is the fact that the cognition and activity levels of patients receiving hemiarthroplasty vary widely and may affect the reporting of pain.

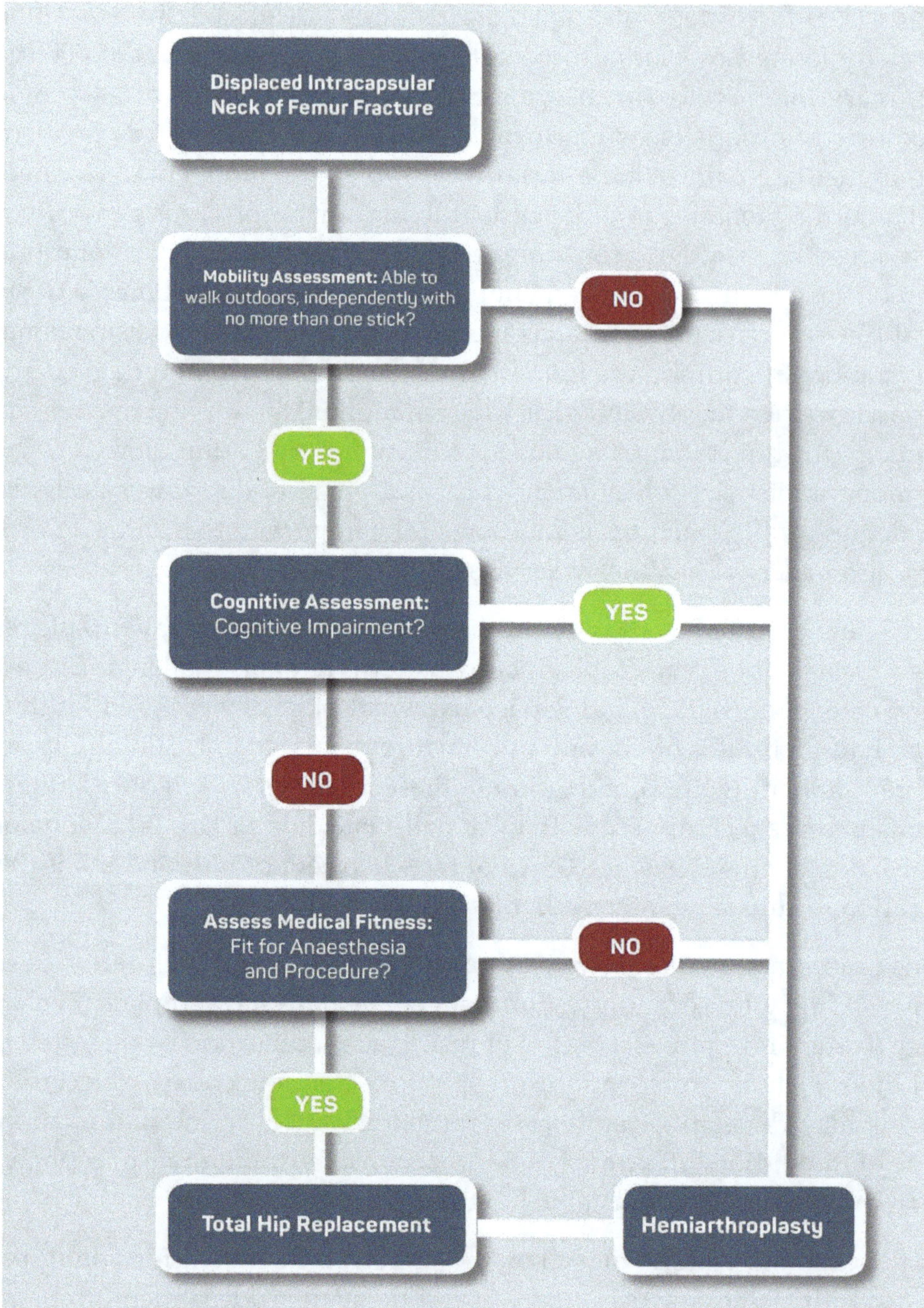

Chart 1. Proposed algorithm in addressing femoral neck fractures in the trauma setting.

The recently published HEALTH trial protocol [26] outlines a prospective randomised control trial to evaluate the outcomes of THR versus hemiarthroplasty in the treatment of femoral neck fractures. This study aims to assess the outcomes of both treatment modalities up to 2 years postoperatively. A recent publication in the *Journal of Arthroplasty* by Grosso et al. demonstrated a low conversion rate of hemiarthroplasty to THR when a hemiarthroplasty was performed for a displaced neck of femur fracture in patients over 75 years. In this study, a 2.5% conversion rate at an average of 1.9 years post-index procedure was recorded, with acetabular wear, which is the leading cause [27]. Uncertainty remains as to which type of prosthesis is most appropriate for the treatment of fractures in these elderly patients. This leads to significant regional variations in treatment: THR is up to three times more likely to be performed in the treatment of hip fractures in Sweden than in England and twice as likely as in Canada [28].

2. Preoperative evaluation

A detailed history and clinical examination is necessary in all cases of hip fractures. Particular care must be made to identify pre-existing medical comorbidities and regular anticoagulants being taken by the patient. A comprehensive discussion should take place with the patient and their relatives in relation to any proposed management strategy. Morbidity and mortality associated with femoral neck fracture care should be discussed. Mortality is 10% within the first 30 days reflecting the compromised status of many of these patients. Mortality rates rise to approximately 40% at 12 months.

Examination may reveal a shortened, externally rotated lower extremity. The neurovascular status of the lower limb should be evaluated and documented, and a secondary survey should be completed to rule out associated injuries.

Appropriate imaging should take the form of plain film radiographs of the pelvis and femur in anterior-posterior and lateral planes. The pelvis should be held in neutral with both femurs clearly visible and the feet held in internal rotation. Preoperative estimates of magnification on X-rays are frequently incorrect and can lead to mismatching of implant sizes, limb length discrepancies, and disturbance of the biomechanical parameters of the hip joint. The magnification factor for pelvic imaging normally ranges from 109 to 128%. Radioopaque calibration spheres can be sited midline to femurs and proximally towards the pubic symphysis to aid in digital templating of the preoperative X-rays. The contralateral hip should be used as a surrogate for templating in the trauma setting. Digital templating is essential to determine the location of the neck cut, size of the prosthesis, appropriate offset, and depth of insertion. If there is a concern for pathological fracture, appropriate imaging of the whole femur should be obtained in the first instance, and intraoperative histological samples should be sent for analysis.

All patients with a hip fracture should have a preoperative electrocardiogram, and in those over the age of 65, a chest X-ray should also be performed. It has been determined by the Association of Anaesthetists of Great Britain and Ireland (AAGBI) that a preoperative echocardiogram should not delay the passage of a patient with a hip fracture to theatre and should rather be performed, if necessary, during the postoperative period. Routine preoperative blood tests may reveal preoperative anaemia which occurs in 30–40% of patients and may be attributable to the fracture itself, haemodilution or a pre-existing condition. The acute response to trauma may lead to neutrophilia or leucocytosis. It is noteworthy that electrolyte imbalances are not uncommon in this cohort of patients, especially hyponatremia and hypokalemia. Hyperkalemia may also be an indicator of rhabdomyolysis occurring secondary to a prolonged period of immobilisation following the initial traumatic event.

Neuraxial anaesthesia is often the preferred form of anaesthesia for treatment of femoral fractures. The suspicion of aortic stenosis on clinical examination often precludes neuraxial anaesthesia. Despite this, general anaesthesia is also a safe option, and the Sprint Audit has shown no significant difference in mortality between these modes of anaesthesia [29]. Combined neuraxial anaesthesia and general anaesthesia has shown a trend towards increased mortality. This is most likely related to the 'double hit' hypotensive effects of both modalities of anaesthesia.

3. Hemiarthroplasty versus total hip replacement

In the vast majority of cases, the accepted treatment for displaced neck of femur fractures in the elderly is a unipolar or bipolar hemiarthroplasty, especially in elderly patients with low functional demands. Compared with THR, hemiarthroplasty has the advantage of being a simpler, standardised procedure with shorter operating times, and less blood loss. In the acute trauma setting, many orthopaedic surgeons are more comfortable performing hemiarthroplasty rather than THR. Therefore, THR may not be readily available to the trauma patient, and surgical delay is likely to increase morbidity and mortality. Recent studies conclude that THR in the trauma setting is associated with improved functional outcomes and lower reoperation rates when compared with hemiarthroplasty, albeit with a higher dislocation rate [30–32]. Instability post THR is multifactorial, and contributory factors include surgical approach, bearing diameter, restoration of hip biomechanics, cognitive dysfunction, and presence of neuromuscular disease. Where the posterior approach has been utilised, meticulous capsular repair is essential to minimise instability. Some authors advocate the anterolateral approach when treating a femoral neck fracture with THR. This reduces the dislocation rate at the expense of potential abductor dysfunction and a postoperative Trendelenburg gait. The use of large head sizes has also reduced dislocation rates, with the literature suggesting that the benefit is greatest when utilising the posterior approach.

It is essential to adhere to strict selection criteria when determining suitability of patients with hip fractures for THR in order to minimise complication rates. In 2011 the National Institute for Health and Care Excellence (NICE) published their guidelines and recommended THR for patients with adequate cognitive and physical function who are fit to undergo anaesthesia and major surgery. Perry et al. evaluated UK Hip Fracture Database information to ascertain compliance with NICE guidelines for THR [33]. Their study evaluated patients over the age of 60 presenting acutely with displaced intracapsular femoral neck fractures. They determined that only 32% of ostensibly eligible patients underwent THR, and, of those who had surgery, 42% did not qualify under the NICE eligibility criteria. Inclusion and exclusion criteria for THR in trauma need to be defined more accurately based on specific rather than arbitrary parameters.

THR performed for trauma has equivalent results to those performed electively. Anakwe et al. matched 100 trauma patients with an elective cohort and demonstrated equivalent functional outcomes [34]. THR may appear as a more expensive treatment for trauma in terms of implant cost, but the overall costs associated with unipolar and bipolar hemiarthroplasties (including revision surgeries) are higher in the long term [35]. Maceroli et al. demonstrated lower mortality rates in patients undergoing THR for femoral neck fractures in centres that performed large numbers of such procedures [36]. Uhler et al. demonstrated that a patient will gain more cumulative utility over the course of 2 years by waiting 48 hours for a THR, despite an increase in short-term morbidity associated with delayed surgery [37]. It seems reasonable therefore to advocate THR for suitable patients where dedicated arthroplasty services are available. **Figure 1** demonstrates a left basicervical neck of femur fracture, with subsequent treatment with a hybrid THR shown in **Figure 2**.

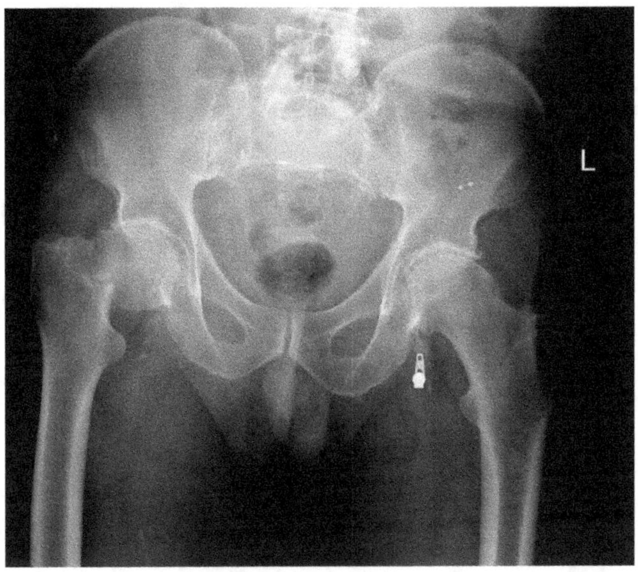

Figure 1. AP radiograph of pelvis showing left basicervical neck of femur fracture.

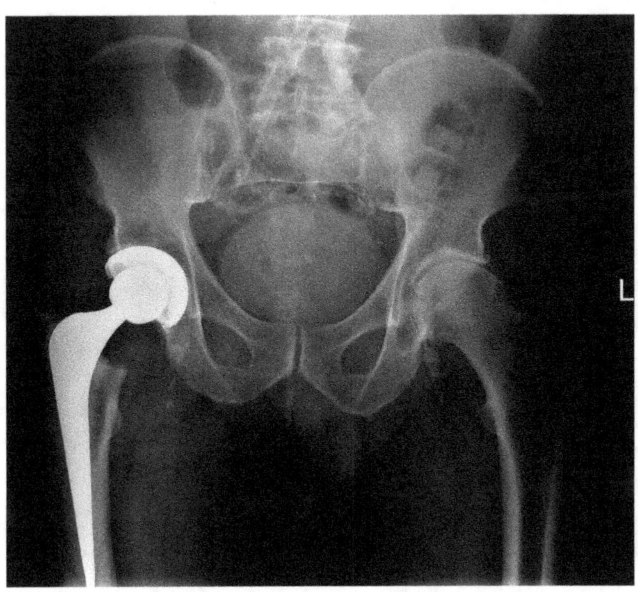

Figure 2. AP pelvis demonstrating subsequent treatment with a hybrid THR in the acute setting.

4. THR for failed neck of femur internal fixation

Following initial treatment with internal fixation, the neck of femur fractures may develop nonunion and osteonecrosis, with reoperation rates of up to 40% reported in the literature. Nikolopoulos et al. demonstrated in a prospective study that patients with displaced neck of femur fractures who underwent internal fixation had a higher rate of avascular necrosis than those that were undisplaced [38]. This group of patients may develop disabling secondary degenerative symptoms necessitating arthroplasty. We highlight this with examples of clinical cases. **Figure 3** shows the collapse of the femoral head following initial sliding screw fixation of a basicervical neck of femur fracture. This was subsequently revised to a hybrid THR as demonstrated in **Figure 4. Figure 5** describes the case of screw cut-out post ORIF of the neck of femur fracture, which was subsequently revised to a modular prosthesis as seen in **Figure 6.**

Tidermark et al. demonstrated suboptimal outcomes in patients with displaced neck of femur fractures treated with internal fixation, showing impaired functional outcomes when compared with a cohort of undisplaced fractures despite radiographic and clinical evidence of union [39].

In treating nonunion the surgical team must consider the presence of infection. Clinical evaluation and serial erythrocyte sedimentation rate (ESR) and C-reactive protein (CRP) levels are useful diagnostic tools and if abnormal might prompt joint aspiration or bone biopsy and culture. If preoperative or intraoperative findings suggest infection, a two-stage revision with removal of metalwork and excision of the femoral head is usually performed. An antibiotic-impregnated spacer is implanted in the first instance, and subsequent arthroplasty is performed at an appropriate later date.

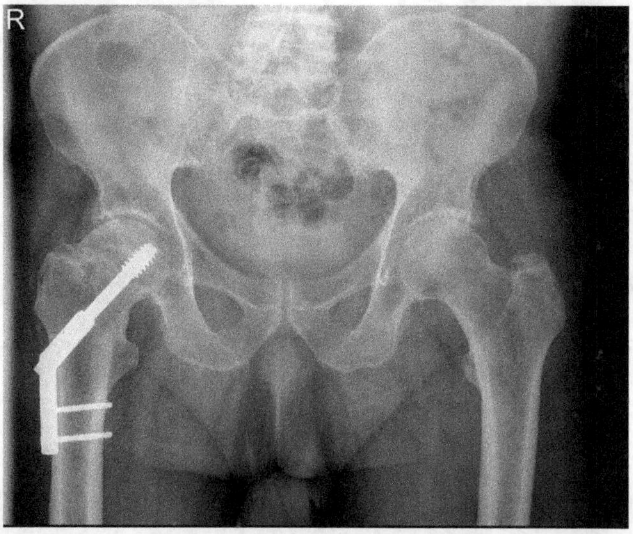

Figure 3. AP radiograph of pelvis demonstrating collapse of femoral head post dynamic hip screw fixation of basicervical neck of femur fracture.

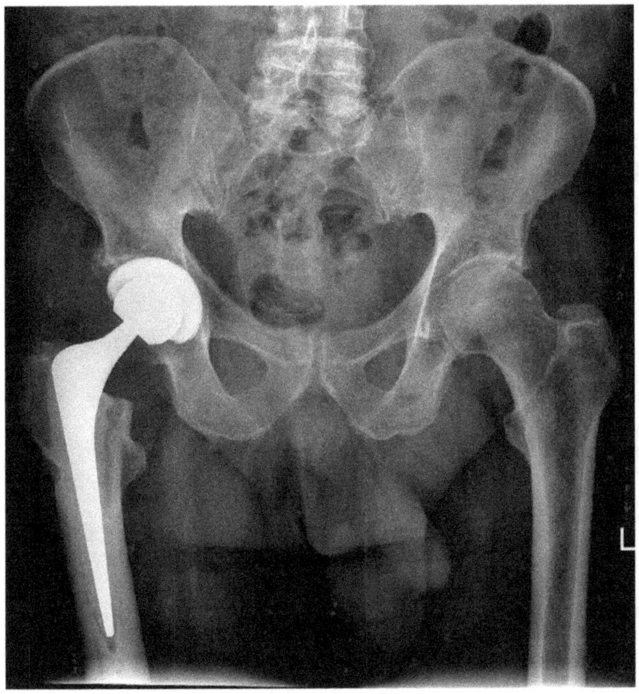

Figure 4. Demonstrating subsequent revision to hybrid THR following failed internal fixation.

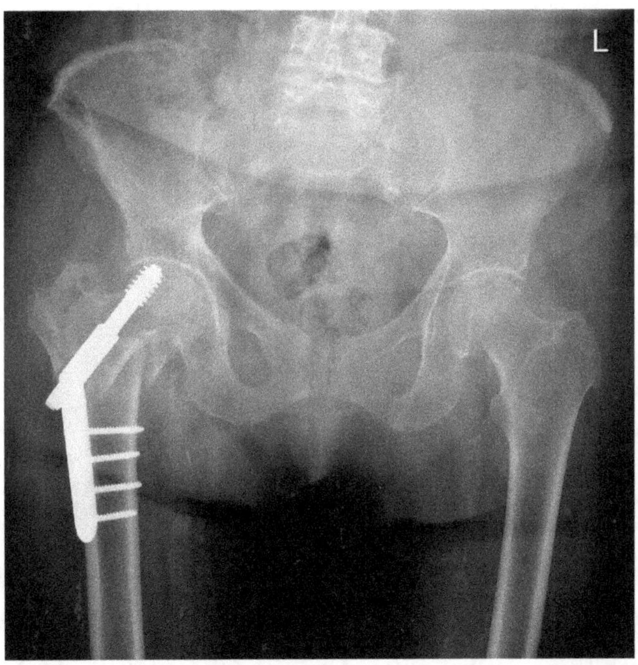

Figure 5. AP radiograph demonstrating screw cut out of post ORIF of neck of femur fracture.

Preoperative templating, paying particular attention to the length of the proposed femoral component is essential to bypass bone defects or screw tracks. An attempt should be made to recreate the patients' normal anatomy; it is essential to restore offset, length, and centre of rotation. If acetabular bone loss is noted as autogenous bone graft, allograft or a fixation device may be necessary to reconstruct or span a marginal, cavitary, or combined defect.

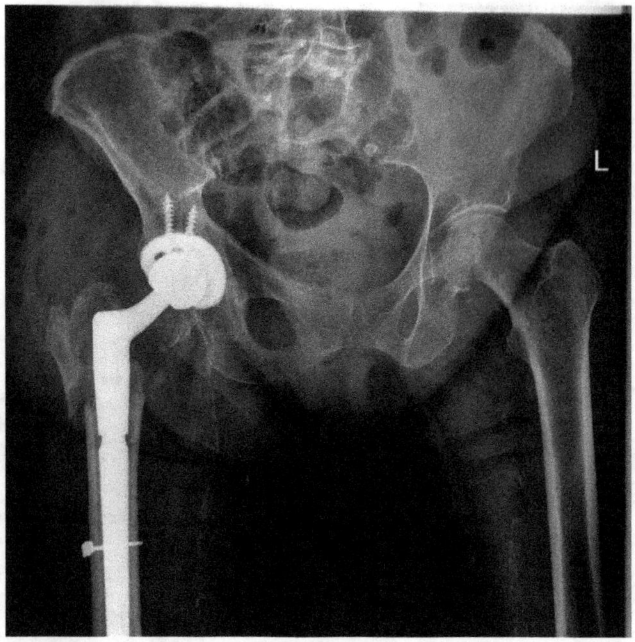

Figure 6. Demonstrating subsequent revision to a modular prosthesis.

During the preparation of the femur, it is recommended to leave the internal fixation device in situ and to avoid excessive traction and leg rotation until dislocation to minimise the risk of intraoperative fracture. Cemented or uncemented components can be used depending on user preference and in conjunction with intraoperative evaluation of acetabular and femoral bone quality.

In such cases the acetabulum may not be degenerative and thus less sclerotic than usually encountered in elective arthroplasty. Reaming therefore should be performed with caution, being mindful of the risk of medial wall penetration. In performing a THR in a cognitively impaired patient, an extended stability or constrained liner and a larger diameter bearing should be considered.

5. THR for failed intertrochanteric fracture fixation

Patients with failed internal fixation of intertrochanteric fractures present with significant functional disability and pain. In these patients revision of the fixation device will often be considered as a first option, but these surgeries are often complicated by bone loss and the presence of avascular bone at the nonunion site. Hip arthroplasty offers a good salvage option for selected patients as it obviates the need for fracture healing and establishes immediate skeletal continuity allowing early, progressive weight bearing. **Figure 7** shows a nonunion of a subtrochanteric femur fracture following cephalomedullary fixation which was successfully revised to a modular THR as seen in **Figure 8**.

Technical issues such as difficulty of implant removal, bone loss, trochanteric nonunion, anticipated haemorrhage and suboptimal bone quality must be considered. A common mode of

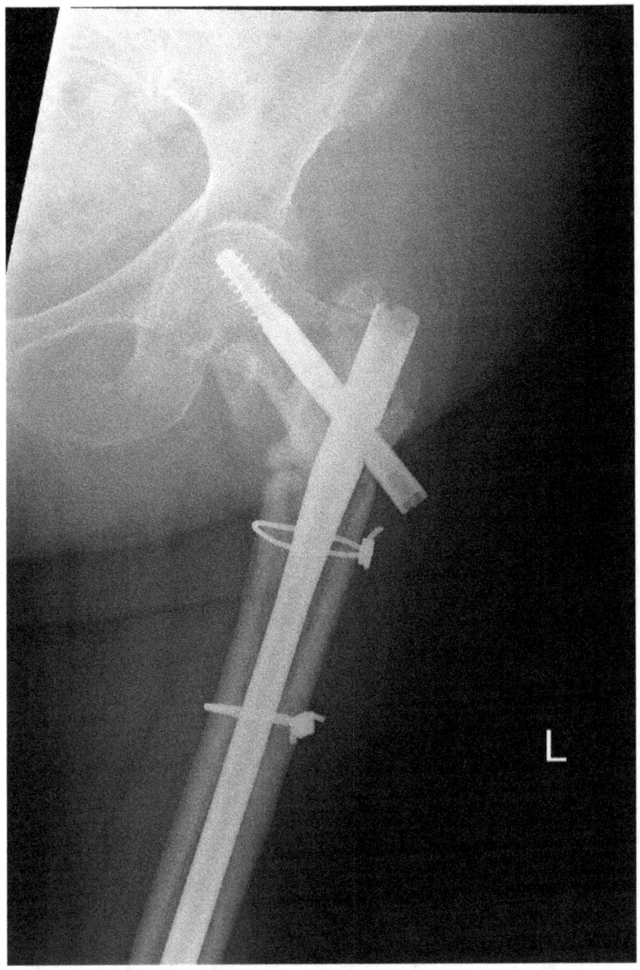

Figure 7. AP radiograph demonstrating non union of a subtrochanteric femur fracture following cephalomedullary fixation.

failure in intertrochanteric fractures is cut-out of the lag screw which consequently damages the acetabular cartilage and often necessitates acetabular replacement during the conversion arthroplasty.

It is imperative that the surgeon eliminates infection as a cause of failure and preoperative evaluation should include measurements of CRP and ESR levels and aspiration or biopsy if inflammatory marker levels are concerning. If infection is demonstrated, a two-stage procedure should be performed with the removal of components and the femoral head during the first stage, with the use of an antibiotic-impregnated cement prosthesis.

During revision of a failed intertrochanteric fracture, it is again advisable to leave the fixation in place until surgical dislocation of the hip is performed. Access is often determined by trochanteric anatomy: gained either between ununited fragments or with mobilisation of malunited fragments. If some continuity is maintained with the fibres of vastus lateralis, the exposure resembles a trochanteric slide. In these cases, the risk of mechanical complications such as fractures and cortical perforations is increased due to reduced bone quality, loss of bone stock, presence of screw holes from previous fixation devices, and distorted bony landmarks. If trochanteric nonunion is encountered, fibrous tissue is debrided from the cancellous surface

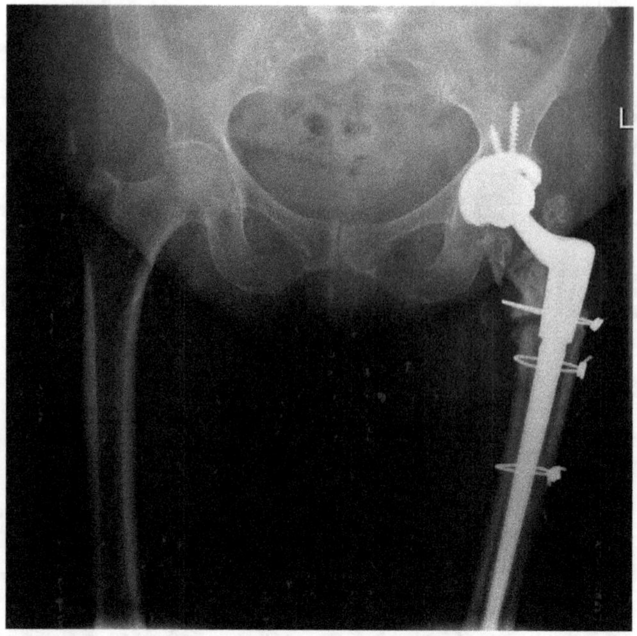

Figure 8. Demonstrating subsequent revision to a modular prosthesis.

of the fragments, and a high-speed burr can be used to expose bleeding cancellous bone. The excised femoral head is often a useful source of autograft, and applying an acetabular reamer to the femoral head will rapidly morselise the fragment. Patients with cephalomedullary nails in situ may exhibit neocortex formation and sclerosis around the nail, and broaching the canal in these cases can be facilitated by using a high-speed burr. Calcar replacing and fully coated stems may be considered in those with loss of proximal bone. Modular implants may also play a role in the setting of severe proximal bone loss. Reattachment of the trochanter in cases of nonunion is a crucial step towards regaining stability, and trochanteric cable plates are particularly useful in many of these cases.

Lee et al. recommended the use of total hip arthroplasty for failed internal fixation of intertrochanteric fractures. They report a 3% 1 year mortality rate in the conversion group. At 3 years of follow-up, there was no significant difference in clinical scores or component loosening when compared to a matched cohort who received hemiarthroplasties [40].

6. THR for pathological or impending fracture

Of patients with advanced cancer, 50% develop bony metastases, and 30% of metastatic deposits occur within the proximal femur. Due to the high mechanical forces directed through the hip, surgery is often required for pain palliation, to restore function and to allow immediate unrestricted weight bearing. Current treatment options include intramedullary nailing, osteosynthesis with a plate-screw construct and endoprosthetic replacements—taking the form of hemiarthroplasties, total hip arthroplasties, and proximal femoral replacements.

For patients expected to live greater than 6 months, the literature supports curettage of the lesion with cemented hemiarthroplasty [41–43]. Those patients demonstrating a radioresistant tumour may necessitate en bloc excision and proximal femoral replacement [44]. Intramedullary fixation should be utilised in those with a life expectancy less than 6 months as it has been demonstrated to provide reliable fracture fixation up to 12 months post-procedure [45, 46]. The use of a hemiarthroplasty to treat pathologic or impending pathologic fractures of the proximal femur has an acceptable rate of complications, reoperations, and functional outcomes as demonstrated by Houdek et al., who studied 199 patients treated with a hemiarthroplasty for metastatic femoral neck disease. They demonstrated a 1% conversion rate to THR due to degenerative changes and groin pain. [47].

With advances in medical management of metastatic disease and concomitant increase in patient's life expectancy, the durability of these implants has become increasingly important. Due to the poor survival rates in this cohort of patients, it has been difficult to compare implant survival rates for patients with metastatic disease with those utilised in primary joint replacement. However, in series comparing THR with osteosynthesis in the setting of pathologic fracture, THR has demonstrated a lower rate of mechanical failure as well as a higher rate of implant survival [48].

7. Conclusion

In conclusion, in the setting of the neck of femur fracture, a cemented hemiarthroplasty is an appropriate treatment for elderly patients. However, studies have suggested that patients treated with THR experience improved functional outcomes but at the expense of a greater dislocation rate. The selective use of THR in cognitively intact, active patients is well supported. In the setting of failed internal fixation, an arthroplasty, while technically demanding, represents an acceptable salvage procedure for the neck of femur and intertrochanteric fractures. However, in both scenarios it is essential that infection is excluded as a precipitant of fixation failure prior to arthroplasty. In cases of pathologic fracture, arthroplasty can represent an appropriate treatment option following careful evaluation of the patient's life expectancy.

Conflict of interest

The authors declare no conflict of interest in the preparation of this chapter. No funding was received by the authors.

Author details

Mark Curtin[1*], Eoghan Pomeroy[1] and James Broderick[2]

*Address all correspondence to: markcurtin10@gmail.com

1 Department of Trauma and Orthopaedics, Beaumont Hospital, Dublin, Ireland

2 Department of Trauma and Orthopaedics, Galway University Hospital, Galway, Ireland

References

[1] Cornwall R, Gilbert MS, Koval KJ, Strauss E, Siu AL. Functional outcomes and mortality vary among different types of hip fractures: A function of patient characteristics. Clinical Orthopaedics and Related Research. Aug 2004;**425**:64

[2] Lewinnek GE, Kelsey J, WHITE III AA, Kreiger NJ. The significance and a comparative analysis of the epidemiology of hip fractures. Clinical Orthopaedics and Related Research. 1980;**152**:35-43

[3] Hung WW, Egol KA, Zuckerman JD, Siu AL. Hip fracture management: Tailoring care for the older patient. JAMA. 2012;**307**(20):2185-2194

[4] Haidukewych GJ, Berry DJ. Hip arthroplasty for salvage of failed treatment of intertrochanteric hip fractures. JBJS. 2003;**85**(5):899-904

[5] Haidukewych GJ, Berry DJ. Salvage of failed internal fixation of intertrochanteric hip fractures. Clinical Orthopaedics and Related Research. 2003;**412**:184-188

[6] Sancheti KH, Sancheti PK, Shyam AK, Patil S, Dhariwal Q, Joshi R. Primary hemiarthroplasty for unstable osteoporotic intertrochanteric fractures in the elderly: A retrospective case series. Indian Journal of Orthopaedics. 2010;**44**(4):428

[7] Lindskog DM, Baumgaertner MR. Unstable intertrochanteric hip fractures in the elderly. Journal of the American Academy of Orthopaedic Surgeons. 2004;**12**(3):179-190

[8] Marsh JL, Slongo TF, Agel J, Broderick JS, Creevey W, DeCoster TA, et al. Fracture and dislocation classification compendium-2007: Orthopaedic Trauma Association classification, database and outcomes committee. Journal of Orthopaedic Trauma. 2007;**21** (10 Suppl):S1-S133

[9] Larsson S. Treatment of osteoporotic fractures. Scandinavian Journal of Surgery. 2002;**91**:140-146

[10] Bannister GC, Gibson AGF, Ackroyd CE, Newman JH. The fixation and prognosis of trochanteric fractures: A randomised prospective controlled trial. Clinical Orthopaedics and Related Research. 1990;**254**:242-246

[11] Chinoy MA, Parker MJ. Fixed nail plates versus sliding hip systems for the treatment of trochanteric femoral fractures: A meta analysis of 14 studies. Injury. 1999;**30**(3):157-163

[12] Flores LA, Harrington IJ, Heller M The stability of intertrochanteric fractures treated with a sliding screw-plate. Bone & Joint Journal. 1990;**72**(1):37-40

[13] Sernbo I, Fredin H. Changing methods of hip fracture osteosynthesis in Sweden: An epidemiological enquiry covering 46,900 cases. Acta Orthopaedica Scandinavica. 1993;**64**(2):173-174

[14] Larsson S, Friberg S, Hansson LI. Trochanteric fractures mobility, complications, and mortality in 607 cases treated with the sliding-screw technique. Clinical Orthopaedics and Related Research. 1990;**260**:232-241

[15] Bess RJ, Jolly SA. Comparison of compression hip screw and gamma nail for treatment of peritrochanteric fractures. Journal of the Southern Orthopaedic Association. 1997;**6**(3):173-179

[16] Halder SC. The gamma nail for peritrochanteric fractures. Bone & Joint Journal. 1992;**74**(3):340-344

[17] Davis TR, Sher JL, Horsman A, Simpson M, Porter BB, Checketts RG. Intertrochanteric femoral fractures. Mechanical failure after internal fixation. Bone & Joint Journal. 1990;**72**(1):26-31

[18] Thomas AP. Dynamic hip screws that fail. Injury. 1991;**22**(1):45-46

[19] Kyle RF, Gustilo RB, Premer RF. Analysis of six hundred and twenty-two intertrochanteric hip fractures. Orthopaedic Trauma Directions. 2010;**8**(06):25-29

[20] Watson JT, Moed BR, Cramer KE, Karges DE. Comparison of the compression hip screw with the Medoff sliding plate for intertrochanteric fractures. Clinical Orthopaedics and Related Research. 1998;**348**:79-86

[21] Michael RC. Prospective randomised controlled trial of an intramedullary nail versus dynamic screw and plate for intertrochanteric fractures of the femur. Journal of Orthopaedic Trauma. 2001;**15**(6):394-400

[22] Simmermacher RKJ, Bosch AM, Van der Werken CHR. The AO/ASIF-proximal femoral nail (PFN): A new device for the treatment of unstable proximal femoral fractures. Injury. 1999;**30**(5):327-332

[23] Bhandari M, Devereaux PJ, Swiontkowski MF, Tornetta P III, Obremskey W, Koval KJ, et al. Internal fixation compared with arthroplasty for displaced fractures of the femoral neck: A meta-analysis. JBJS. 2003;**85**(9):1673-1681

[24] Parker MJ, Khan RJK, Crawford J, Pryor GA. Hemiarthroplasty versus internal fixation for displaced intracapsular hip fractures in the elderly. Bone & Joint Journal. 2002;**84**(8):1150-1155

[25] Poolman RW, Struijs PA, Krips R, Sierevelt IN, Lutz KH, Bhandari M. Does a "Level I Evidence" rating imply high quality of reporting in orthopaedic randomised controlled trials? BMC Medical Research Methodology. 2006;**6**(1):44

[26] Bhandari M, Devereaux PJ, Einhorn TA, Thabane L, Schemitsch EH, Koval KJ, et al. Hip fracture evaluation with alternatives of total hip arthroplasty versus hemiarthroplasty (HEALTH): Protocol for a multicentre randomised trial. BMJ Open. 2015;**5**(2):e006263

[27] Grosso MJ, Danoff JR, Murtaugh TS, Trofa DP, Sawires AN, Macaulay WB. Hemiarthroplasty for displaced femoral neck fractures in the elderly has a low conversion rate. The Journal of Arthroplasty. 2017;**32**(1):150-154

[28] Hopley C, Stengel D, Ekkernkamp A, Wich M. Primary total hip arthroplasty versus hemiarthroplasty for displaced intracapsular hip fractures in older patients: Systematic review. BMJ. 2010;**340**:c2332

[29] White SM, Moppett IK, Griffiths R, Johansen A, Wakeman R, Boulton C, et al. Secondary analysis of outcomes after 11,085 hip fracture operations from the prospective UK Anaesthesia Sprint Audit of Practice (ASAP-2). Anaesthesia. 2016;**71**(5):506-514

[30] Su EP, Su SL. Femoral neck fractures. The Bone & Joint Journal. 2014;**96**(11 Supple A): 43-47

[31] Zi-Sheng A, You-Shui G, Zhi-Zhen J, Ting Y, Chang-Qing Z. Hemiarthroplasty vs. primary total hip arthroplasty for displaced fractures of the femoral neck in the elderly: A meta-analysis. The Journal of Arthroplasty. 2012;**27**(4):583-590

[32] Gao H, Liu Z, Xing D, Gong M. Which is the best alternative for displaced femoral neck fractures in the elderly?: A meta-analysis. Clinical Orthopaedics and Related Research. 2012;**470**(6):1782-1791

[33] Perry DC, Metcalfe D, Griffin XL, Costa ML Inequalities in use of total hip arthroplasty for hip fracture: Population based study. Bmj. 2016;**353**:i2021

[34] Anakwe RE, Middleton SD, Jenkins PJ, Butler AP, Aitken SA, Keating JF, et al. Total hip replacement in patients with hip fracture: A matched cohort study. Journal of Trauma and Acute Care Surgery. 2012;**73**(3):738-742

[35] Ossendorf C, Scheyerer MJ, Wanner GA, Simmen HP, Werner CM. Treatment of femoral neck fractures in elderly patients over 60 years of age-which is the ideal modality of primary joint replacement? Patient Safety in Surgery. 2010;**4**(1):16

[36] Maceroli MA, Nikkel LE, Mahmood B, Elfar JC. Operative mortality after arthroplasty for femoral neck fracture and hospital volume. Geriatric Orthopaedic Surgery & Rehabilitation. 2015;**6**(4):239-245

[37] Uhler LM, Schultz WR, Hill AD, Koenig KM. Health utility of early hemiarthroplasty vs. delayed total hip arthroplasty for displaced femoral neck fracture in elderly patients: A Markov model. The Journal of Arthroplasty. 2017;**32**(5):1434-1438

[38] Nikolopoulos KE, Papadakis SA, Kateros KT, Themistocleous GS, Vlamis JA, Papagelopoulos PJ, et al. Long-term outcome of patients with avascular necrosis, after internal fixation of femoral neck fractures. Injury. 2003;**34**(7):525-528

[39] Tidermark J, Zethraeus N, Svensson O, Törnkvist H, Ponzer S. Quality of life related to fracture displacement among elderly patients with femoral neck fractures treated with internal fixation. Journal of Orthopaedic Trauma. 2002;**16**(1):34-38

[40] Lee YK, Kim JT, Alkitaini AA, Kim KC, Ha YC, Koo KH. Conversion hip arthroplasty in failed fixation of intertrochanteric fracture: A propensity score matching study. The Journal of Arthroplasty. 2017;**32**(5):1593-1598

[41] Wedin R, Bauer HC. Surgical treatment of skeletal metastatic lesions of the proximal femur. Bone & Joint Journal. 2005;**87**(12):1653-1657

[42] Harvey N, Ahlmann ER, Allison DC, Wang L, Menendez LR. Endoprostheses last longer than intramedullary devices in proximal femur metastases. Clinical Orthopaedics and Related Research. 2012;**470**(3):684-691

[43] Park DH, Jaiswal PK, Al-Hakim W, Aston WJS, Pollock RC, Skinner JA, et al. The use of massive endoprostheses for the treatment of bone metastases. Sarcoma. 2007;**2007**:62151

[44] Hwang N, Nandra R, Grimer RJ, Carter SR, Tillman RM, Abudu A, et al. Massive endoprosthetic replacement for bone metastases resulting from renal cell carcinoma: Factors influencing patient survival. European Journal of Surgical Oncology (EJSO). 2014;**40**(4):429-434

[45] Moholkar K, Mohan R, Grigoris P. The Long Gamma Nail for stabilisation of existing and impending pathological fractures of the femur. An analysis of 48 cases. Acta Orthopaedica Belgica. 2004;**70**(5):429-434

[46] Piccioli A, Rossi B, Scaramuzzo L, Spinelli MS, Yang Z, Maccauro G. Intramedullary nailing for treatment of pathologic femoral fractures due to metastases. Injury. 2014;**45**(2):412-417

[47] Houdek MT, Wyles CC, Labott JR, Rose PS, Taunton MJ, Sim FH. Durability of Hemiarthroplasty for Pathologic Proximal Femur Fractures. The Journal of Arthroplasty. 2017;**32**(12):3607-3610

[48] Harvey N, Ahlmann ER, Allison DC, Wang L, Menendez LR. Endoprostheses last longer than intramedullary devices in proximal femur metastases. Clinical Orthopaedics and Related Research. 2012;**470**(3):684-691

3

Physical Therapy Based on Closed Kinematic Chain Patterns for Patients after Total Hip Replacement

Jan Vagner, Ingrid Palaščáková Špringrová, Pavel Přikryl, Šárka Tomková and Rafi Moheb

Abstract

In this chapter I will focus on the importance of properly managed movement therapy for patients after total hip replacement. It is necessary to find correct movement patterns which can help patient to become more independent in ADL and locomotion. It seems to be much more effective to choose therapy based on closed kinematic chains (CKC). In CKC we have bigger amount of motor units and it is easier to maintain postural reactivity. The main aim is to use similarity in movement patterns. In therapy we choose patterns that are similar to ADL activities. Acral Coactivation Therapy (ACT) is a movement therapy that works with these principles. The effects of the therapy are seen in different areas: improvement of patient's ADL skills, better postural reactivity and stability (lumbo-pelvic stability), decrease subjective level of pain. In the subacute and chronic phase of therapy, we can follow up previous aims and focus on restoring full function and condition.

Keywords: total hip replacement, closed kinematic chain, Acral Coactivation Therapy, balance therapy, motion abilities for ADL, reduce pain

1. Introduction

This chapter deals with movement therapy management in patients after total hip joint replacement (THR). Primarily it is about setting movement patterns which are the most beneficial for patients in terms of postural reactivity, next about reducing subjective perception of pain, renewing functional abilities from the perspective of activities of daily living (ADL) and last but not least about satisfaction with surgery.

Degenerative changes of weight-bearing joints rank, without hesitation, among diseases of civilization of the musculoskeletal system. In the final stage of this disease the patients are significantly limited, in particular their movement abilities in ADL, and they suffer from strong pain which is frequently alleviated by pharmaceutical drugs. In the final stage total replacement of the afflicted joint, a hip joint in this case, is indicated in the patients. There is no doubt that postoperative care of the patients is a multi-branch matter and that rehabilitation managed by a qualified physiotherapist is its integral part [1, 2].

In total hip replacement the joint capsule is damaged, which results in the reduction of statesthetic and kinetic proprioception and aggravation of postural stability mainly in vertical positions and deterioration of locomotion skills. Postoperative recovery is accompanied by other problematic factors, e.g. pain caused by the surgical intervention itself or limited mobility of the operated limb due to anti-luxation regime. All the named factors reflect on the patient's final movement expression.

The aim of the managed postoperative rehabilitation should be not only motor recovery of the operated lower limb but also setting stereotyped physiological movement concerning ADL. The selected movement patterns, which the patient performs within the therapy, should reflect on their daily performance. The therapy should not lack a principle of similarity, i.e. the patients are provided with such movement patterns that can be integrated in activities of daily living.

Many authors consider learning and mastering closed kinetic chain (CKC) activities as a factor indispensable for carrying out physiological movements in an open kinetic chain (OKC). It means that the therapy itself should always start in a position which is relatively easy for muscle chains activation, i.e. applying pressure. Closed kinetic chain movements optimize activity of the engaged muscle groups which besides other things helps reduce subjective pain perception [3–7].

For the purposes of our study we chose the Acral Coactivation Therapy (ACT) that meets all the above mentioned criteria for the management of high quality rehabilitation of the patients after total hip joint replacement.

This study also aims at pointing out that minimum objectivization means are used in the branch of rehabilitation, which results in interpretation of movement therapy as an empirical branch lacking objective values. The patients′ subjective feedback concerning evaluation of therapy results is certainly important, however, efficacy of therapy cannot be objectively assessed without recorded data. For this reason we chose a measurement system of a force plate by Tekscan or specific questionnaires tailor-made for patients with a given diagnosis in order to make the results objective.

2. The Acral Coactivation Therapy (ACT) characteristics

The Acral Coactivation Therapy is a physiotherapeutic method based on neurophysiology. The founder of the ACT is PhDr. Ingrid Palaščáková Špringrová Ph.D. and the basic ideas are inspired by Roswitha Brunkow's method.

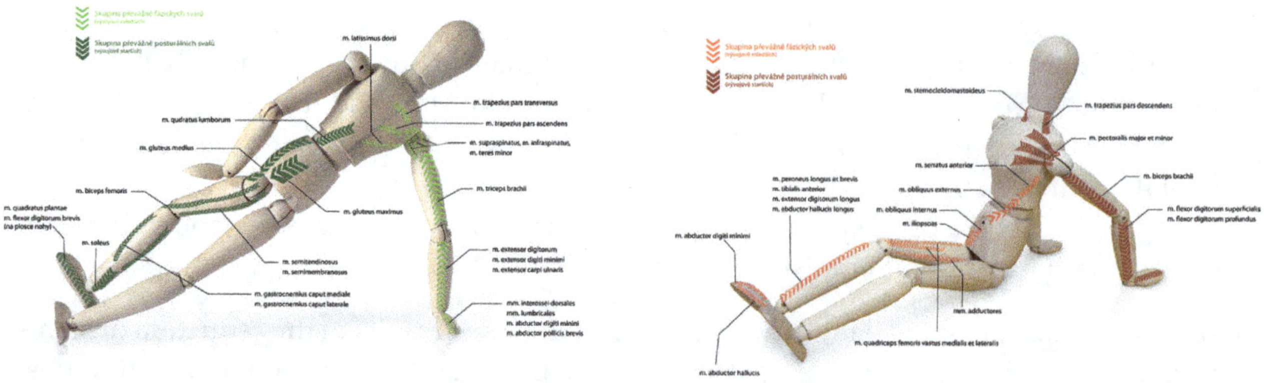

Figure 1. Dorsal and ventral muscle chain.

One of the basic ACT principles is applying pressure on the acral parts of extremities (both upper and lower). Applying pressure on the acral parts leads to straightening the spine and activating posture against external forces. Setting and maintaining correct posture is fundamental for creating a physiological movement programme, thus part and parcel of a movement itself. Muscle contraction proceeds in the disto-proximal direction, i.e. from the acral parts toward the trunk. Applying pressure aims at co-activation of muscle chains (see **Figure 1**). In order to improve movement pattern quality, thus better co-activation of muscle chains, manual techniques are used. Muscle tone balance of co-activated muscle chains is achieved by exteroceptive and proprioceptive inputs [7].

The ACT works on the principle of repetition of a movement pattern based on applying pressure on the acral parts. These conscious repetitive presses form the basic element of mastering the practised movement skills (motor learning). Mastering new skills by means of conscious repetition of movement patterns is one of the basic principles of the ACT. Motor learning can be simply characterized as a set of processes connected with training or experience leading to relatively constant changes of the ability to react [7, 8].

The acres are significantly represented in human brain matter so they initiate motor activity in the ACT. Unlike proximally placed muscle groups, which are significantly represented in the pre-motor brain area, the acres are located mainly in the primary motor cortical areas [7, 8–10].

During the workout patients carry out planned (intentional) movements. It is presumed that applying pressure activates the limbic system. Motivation is indispensable for movement as well. Activation of the limbic system is followed by a sensory analysis of the movement, the function of which is to draw up an ideal plan of the press. While pressing up the central nervous system (CNS) uses peripheral information and assesses quality of the press, in particular straightening the spine apparatus. If the spinal alignment is not correct (the spine is not straightened), the posture is adjusted, i.e., the angle of the acres is changed. After adjusting posture, pressure is applied again and a new movement pattern with the identical objective of straightening the spine apparatus is ingrained [7, 9, 11, 12].

The ACT therapy exploits positions from ontogenetic development of human motor activity. The early motor activity of newborns manifests itself in open kinetic chains. However, during development the postural activity caused by confrontation of the CNS and external

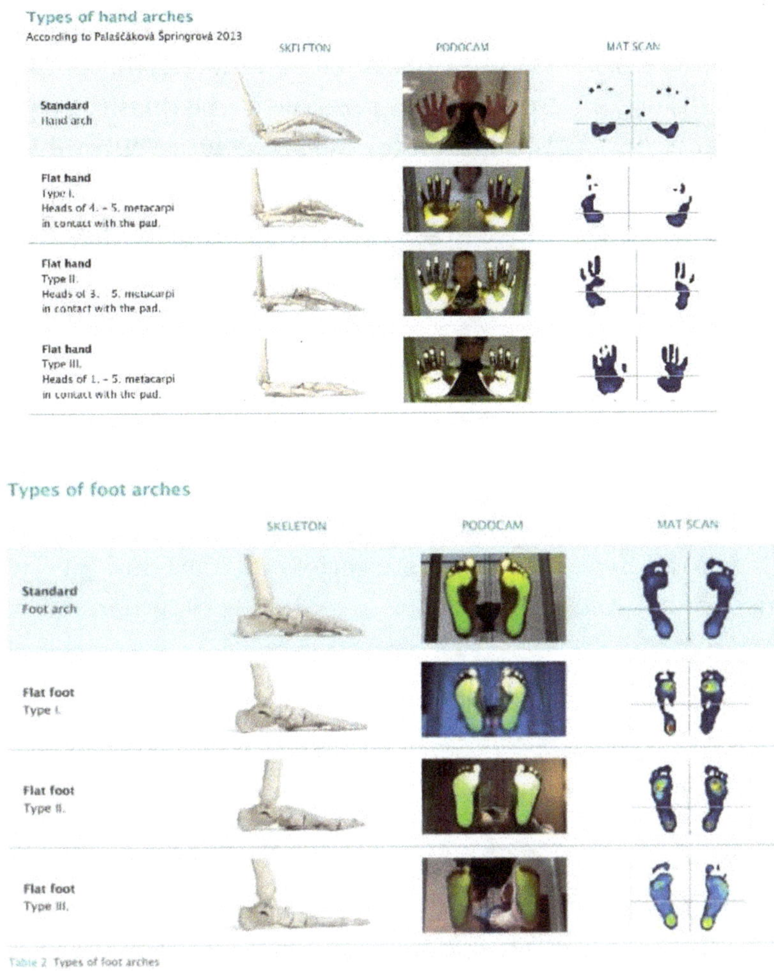

Figure 2. Evaluation of arches of the hand and the foot by means of the ACD.

stimuli increases. Movement patterns in closed kinetic chains are involved. Due to increasing demand on movement patterns the CNS is forced to choose an adequate movement pattern in terms of its economy and function [7, 13–15].

The closed kinetic chain activities provide the basis for postural presumptions of all motor activities of a child. The open kinetic chain motor activity is focused mainly on movements with a particular purpose, i.e. teleological movements [3, 4, 7, 13].

Many authors consider learning and mastering closed kinetic chain (CKC) activities as a factor indispensable for carrying out physiological movements in an open kinetic chain (OKC). It means that the therapy itself should start in a position which is relatively easy for muscle chain activation, i.e. applying pressure. Closed kinetic chain movements optimize activity of the engaged muscle groups. Correct involvement of muscle groups as well as centration of key joints in closed kinetic chains requires correct physiological position of the trunk and the limbs. The ACT method uses mainly closed kinetic chain movements since many authors consider them more functional, thus more effective in the therapy [3–5, 7].

The Acral Coactivation Diagnostics (ACD) is irreplaceable in the Acral Coactivation Therapy. It includes evaluation of position of upper and lower extremities and straightening of the spine. The ACD exploits measuring instruments, e.g. PodoCam or Tekscan, thanks to which position of the acral parts of limbs can be objectively evaluated. If a pathological position of arches (of a hand or a foot) occurs, a press is not possible in the quality ensuring physiological muscle coactivation that results in straightening the spine and centration of root joints. The ACT uses also entry and exit questionnaires including, beside other things, basic case history, visual analog scale (VAS) and questions targeted at early motor development [7] (**Figure 2**).

3. Methodology of the study

Thirty patients of the Department of Orthopedics and Traumatology of Přerov Hospital (SMN Přerov), branch of the business Středomoravská nemocniční a.s., took part in the study. In order to be included in the study the patients had to meet the following criteria: they had not undergone any endoprosthesis or lower extremities surgery in the past and they were not diagnosed with any mental illness or neurological disorder of central or peripheral nervous system.

"Only" 30 patients out of total 352 applicants who had undergone total hip joint replacement in Přerov Hospital met these criteria. Collecting data for this study took 12 months.

3.1. The CKC group (CKC=closed kinetic chain)

The CKC group consisting of 15 patients (7 men and 8 women) of the Department of Orthopedics and Traumatology of SMN Přerov went through postoperative rehabilitation according to the Acral Coactivation Therapy principles. The average age of the patients was 59 ± 13.9 years.

3.2. The OKC group (OKC=open kinetic chain)

Also the OKC group included 15 patients (8 men and 7 women) of the Department of Orthopedics and Traumatology of SMN Přerov who underwent postoperative therapy, which is based mostly on open kinetic chain exercises, according to the standard procedures of SMN Přerov. The average age of the patients was 58 ± 9.7 years.

The probands were divided into individual groups by means of adaptive randomization. At the beginning of the study both groups of the patients did not differ considerably in terms of the observed parameters (**Table 1**). At-entry differences of the observed groups did not show any statistical significance.

3.3. The CKC group therapy

The CKC group therapy followed the basic principles of the Acral Coactivation Therapy. The rehabilitation plan consisted of (on average) six 30-min workout units under the guidance of a qualified physiotherapist who supervised quality of the carried out motor patterns. The therapy itself began the second postoperative day and continued until the patients were discharged and took part in subsequent rehabilitation treatment.

	CKC group (μ)	P	OKC group (μ)
Age	59	SID	58
B.E.S.S.	5.3	SID	5.3
FT	36.1	SID	35.5
HHS	48.1	SID	52.8

Table 1. Entry parameters.

The managed therapy took place only during working hours of the physiotherapist (i.e. working days). In order to improve quality the patients got an aid: Functional Hand Arch Support (only for the purpose of the managed therapy). These gloves, specially tailored for the ACT method, maintain optimum setting of arches of the hand. Outside the time set aside for the therapy (i.e. at weekends, in free time) the probands carried out autotherapy according to the ACT without the physiotherapist's intervention. For these purposes the patients got the publication of The Acral Press Up Exercises for Straightened Spine where the ACT positions used in the therapy were marked. First, the patients carried out all the safe exercises in the managed therapy conducted under the guidance of a physiotherapist to avoid wrong fixation of motor patterns and subsequent errors in autotherapy. The therapy took place in SMN Přerov in the gym of the department of orthopedics and traumatology. This place was calm with suitable conditions for working out. Selected positions from the CKC group therapy are depicted in **Figures 3–10**.

3.4. List of CKC group static positions and their variants

When selecting static positions for therapy in a closed kinetic chain we took into consideration regime measures (anti-luxation regime) that the patients had to observe. The applied positions were chosen from the publication of The Acral Press Up Exercises for Straightened Spine in order to make autotherapy easier [16].

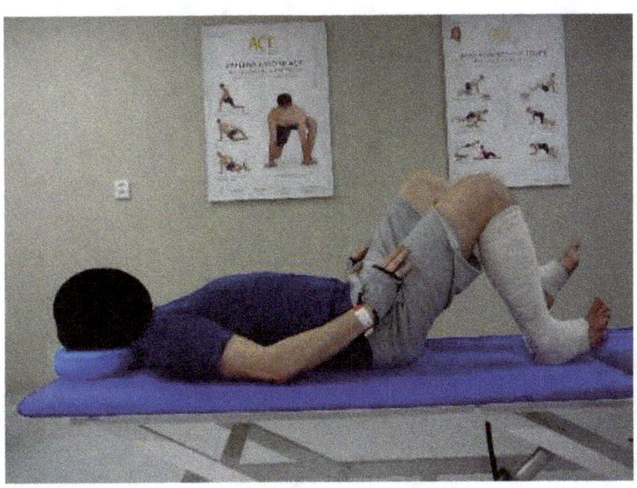

Figure 3. A press up in the supine position variant of flexion: Static coactivation.

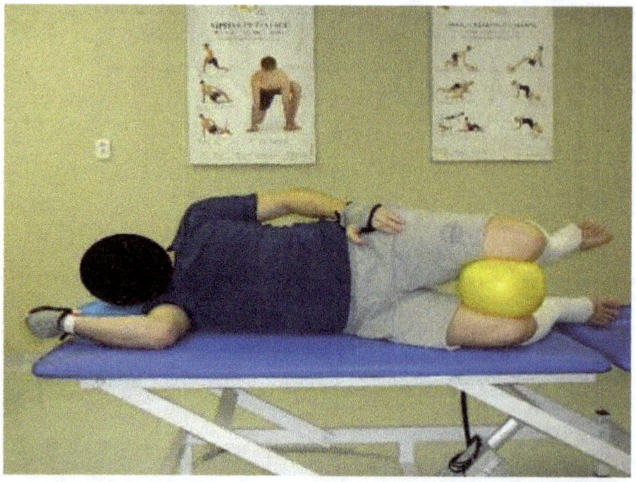

Figure 4. A press up on the healthy hip: Static coactivation.

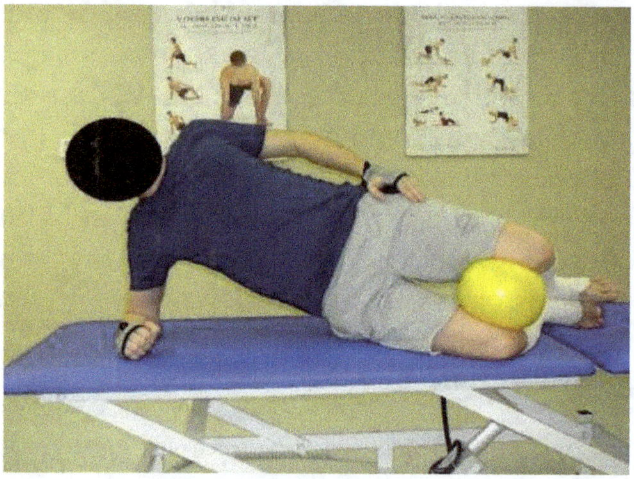

Figure 5. A press up in the low oblique sitting: Static coactivation.

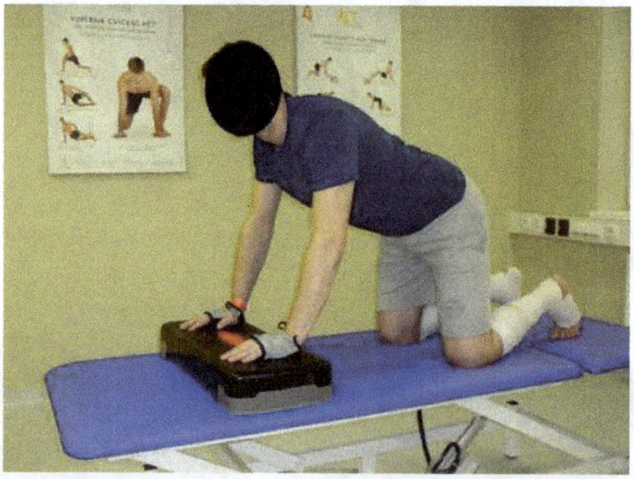

Figure 6. A press up on all fours: Static coactivation.

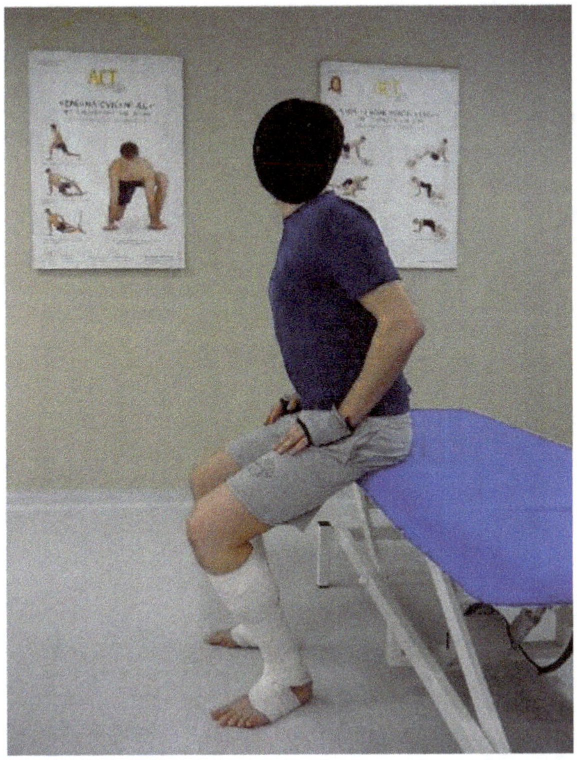

Figure 7. A press up in the sitting position, initial stage of dynamic transition from the sitting to the standing position.

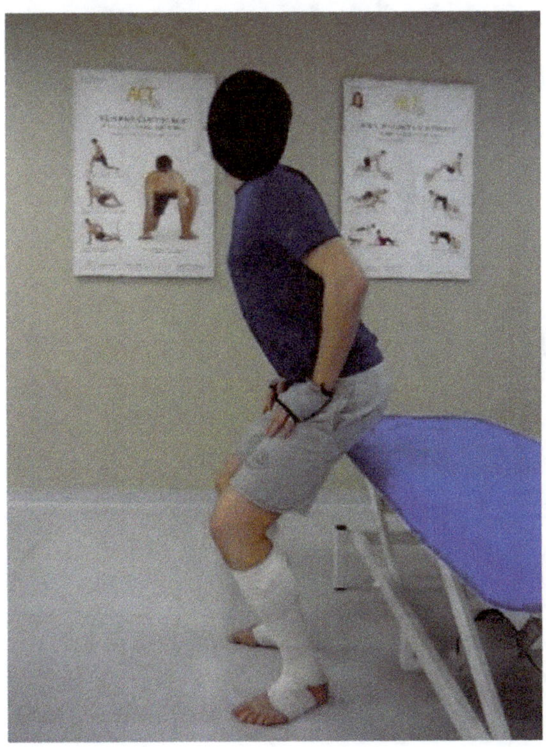

Figure 8. A final stage of dynamic transition from the sitting to the standing position.

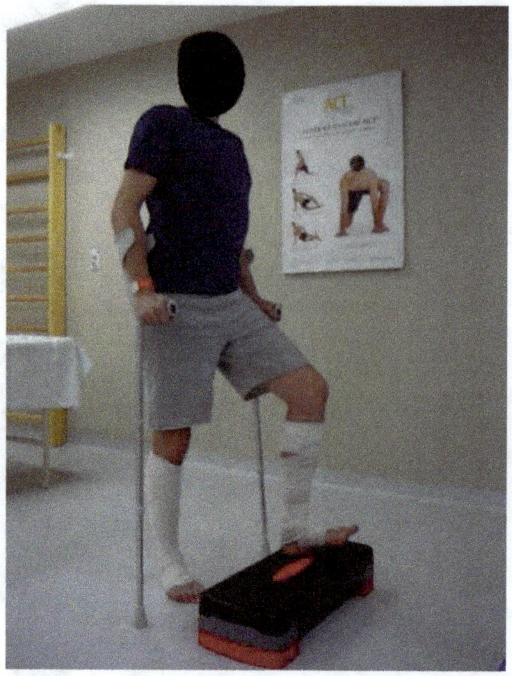

Figure 9. A press up in the standing position with 2 forearm crutches; putting a foot forward on the step: Static coactivation.

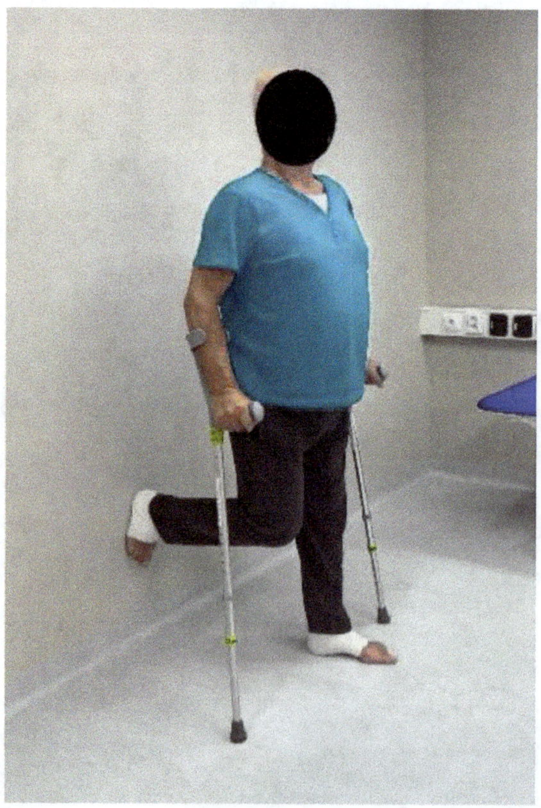

Figure 10. A press up in the standing position with 2 forearm crutches, extension against the wall: Static coactivation.

1. A press up in the supine position and its variants:

- gait movement pattern: alternating flexion and extension of lower extremities in the CKC (after mastering the OKC exercises)
- alternating flexion of lower extremities in the CKC

2. A press up in the side-lying position (lying on the healthy hip) with neutral position of lower extremities and its variants:

- abduction of the operated leg in the CKC after mastering OKC exercises

3. A press up in the side-lying position while pressing up the upper body with an arm.
4. A press up in the prone position and its variants:

- alternating knee joint flexion

5. A press up in the position on all fours and its variants:

- alternating flexion and extension of lower extremities
- pressing up on all fours while lifting the knees above the floor
- abduction of lower extremities while lifting the knees above the floor

6. A press up in the upright kneeling position.
7. A press up while sitting on the chair and its variants:

- gait movement pattern: alternating flexion and extension of lower extremities in the CKC (after mastering the OKC exercises)

8. A press up while standing with two forearm crutches and its variants:

- putting a foot forward on the step (alternating lower extremities) with subsequent support
- training of extension while leaning against the wall (alternating lower extremities)

3.5. List of dynamic transitions in the CKC group

The patients carried out dynamic transitions from individual press up (static) positions. These were functional dynamic changes in positions according to the ACT principles. Two sets of dynamic transitions selected in advance were applied. Dynamic transitions were chosen on the basis of the similarity principle in order to evoke the movement patterns the patients used in ADL. The therapy was aimed at integration of physiological movement patterns into motor expression of the patients in ADL [16].

Dynamic transitions for verticalization from the supine to the standing position (i.e. getting up from the bed).

1. A press up from the supine to the side-lying position.
2. A press up from the lateral to the side-lying position while pressing up the upper body with an arm and having lower extremities hanging off the bed.
3. A press up from the side-lying position while pressing up the upper body with an arm to the sitting position with lower extremities hanging off the bed.
4. A press up from the sitting position with lower extremities hanging off the bed to the standing position (hands on thighs – the CKC).

Dynamic transitions for verticalization from the supine to the standing position (from the floor).

1. A press up from the supine to the lateral position.
2. A press up from the lateral to the prone position.
3. A press up from the prone position to the position on all fours.
4. A press up from the position on all fours to the upright kneeling position.
5. A press up from the upright kneeling position to putting the foot forward (i.e. the healthy leg); with support of 1 forearm crutch if needed.
6. A press up from the position of having a foot forward to the standing position (with support of a chair or a forearm crutch if needed).

3.6. The OKC group therapy

Also the patients in this group went through managed (on average) six 30-min workout units. These patients worked out according to the standardized SMN Přerov rehabilitation plan intended for patients after total hip joint replacement. The exercises were analytical exercises mostly in an open kinetic chain, without a direct link to the ADL therapy. The beginning and the end of the therapy collided with the CKC group. In order to maintain the same conditions this group worked out in the same gym of the department of orthopedics and traumatology of Přerov Hospital as well. In their free time the probands performed autotherapy based on a list of standardized SMN Přerov exercises intended for patients after total hip joint replacement (see below). First, the patients carried out all the exercises under the guidance of a physiotherapist, next the exercises became part of their autotherapy.

3.7. The list of exercises for patients after total hip joint replacement according to the SMN Přerov standards

1. In the supine position

- point and flex your feet rhythmically
- flex your feet, straighten your knees and squeeze your buttocks
- move the extended leg sideways (on the bed) and back to the body axis

- bend the knee (i.e. move the heel along the bed)
- bend the knees, put a pillow between them and squeeze you knees together
- bend your knees, lift your buttocks (hold for a few seconds), your arms rest along your body
- lie on your side and raise your top leg

2. In the prone position

- squeeze your buttocks and push your pelvis toward the floor
- push your toes to the floor and straighten your knees
- alternate flexion and extension of your knees
- lift the entire extended leg

3. Sitting with legs hanging off the bed

- straighten your knee while pushing your thigh toward the bed (hold for a few seconds)
- put your hands on your thighs, squeeze your buttocks and then release
- raise your feet slightly

4. Standing at the head of the bed:

- stand on your toes
- move your operated leg sideways and back
- flex your operated hip (no more than 90 degrees)
- extend your operated leg backwards

3.8. Common therapy

Both groups of probands went through the same locomotion training using stairs and mobility aids, i.e. two forearm crutches in this case. Another common therapy element was practising forward bends (picking things up off the floor) while extending the operated hip joint.

3.8.1. Evaluation of postural stability by means of MobileMat™ Programme

Postural stability and reactivity was evaluated by means of a force plate by Tekscan using the MobileMat™ programme. This programme works on the Balance Error Scoring System (B.E.S.S.) principle developed by researchers Guskiewitz, Riemann and Shields.

MobileMat™ programme was developed mainly in order to improve the accuracy of B.E.S.S. evaluation, which can be influenced by a human factor, i.e. subjective inputs of a testee. It is a computer-based evaluation of B.E.S.S. The studies show that the MobileMat™ programme can run a more precise analysis of B.E.S.S., in particular lifting a part of the foot off the force plate, lifting an arm from the base position or changing the position of a non-weight bearing hip (i.e. when standing only on the other leg). However, MobileMat™ programme cannot evaluate if the testee closes their eyes. In this case, this factor is supervised by a qualified physiotherapist [17–19].

Evaluation of postural stability took place in a calm environment of the department of orthopedics and traumatology in the gym of SMN Přerov. The measurement included three positions that were repeated three times by the probands. With regard to an early postoperative stage alternative positions were chosen (see below) which could be carried out by the patients without being exposed to dangerous positions or inadequate physical load of the operated leg. The patients held each position for 20 seconds and had their eyes closed during the whole measurement.

3.8.1.1. Selected positions

1. Standing with feet hip-width apart on both feet; the entire feet are in touch with the Tekscan force plate; standing straight with the hands on the hips.
2. Standing on both lower extremities, in tandem left forward position; the entire feet are in touch with the Tekscan force plate; standing straight with the hands on the hips.
3. Standing on both lower extremities, in tandem right forward position; the entire feet are in touch with the Tekscan force plate; standing straight with the hands on the hips.

Two physiotherapists made measurement while one of them operated the computer and the other one supervised correct posture of the probands in the selected positions. Due to personnel reasons the persons who were not familiar with classification of the probands into the test groups could not make measurement. Evaluation was carried out properly without any intervention leading to distorting results. Measurement was performed 1 day before surgery, the fourth postoperative day and finally on the tenth postoperative day (i.e. the last day of the managed rehabilitation). During evaluation of postural stability the measured values of the individual positions were counted up and the arithmetic mean was calculated.

Both groups had the same average values, i.e. 5.3 postural errors, during entry measurement. In the postoperative stage the CKC group showed 5.1 errors per patient, while the OKC group had 3.5 errors on average. The measured values were entered in a table (see **Table 2**). **Graph 1** shows the differences in the reached B.E.S.S. values of the observed groups.

The final measurement showed a significant statistical difference ($p = 0.008975$) between the entry values of the individual groups. The CKC group reached 1.2 error, while the OCK group had 4.1 errors on average. This difference shows also high effect size (Cohen's $d = 0.875$). Non-parametric Mann–Whitney U test was used to determine statistical significance of two selected files.

3.8.2. Evaluation of the patient functional movement skills

A day before surgery a qualified physiotherapist evaluated functional skills of the patients according to the Functional Test Questionnaire (see **Table 3**). This specific questionnaire was

	CKC group (μ)	P	OKC group (μ)
B.E.S.S. 1	5.3	SID	5.3
B.E.S.S. 2	5.1	SID	3.5
B.E.S.S. 3	1.2	SSD	4.1

Table 2. B.E.S.S. evaluation.

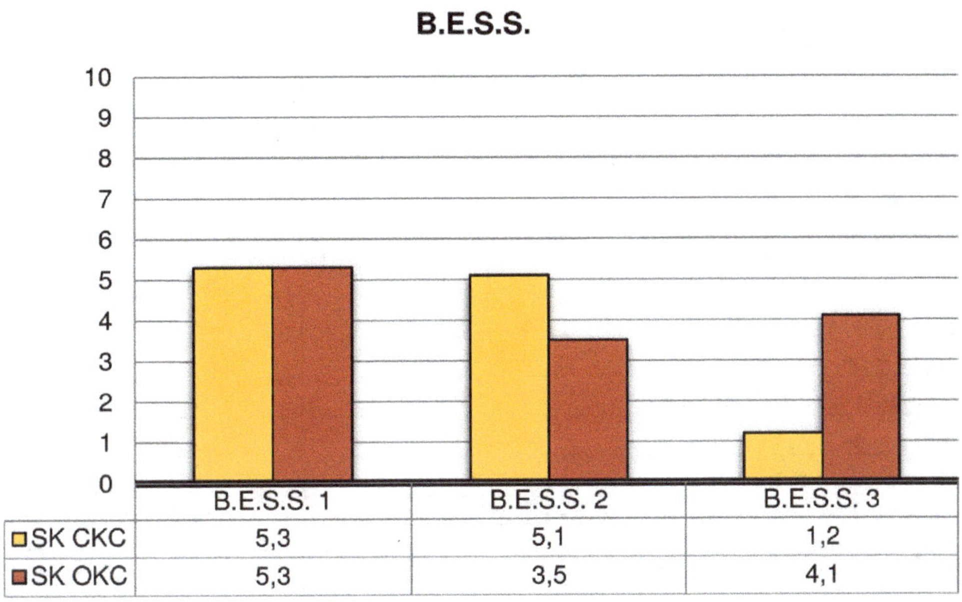

Graph 1. Results of the balance error scoring system explanatory notes: B.E.S.S. 1-evaluation of postural errors according to the balance error scoring system in the MobileMat™ programme (preoperative measurement), B.E.S.S. 2-evaluation of postural errors according to the balance error scoring system in the MobileMat™ programme (postoperative measurement), B.E.S.S. 3-evaluation of postural errors according to the balance error scoring system in the MobileMat™ programme (after termination of the managed rehabilitation), SK CKC-the CKC group, SK OKC-the OKC group.

developed solely for the purpose of this study. The Functional Test Questionnaire included those movement patterns that the patients used in ADL. Evaluation of functional movement skills consisted in assessment of a manner of execution of the selected movement patterns. Finally, these results were quantified in the questionnaires. The highest achievable score was 50.

Functional skills were evaluated again on the fourth postoperative day in order to visualize the differences between the preoperative and postoperative physical condition of the patients. Exit measurement took place on the tenth postoperative day (i.e. the last day of the managed rehabilitation). The testing was done by one qualified physiotherapist in order to avoid data distortion.

Before surgery the CKC group patients reached 36.1 points on average. The fourth postoperative day the average value of functional skills fell to 11.1 points. However, the patients reached 38.1 points on average within the final measurement. The OKC group showed an

	before surgery	after surgery	after rehabilitation
Turning from the supine to the side-lying position (on the healthy hip)			
Without any aids (without a wedge) 5 p.			
With a pillow, without difficulties 3 p.			
With a pillow, with difficulties 1 p.			
Cannot manage to do it 0 p.			
Turning from the supine to the prone position			
Without any aids (without a wedge) 5 p.			
With a pillow, without difficulties 3 p.			
With a pillow, with difficulties 1 p.			
Cannot manage to do it 0 p.			
Verticalization from the supine to the sitting position with legs hanging off the bed			
Without any aids (without a wedge) 5 p.			
With a pillow, without difficulties 3 p.			
With a pillow, with difficulties (using a bar) 1 p.			
Cannot manage to do it 0 p.			
Verticalization from the sitting to the standing position			
Without any aids (without crutches) 5 p.			
With support of 1 crutch 3 p.			
With support of 2 crutches 1 p.			
Cannot manage to do it 0 p.			
Picking things up off the floor			
Can manage to do it without any aids 10 p.			
Can manage to do it with 1 forearm crutch 5 p.			
Can manage to do it with support of the furniture 2 p.			
Cannot manage to do it 0 p.			
Verticalization from the floor			
Can manage to do it without any aids 20 p.			
Can manage to do it with 1 forearm crutch 10 p.			
Can manage to do it with support of the furniture 5 p			
Cannot manage to do it 0 p.			

Table 3. Functional tests.

average value of 35.5 points of functional skills at the beginning of the research. The average reached value after surgery was 7.3 points. However, the OKC group reached only 17.1 points on average within the final measurement.

Table 4 shows results of the individual measurements. In order to visualize the results a graph (see **Graph 2**) was developed in order to depict changes in the result values of both groups.

The difference between exit values (i.e. those measured after termination of rehabilitation) of the individual groups was statistically significant (p = 0.00001). This result showed also a significant effect size (Cohen's d = 4.04). Non-parametric Mann–Whitney U test was used to determine statistical significance of two selected files.

	CKC group (μ)	P	OKC group (μ)
FT 1	36.1	SID	35.5
FT 2	11.1	SID	7.3
FT 3	38.1	SSD	17.1

Table 4. Evaluation of movement skills (Functional tests).

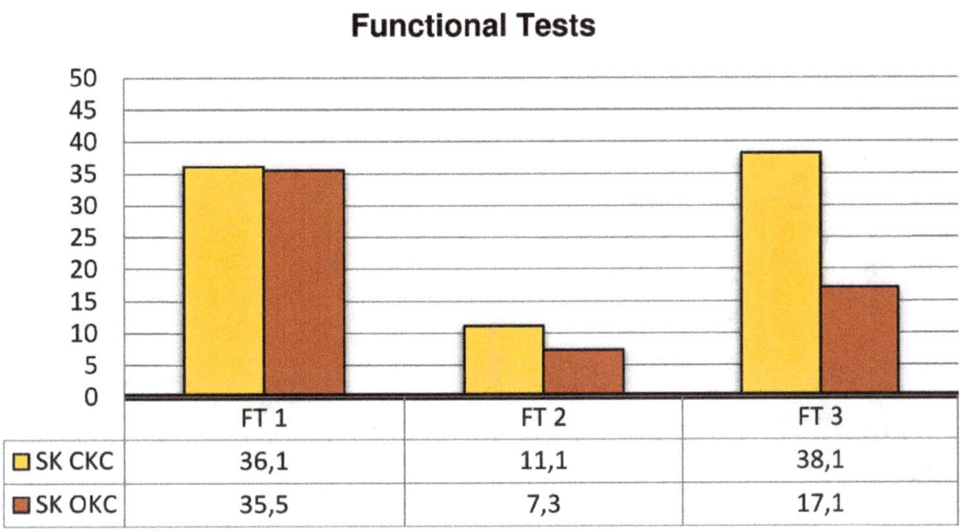

Graph 2. Results of the functional tests explanatory notes: FT 1-functional tests (preoperative measurement), FT 2-functional tests (postoperative measurement), FT 3-functional tests (final measurement after rehabilitation), SK CKC-the CKC group, SK OKC-the OKC group.

3.8.3. Objectivization of the closed kinetic chain therapy results based on the Harris hip score

The patients who took part in the study filled in a Harris Hip Score questionnaire before their surgery. This is a specialized questionnaire assessing skills within ADL in patients with hip joint diseases (arthrosis, necrosis of the ball). William H. Harris developed this questionnaire in order to evaluate level of pain and movement skills of patients before and after surgery. For the purpose of our study a modified version of the questionnaire was used, i.e. evaluation of the range of motion of the hip joint. The highest achievable score is 100. If a patient reaches 70 points or less, their physical condition is considered bad. Willim H. Harris considered a surgery successful when the score reached after surgery was at least 20 points higher than before surgery [20–24].

The patients filled in the Harris Hip Score questionnaire again on the fourth postoperative day in order to visualize the difference between the preoperative and postoperative physical condition. The final evaluation took place on the last day of the managed rehabilitation, i.e. on the tenth postoperative day.

	CKC group (μ)	P	OKC group (μ)
HHS 1	48.4	SID	52.8
HHS 2	40.5	SID	40.5
HHS 3	78.4	SSD	54.2

Table 5. Harris Hip Score values.

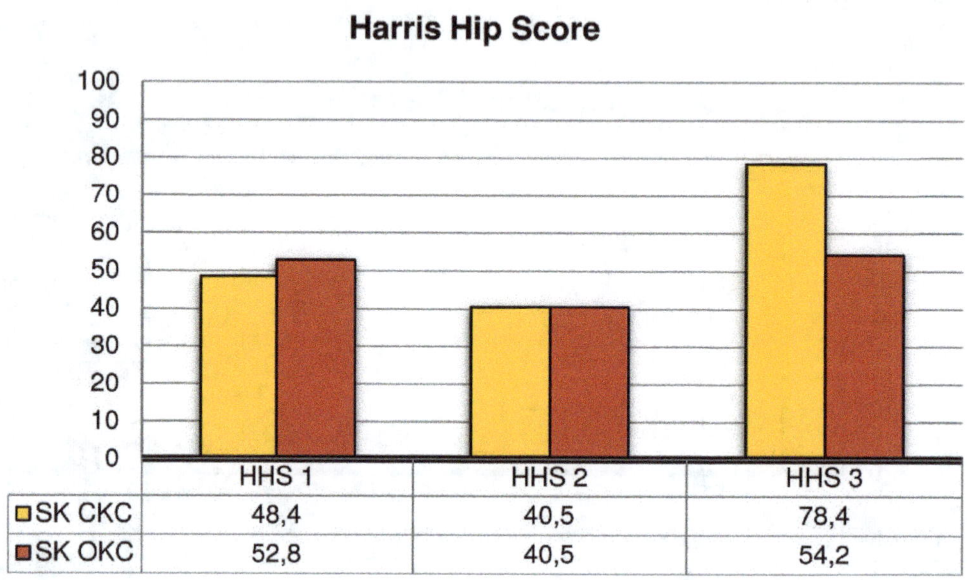

Graph 3. Harris hip score results explanatory notes: HHS 1 - Harris hip score (preoperative measurement), HHS 2 - Harris hip score (postoperative measurement), HHS 3 - Harris hip score (final measurement after rehabilitation), SK CKC – The CKC group, SK OKC – The OKC group.

Within the entry measurement of the Harris Hip Score the CKC group reached 48.4 points on average. The OKC group's average score in the questionnaire was 52.8. Both groups reached equal values in the postoperative measurement, i.e. 40.5 points per patient on average. The measured values were entered in a table (see **Table 5**). **Graph 3** shows the differences between the reached values of the individual group.

The exit measurement showed a significant statistical difference ($p = 0.00001$), where the CKC group reached 78.4 points and the OKC group 54.2 points on average. This difference showed also a high effect size (Cohen's $d = 3.63$). Non-parametric Mann–Whitney U test was used to determine statistical significance of two selected files.

3.8.3.1. Two-year study assessing Harris hip score results

The Harris Hip Score questionnaire has been used in the department of orthopedics and traumatology of SMN Přerov since the beginning of 2015 and it replaced the Staffel Score questionnaire used formerly, which is not globally recognized and is less specific in terms of evaluation activities of daily living.

	168 CKC group patients (μ)
HHS 1	43.3
HHS 2	74.3
HHS 3	94

Table 6. Harris Hip Score results of two-year observation.

On the grounds of the two-year research efficacy of the therapy based on the ACT principles, i.e. therapy in a closed kinetic chain, was assessed. In order to get long-term results the time during which the patients filled in the questionnaire was modified.

The first time the patients filled in the questionnaires was standard, i.e. 1 day before surgery, next after termination of the managed rehabilitation in the department of orthopedics and traumatology of SMN Přerov (6 therapies on average) and the last time was 4 months after hip joint replacement, i.e. within a regular orthopedic check-up. The patients were observed from the beginning of 2015 until the end of 2016. During this period 168 patients who underwent total hip joint replacement went through the therapy based on the ACT principles. The measured values were entered into a table (see **Table 6**). Before surgery the patients had 43.3 points of Harris Hip Score, after termination of the managed rehabilitation they reached 74.3 points on average. After leaving the department of orthopedics and traumatology of SMN Přerov the patients started subsequent rehabilitation treatment, they followed up the existing therapy and went on improving their functional and conditional skills. Within the regular orthopedic check-up, i.e. during the fourth month after surgery, the patients reached on average 94 points in the Harris Hip Score questionnaire.

The benefit of the therapy applied in a CKC consists mainly in relatively easy performance and understanding of exercises which can be modified according to the skills and needs of an individual. The therapy based on the ACT principles helps to reduce subjective perception of pain and to improve motor skills in patients. Patient satisfaction with surgery depends on improvement of the quality of their life, i.e. on reduction or elimination of pain and renewal of motor skills they could do with a healthy hip joint [25–29].

4. Conclusion

The results of this study show that the managed rehabilitation in a closed kinetic chain has demonstrably better results compared to the therapy conducted in an open kinetic chain. The similarity principle, which integrates functional movement patterns into patients′ activities of daily living, is considered the key element. The patients agree that if the movement therapy is aimed at improvement of specific motion skills applicable in ADL, their motivation to perform the exercises is higher. Correctly set up CKC therapy leads to reduction of subjective perception of pain, which has already been proved in various studies. The results of our study show not only significant improvement of functional skills of patients in ADL but also significant reduction of a number of postural errors concerning standing positions and locomotion.

Patients undergo total hip joint replacement in particular in order to improve the quality of their life. On the grounds of our study's results it can be stated that the ACT based therapy, compared with the open kinetic chain therapy, influences the quality of the patients' life after total hip joint replacement in a significant way.

Acknowledgements

I would like to thank to my co-workers from the department of rehabilitation and the department of orthopedics and traumatology of SMN Přerov for their cooperation on development of this study.

Author details

Jan Vagner[1*], Ingrid Palaščáková Špringrová[2], Pavel Přikryl[3], Šárka Tomková[4] and Rafi Moheb[5]

*Address all correspondence to: mgrjanvagner@gmail.com

1 Rehabilitation Department, Středomoravská nemocniční a.s, Přerov Hospital, Czech Republic

2 ACT centrum s.r.o., Postgraduate Education Centre, establishment accredited by the Ministry of Health of the Czech Republic, Praha, Czech Republic

3 Department of Orthopaedics and Traumatology, Středomoravská nemocniční a.s, Přerov Hospital, Czech Republic

4 Faculty of Health in Bánska Bystrica, St Elizabeth College of Health and Social Work in Bratislava, Slovak Medical University in Bratislava, Slovakia

5 Department of Orthopaedics, Kroměříž Hospital, Czech Republic

References

[1] Cannale TS, Beaty JH. Campbell's Operative Orthopaedics, 12th ed. Philadelphia: Mosby; 2013. 4253 p. ISBN 978-0-323-07243-4

[2] Dungl P. A Kol. Ortopedie. Praha: Grada Publishing, a.s; 2005. 1273 p. ISBN 80-247-0550-8

[3] Dvořák D. Některé teoretické poznámky k problematice otevřených a uzavřených biomechanických řetězců. In: Rehabilitace a fyzikální lékařství. Praha; ČSL JEP: 2005a;**12**(1): 12-17. ISSN 1211-2658

[4] Dvořák D. Otevřené a uzavřené biomechanické řetězce v kinezioterapeutické praxi. In: Rehabilitace a fyzikální lékařství. Praha: ČSL JEP; 2005b:**12**(1):18-22. ISSN 1211-2658

[5] Enoka RM. Neuromechanics of Human Movement (4th). Champaign, United States: Human Kinetics Publishers; 2008. 560 p. ISBN 978-07-360-6679-2

[6] Nankaku M. Effects of vertical motion of the centre of mass on walking efficiency in the early stages after total hip arthroplasty. In Hip International [online]. 2012;**22**(5): 521-526. Available from: http://www.hip-int.com/article/effects-of-vertical-motion-of-the-centre-of-mass-on-walking-efficiency-in-the-early-stages-after-total-hip-arthroplasty. ISSN 1724-6067

[7] Palaščáková Špringrová I. Akrální koaktivační terapie (ACT®) vycházející ze základ ních principů Roswithy Brunkow. Čelákovice; Rehaspring; 2011. 142 p. ISBN 978-80-260-0 912-2

[8] Ambler Z. Základy neurologie (Učebnice pro lékařské fakulty. Šesté, přepracované a doplněné vydání). Praha: Galén; 2006. 351 p. ISBN 978-80-246-1258-5

[9] Králíček P. Úvod do speciální neurofyziologie (Třetí, přepracované a rozšířené vydání). Praha: Galén; 2011. 235 p. ISBN 978 80-7262-618-2

[10] Vařeka I. Posturální stabilita (1. část). Terminologie a biomechanické principy. In Rehabilitace a fyzikální lékařství. Praha: ČSL JEP; 2002;**9**(4):115-121. ISSN 1211-2658

[11] Dvořáková H. Didaktika tělesné výchovy nejmenších dětí. Praha; Univerzita Karlova v Praze, Pedagogická fakulta: Praha; 2007. 124 p. ISBN 978-80-7290-298-9

[12] Rokyta R, et al. Fyziologie pro bakalářská studia v medicíně, přírodovědných a tělovýchovných oborech. Praha: ISV nakladatelství; 2000. 359 p. ISBN 80-85866-45-5

[13] Kolář P. et al. Rehabilitace v klinické praxi. Praha: Galén; 2009. 711 p. ISBN 978-80-7262-657-1

[14] Vařeka I. Revize výkladu průběhu motorického vývoje-novorozenecké období a homokinetické stádium. In Rehabilitace a fyzikální lékařství. Praha: ČSL JEP; 2006a;**13**(2):74-81. ISSN 1211-2658

[15] Vařeka I. Revize výkladu průběhu motorického vývoje-novorozenecké monokinetické stadium až batolecí období. Rehabilitace a fyzikální lékařství. Praha; ČSL JEP. 2006b;**13**(2):82-91. ISSN 1211-2658

[16] Palaščáková Špringrová I. Straight back with Acral dynamic-support exercises. Čelákovice; ACT centrum s.r.o. 2014. 78 p. ISBN 978-80-260-5871-7

[17] Bell DR et al. Systematic review of the balance error scoring system. Sports Health [online]. May-June 2011;**3**(3):287-295. Available from: http://www.ncbi.nlm.nih.gov/pmc/articles/PMC3445164/ ISSN 1941-0921

[18] Borský M, Crowe P. MatScan® SAM (Sway Analysis Module), Systém pro posturální analýzu (český překlad SAM a doplnění). Zlín; Proteching B. 2012:37

[19] Caccese JB, Kaminski TW. Comparing computer-derived and human-observed BESS scores. In Journal of Sport Rehabilitation; October 2014. 68 p. ISBN 1056-6716

[20] Blomfeldt R et al. A randomised controlled trial comparing bipolar hemiarthroplasty with total hip replacement for displaced intracapsular fractures of the femoral neck in elderly patiens. The Bone and Joint Journal [online]. February 2007;**89**(2):160-165.

Available from: http://www.bjj.boneandjoint.org.uk/content/jbjsbr/89-B/2/160.full.pdf ISSN 2049-4408

[21] Dorr LD et al. Early pain relief and function after posterior minimally invasive and conventional total hip arthroplasty. In The Journal of Bone & Joint Surgery [online]. June 2007;**89**(6):1153-1160. Available from: http://jbjs.org/content/89/6/1153.full.pdf. ISSN 1535-1386

[22] Langton J et al. Early failure of metal-on-metal bearings in hip resurfacing and large-diameter total hip replacement. In The Bone and Joint Journal [online]. January 2010;**92**(1):38-46. Available from: http://www.bjj.boneandjoint.org.uk/content/jbjsbr/92-B/1/38.full.pdf. ISSN 2049-4408

[23] Ogonda L et al. A minimal-incision technique in Total hip Arthroplasty does not improve early postoperative outcomes In The Journal of Bone & Joint Surgery [online]. April 2005;**87**(4):701-710. Available from: http://jbjs.org/content/87/4/701.full.pdf. ISSN 1535-1386

[24] Söderman P et al. Is the Harris hip score system useful to study the outcome of total hip replacement? In Clinical Orthopaedics and Related Research [online]., March 2001;**348**(1):189-197. Available from: https://www.researchgate.net/publication/12083562_Is_the_Harris_Hip_Score_System_Useful_to_Study_the_Outcome_of_Total_Hip_Replacement. ISSN 1528-1132

[25] Beaulé PE et al. The value of patient activity level in the outcome of Total hip Arthroplasty. The Journal of Arthroplasty [online]. June 2006;**21**(4):547-552. Available from: http://www.arthroplastyjournal.org/article/S0883-5403(05)00580-2/fulltext. ISSN 1532-8406

[26] Noble PC et al. The John Insall award: Patient expectations affect satisfaction with Total knee Arthroplasty. Clinical Orthopaedics and Related Research [online]. November 2006;**452**(1):35-43. Available from: https://www.researchgate.net/publication/6824053_The_John_Insall_Award_Patient_Expectations_Affect_Satisfaction_with_Total_Knee_Arthroplasty. ISSN 1528-1132

[27] Vagner J et al. Vzpěrné pohybové vzory a jejich vliv na bolest u pacientů po implantaci totální endoprotézy kyčelního kloubu. Rehabilitace a fyzikální lékařství. 2017;**24**(1):4-10. ISSN 1211-2658

[28] Skikić EM et al. Brunkow exercises and low back pain. Bosnian journal of basic medici science [online]. October 2004;**4**(4):37-41. Available from: http://old.bjbms.org/archives/2004-4/9.Bos.J.2004.4..pdf. ISSN 1512-8601

[29] Zeman P, Rafi M, et al. Clinical results of endoscopic treatment of greater trochanteric pain syndrome. Acta Chirurgiae Orthopaedicae et Traumatologiae ČECHOSL. 2017;**84**(3):168-174. ISSN 0001-5415

4

Total Hip Replacement in Developmental Dysplasia of the Hip: Pitfalls and Challenges

Özgür Korkmaz and Melih Malkoç

Abstract

Introduction: Surgical treatment methods for developmental dysplasia of the hip (DDH) in the elderly patients contain pelvic or periacetabular osteotomy and hip arthroplasty. Total hip arthroplasty (THA) is the last and definitive surgical treatment modality for the end stage developmental dysplasia of the hip.

Deformity classification and reconstruction: Crowe classification system describes the degree of dysplasia and gives information about the reconstruction procedure with hip arthroplasty. Classification is based on the magnitude of proximal femoral migration relative to the acetabulum. Acetabular component must be implanted to the true acetabulum for the optimal range of motion and stability of the reconstructed hip. The femoral component must be placed in neutral or slight anteversion but narrow femoral canal can be a problem for the reconstruction of femur.

Conclusion—key results: The results of total hip arthroplasty in developmental dysplasia of the hip have been satisfactory for stability, mobility, and pain relief. The survivorship of cemented arthroplasty in dysplastic hips is inferior because of the young age of the patients and the complexity of the procedures. Early and midterm results of cementless hip arthroplasty are better. Most important complications after the surgery are dislocation of the reconstructed hip and sciatic nerve injury.

Keywords: hip, arthroplasty, developmental dysplasia

1. Introduction

Hip arthroplasty is the end stage treatment method for developmental dysplasia of the hip (DDH). Pelvic and femoral osteotomies are the first option for surgical treatment. Before performing osteotomies, cartilage space in the hip joint must be determined. It must be verified with X-rays. In the long-term follow-up after pelvic or femoral osteotomies, degenerative changes occur in the hip joint. Also, hip arthroplasty is the last stage treatment modality after osteotomies around hip joint.

Hip arthroplasty for developmental dysplasia of the hip is technically complex surgical procedure because of the anatomical changes of acetabulum and proximal part of the femur. Soft tissue contractures and laxity can be present as a result of the acetabular and proximal femoral anatomical differences.

Patients with dysplasia require arthroplasty in younger age than the others with osteoarthritis. For this reason, implant selection is an important issue. Bearing surfaces alternative to metal on polyethylene should be preferred in this young patient population.

2. Anatomical differences in developmental dysplasia of the hip

2.1. Acetabular abnormalities

An acetabulum with dysplasia can be shallow, narrow, and lateralized. Increased anteversion and deficiency of the anterior and superior walls of acetabulum are changes expected to be seen in these patients [1]. The width of acetabulum remains same, but there is an increase in length and decrease in depth [2, 3]. As a result of these deformities, the coverage of the femoral head by the acetabulum has deficiency anteriorly, laterally, and superiorly. Completely dislocated hips have a false acetabulum on ilium with joint capsule. True acetabulum is hypoplastic and invaded with adipose tissue.

2.2. Femoral abnormalities

The dysplastic femur has a small femoral head. Femoral neck anteversion has increased. Generally, femoral neck is shortened with an increased neck-shaft angle [3]. There can be posterior displacement of trochanter major and a narrow femoral canal can be seen [1]. Narrowing of medullary canal around the level of the lesser trochanter is evident in Crowe IV DDH [4].

2.3. Soft tissue abnormalities

The abductor muscles orientation becomes transverse. Hypertrophies can be seen in psoas tendon and hip capsule. The hamstrings, adductors, and rectus femoris muscles shorten. Also, ligamentum teres and labral hypertrophies occur. For patients with unilateral DDH, the sciatic nerve lies close to the ischium and ilium but far from the femur of DDH when compared to healthy side. Sciatic nerve becomes shorter in the affected side, and it can be injured by posterolateral approach [5].

3. Classification of developmental dysplasia of the hip

There are several classification systems for developmental dysplasia of hip. Most popular ones are that were defined by Crowe and Hartofilakidis [6, 7]. There are three grades according to Hartofilakidis classification. The femoral head is covered within the true acetabulum in the first grade. In the second grade, femoral head has an articulation with the false acetabulum, and there is a contact between inferior lip of the false acetabulum and superior lip of the true acetabulum. This type is also called low dislocation. In the third grade, the femoral head is outside the true or the false acetabulum, and there is no articulation between femoral head and acetabulum. It is called high dislocation [7].

Crowe classification is a radiological classification based on proximal migration of the femoral head. There are four categories in this classification. The migration is calculated by measuring the vertical distance between the inter-teardrop line and the medial head-neck junction of hip. The stage of the subluxation is determined by the ratio of this distance to the vertical diameter of the opposite femoral head. If this ratio is less than 50% type 1, between 50% and 75% type II, between 75% and 100% type III, and greater than 100% subluxation type IV [6] (**Figure 1**).

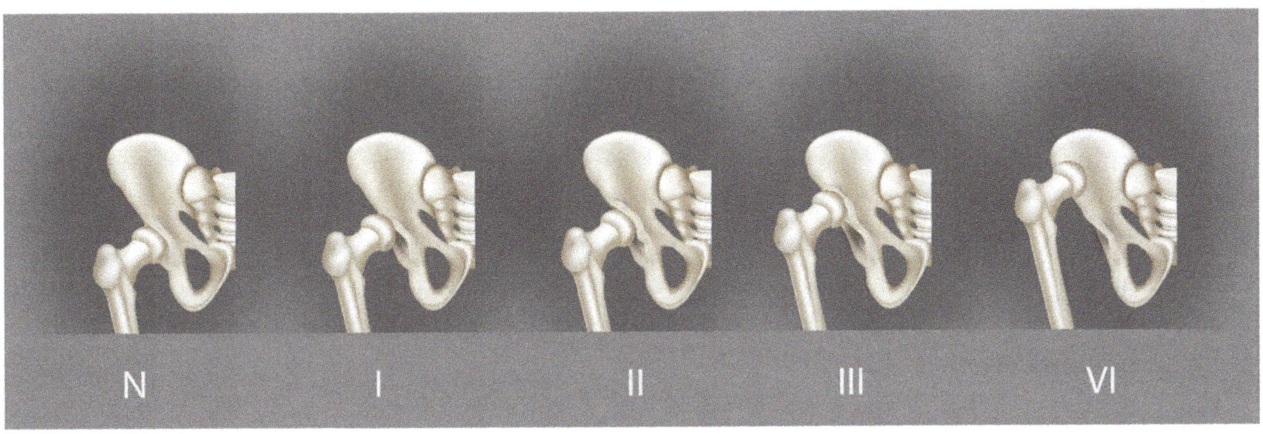

Figure 1. Crowe classification for developmental dysplasia of the hip.

4. Preoperative evaluation

Total hip arthroplasty (THA) is recommended for patients with end-stage disease who have pain and restriction in activities of daily living. Hip range of motion must be evaluated. Limb length inequality of the effected extremity must be measured. Anteroposterior views of the pelvis and hip radiographs should be taken. Lateral views of the hip and Judet views can be helpful to determine the acetabular bone stock. CT scan can be useful to evaluate acetabular bone stock and femoral version [8].

Bone stock of the acetabulum is the first important issue for preoperative planning. If there is enough acetabular bone stock for implantation of the acetabular cup, it will facilitate the surgical process. But if there is not enough bone stock, then bone grafting and reconstruction systems for hip arthroplasty must be considered.

Anteversion of the femoral neck, femoral stenosis, and limb shortening are the main problems that can be faced. If the rotation of the affected extremity is advanced, corrective osteotomy can be planned [9, 10]. Femoral bowing is another difficulty in adaptation of the femoral component. Templating helps to select the ideal femoral component size.

5. Surgical approaches

Hip arthroplasty can be performed through anterolateral, anterior, and posterolateral approach. But extensile exposures are needed when there is difficulty in reaching the bone structures. Transtrochanteric approach is the one that can be used for this condition but nonunion is the most important complication. When femoral shortening is needed, a transfemoral approach and subtrochanteric osteotomy can be considered. There is an increased risk of sciatic nerve injury if leg lengthening is over 3–4 cm [11]. Femoral shortening osteotomy can be performed to avoid sciatic nerve injury [9].

6. Acetabular reconstruction

The aim of the acetabular reconstruction is to place the acetabular component to true acetabulum and to provide the normal biomechanical properties of the hip with normal hip center of rotation. Another important issue is the coverage of the acetabular cup with the acetabular bone. If there is not enough support with the bone, there can be increased stresses at the bone-implant (or bone-cement) interface, and mechanical failure can occur in the early period. For this reason, acetabular cup coverage by the natural bone must be done as much as possible. If acetabular cup coverage is not provided, alternative reconstructive techniques should be performed. The methods of reconstruction are discussed according to Crowe classification.

6.1. Crowe I hips (dysplasia)

These types of dysplastic hips have a minimal acetabular bony deformity. Reconstruction of the acetabulum can be done with the standard acetabular component. The component can be medialized to increase coverage of the implant by the natural bone. Good clinical results may be achieved using standard prosthesis stem sizes and press-fit acetabular component [12]. But small diameter femoral heads can be used for this reason that kinds of small implants must be ready to use in the operating room. Large femoral heads can be used when stability of acetabular component is achieved. Short-term results of large head metal-on-metal total hip arthroplasty in young and active patients with developmental dysplasia of the hip are similar to conventional THA [13]. Resurfacing hip arthroplasty is an option for the surgical treatment. There are several complications that can be seen like femoral neck fractures. But fixation of the acetabular component without adjuvant fixation can be achieved without complete acetabular coverage of the acetabular component [14].

6.2. Crowe II and III hips (low dislocation)

There is bone deficiency in the lateral part of the acetabulum. There is less bone support for the acetabular component. There are several surgical techniques to increase the coverage of the acetabular component. The medial wall of the acetabulum can be reamed deeper, so coverage of the acetabular component can be increased. But if the coverage of the cup is not sufficient by this method, acetabular augmentation, reconstruction of the acetabulum in a superior location, or acetabular reinforcement rings are the other alternatives to provide coverage [15].

Bone grafts and cement are used for acetabular augmentation in the presence of superolateral acetabular defect. Allografts can be used, but patient's original femoral head is generally a good option. With this technique, normal hip center of rotation can be achieved with strong superolateral acetabular bone stock. A total of 60–70% coverage of the cementless acetabular cups can be acceptable [16, 17]. Long-term results of the bone stock of the acetabulum that was reconstructed using femoral head as autograft are favorable [18]. But if the amount of the acetabular component that is covered by graft is not large, there is a risk of graft resorption and collapse [19].

The other alternative technique is reconstruction of the acetabulum in a superior location which is called high hip center. The acetabular component is covered more with bone, and this technique facilitates biological fixation, and generally, there is no need for bone grafts. Main disadvantage of this technique is the need for small acetabular component with small femoral head which restricts range of motion of hip with abnormal hip biomechanics [20]. Midterm results of cementless acetabular component hip arthroplasty with high hip center are satisfactory with low rates of revision surgery [21].

Another technique is medialization of the acetabular component by over reaming the medial wall of the acetabulum. This technique was described first by Dunn and Hess [9]. It is also called acetabuloplasty. Medialization of the hip center of rotation increases coverage of the acetabular component and decreases joint reactive forces. Cup medialization has a compensatory effect on the femoral offset of the hip with less femoral antetorsion [22]. The only disadvantage of this method is the loss of bone stock of the medial acetabulum. The rate of medial protrusion of <60% is recommended for acceptable clinical and radiographic results [23].

The last technique is to use acetabular reinforcement rings for deficient acetabular bone. Ring is implanted to maximize host bone contact. Then, polyethylene cup is cemented in appropriate position for hip biomechanics. Reinforcement rings provide predictable good long-term results [24, 25].

6.3. Crowe IV hips (high dislocation)

In Crowe IV hips, the acetabulum is hypoplastic, but the superior rim of the acetabulum is less eroded than Crowe II and III hips, and bone stock is more than the Crowe II and III hips. Acetabular component can be placed to the anatomic hip center. But small-sized acetabular components can be used because of the hypoplastic acetabulum [26].

7. Femoral reconstruction

There are several deformities that can be seen in the femoral part of hip joint. There is an increased anteversion and valgus deformity. The medullar canal is generally narrower than normal medullar canal. Anterior-posterior diameter of the canal is more extensive than the medial-lateral diameter. The great trochanter can be placed posteriorly than normal hip.

7.1. Crowe I and II hips

In Crowe type I and type II dysplasias, femoral length is not a problem for reconstruction. Generally, there is no need for femoral osteotomy. Small diameter cemented or cementless stems can be used because of the narrower femoral medullar canal. Proximally coated femoral components are good options for the femoral reconstruction without osteotomy. Hip center of rotation can be changed in the reconstruction of acetabular part. For this reason, anteversion of the femoral component is an important issue for the hip stability. Placement of the femoral component is recommended in neutral or slight anteversion. Anteversion of the femoral neck can be significant in some hips, so femoral component anteversion must be aligned to the axis of the knee joint.

7.2. Crowe III and IV hips

After the center of hip rotation is configured in the true acetabulum, reduction of the hip joint in Crowe type III and IV hips is difficult because of the femoral length. Isolated soft tissue release is not enough for the reduction. For this reason, femoral osteotomies should be done. If the reduction of the hip joint is maintained after the soft tissue release, resulting in leg lengthening of more than 4 cm, then sciatic nerve injury may occur [27, 28].

There are two kinds of femoral osteotomies that can be performed in total hip arthroplasty for Crowe Types III and IV hips. First one is trochanteric osteotomy with proximal femoral shortening. Trochanteric osteotomy provides visualization of femur and acetabulum and preserves abductor mechanism with low risk of dislocation [29]. But risk of nonunion of great trochan-

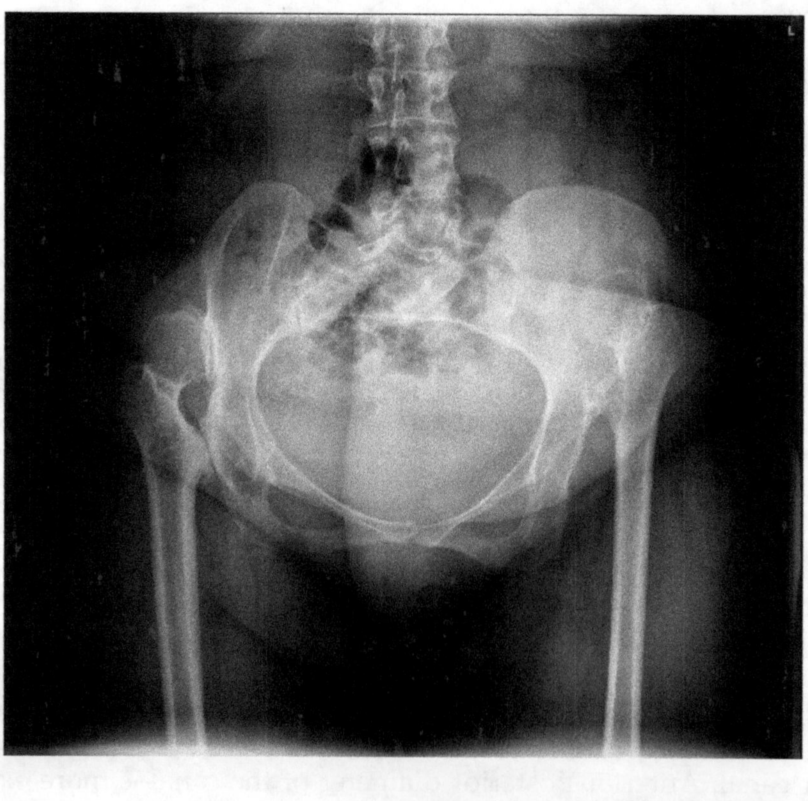

Figure 2. Bilateral Crowe IV developmental dysplasia of the hip. Both acetabula have bone deficiency with narrow femoral canal.

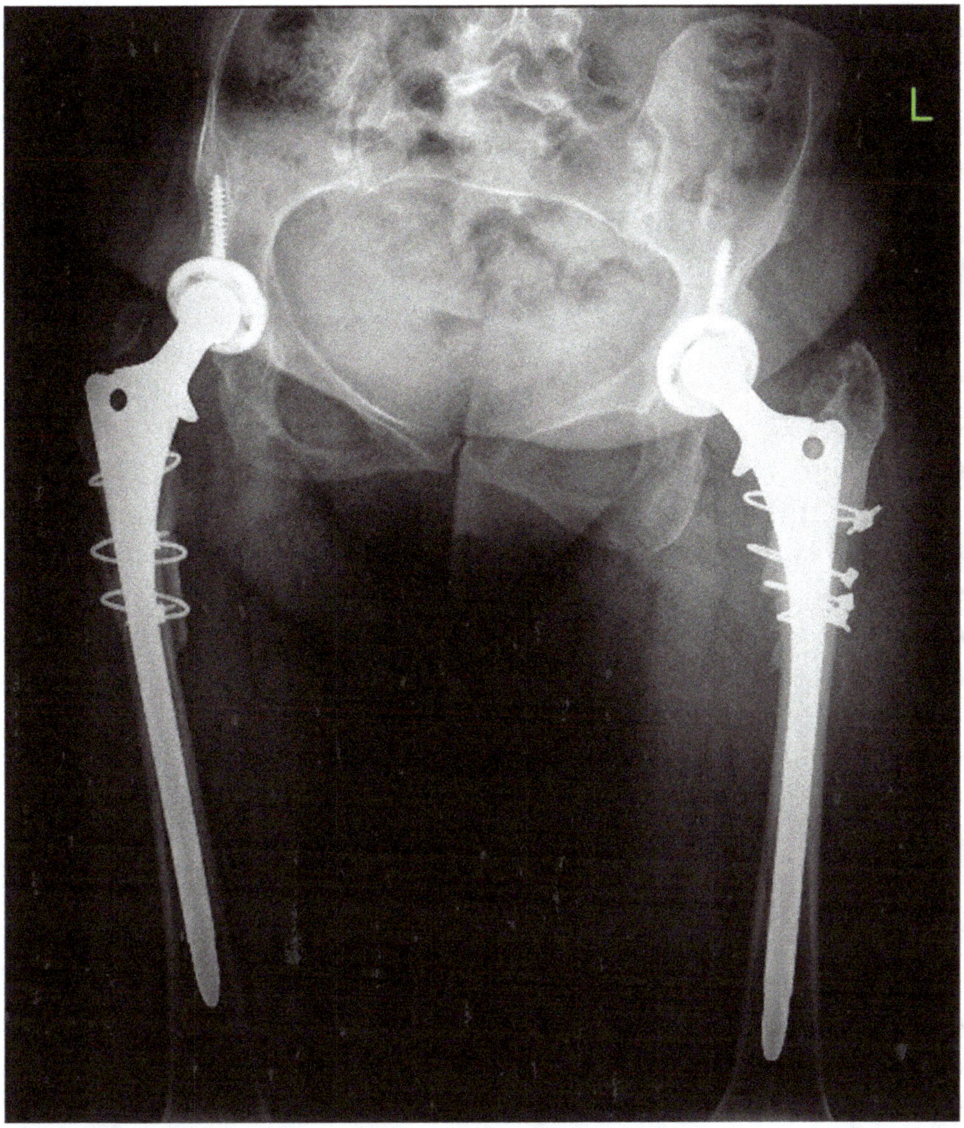

Figure 3. Postoperative radiograph of the pelvis showing bilateral reconstruction. Both acetabular reconstructions are done in a higher position than the true acetabulum because of the acetabular bone deficiency. Bilateral femoral shortening has been performed with usage of resected bone as auto graft.

ter is much with this technique [30, 31]. Subtrochanteric osteotomy preserves the metaphyseal region and has an advantage of correcting the rotational abnormalities with femoral shortening [32, 33]. After subtrochanteric femoral shortening, osteotomy noncemented femoral component can be used but a cemented DDH specific stem is preferable.

Subtrochanteric osteotomy is performed through a lateral approach than a transverse osteotomy is created in the subtrochanteric region. A femoral component is inserted to the proximal part of the osteotomy; then, hip is reduced. At this time, the amount of the femoral shortening can be calculated, and second cut is performed on distal part. Then, distal part of the femoral component is inserted to the distal fragment with adjusting anteversion. Prophylactic cerclage wiring of the fragments can prevent fractures. The resected portion of femur can be used as auto graft over the osteotomy line (**Figures 2** and **3**). Instead of a transverse osteotomy, a chevron-shaped osteotomy which was defined by Becker and Gustillo can be performed for more rotational stability [34].

In some cases, there can be an impingement of the trochanter on the pelvis in abduction or on the posterior acetabulum in external rotation. To solve impingement in abduction, trochanter is osteotomized and reattached distally. Trochanter is osteotomized and reattached laterally for the impingement in external rotation.

8. Bearing surfaces

Generally, there are three types of bearing surface alternatives for hip arthroplasty. Metal on polyethylene is the one that is used mostly. Polyethylene wear is the important issue for osteolysis and revision surgery. Most of the patients with DDH have to be performed hip arthroplasty in younger ages than the primary osteoarthritis. For this reason, other bearing surface alternatives must be chosen for the younger patients. Metal on metal bearing surface has an advantage of larger head sizes with small acetabular components. Larger head sizes provide more range of motion [35, 36]. Adverse allergic reactions and increased ion concentrations in the blood are the main unknown circumstances [37]. Ceramic on ceramic bearing surfaces has low friction but component fracture, development of noise, and less implant size options are the restrictive situations.

9. Total hip replacement in developmental dysplasia of the hip—pitfalls and challenges

9.1. Acetabular part

Cemented acetabular components can be used for the reconstruction of the acetabulum with the acetabular wall defects. Providing appropriate position of the component can be difficult because of the acetabular bone defects. Inappropriate placement of the acetabular cup causes decreased range of motion, less stability, and hip dislocation. Aseptic loosening is the main problem as a result of inappropriate placement of the acetabular cup in the long-term follow-up period. Cemented acetabular components have variable results in the literature. Survival ratio of the acetabular component was found 96% and 91% at 15 years with excellent long-term clinical and radiographic survivorship for acetabular dysplasia [38]. In another study with mean follow-up period of 15.7 year, the survival of the cemented acetabular component was 78%. The main reason of revision surgery was aseptic loosening with ratio of 88.3%. Higher rate of failure of the acetabular component was determined with increasing severity of hip dysplasia according to Crowe and Hartofilakidis classification [39]. Proximal migration of the hip center of rotation and nonanatomic placement of the acetabular component are the main reasons for aseptic loosening of the cemented acetabular component [40]. Nowadays, cemented acetabular reconstruction is not the first line treatment modality because of high revision rates [41, 42].

Coverage ratio of noncemented cups is the main important issue for the survival of the implant. For this reason, we must provide as much as possible surface coverage of the acetabular cup by acetabulum. But acetabular wall fracture can occur while reaming of the acetabulum. Reconstruction plates must be ready in the operating room. Noncemented acetabular components with grafts have same survival rates like the cemented acetabular components, with revision rates of 0–5% [43, 44]. The 20-year survivorship free from acetabular revision was 66% for noncemented acetabular components with femoral head as autograft [45]. In another study, 57% of the acetabular components underwent revision at a mean of 14.6 years because of osteolysis [46]. Twenty percent of the superolateral aspect of the acetabular cup could be left uncovered to prevent the failure risk [47] but there is no exact data about the amount of adequate acetabular cup coverage. Li et al reported results of the hip arthroplasty with more than 30% lateral uncoverage of noncemented acetabular components. There were no prosthesis revision and loosening during the mean 4.8 years follow-up [48]. Tikhilov et al. recommend acetabular component fixation without screws with moderate uncoverage within 25% but they offer two-screw fixation with significant uncoverage to 35% [49].

High hip center is another reconstruction option. The new acetabulum in the high hip center does not have strong osseous structures like true acetabulum. Reaming of the new acetabulum for the acetabular component can be resulted as a perforation of the bone. Superior wall of the acetabulum is not so strong, and acetabular cup stabilization cannot be sufficient. Acetabular cup stabilization can be provided with extra screws. These extra screws can cause neurovascular injury. In some cases, the new acetabulum can be formed in a higher position than the true acetabulum because of the acetabular bone deficiency (**Figure 2**). There are several studies that showed good results with cemented and noncemented acetabular components [21, 50, 51]. Results of a study that was compared the survivorship of the components for anatomical or high-cup placement; 100% in the anatomical placement and 97% for high hip center group [52]. Higher loosening and revision rates for both femoral and acetabular components have been reported with cemented acetabular cups for high hip center [40, 53]. There is a correlation between lateral displacement of the hip center and higher rates of component loosening [40].

Medialization of the acetabular cup can provide more surface coverage of the acetabular component by acetabular bone. To achieve a good stabilization, acetabular component can be 1 size larger than the acetabular reamer size. While impacting the acetabular component, there is a risk for acetabular fracture. If a fracture occurs, we must check the stability of the acetabular component. If the stability of the acetabular component is insufficient, stabilization must be maintained with extra acetabular cup screws. Medialization of the acetabular component by medial wall reaming has been reported low revision rates with both cemented and noncemented components [7, 54]. Medial wall defect of 25% of the acetabular area is recommended [54]. But in another study, higher loosening rates of the cemented components have been determined [55].

9.2. Femoral part

Narrower femoral canal in DDH is the main problem for femoral component. Cemented femoral components have an advantage of low fracture risk during the fixation. Cement mantle must cover one third of the cross-sectional area of the femoral canal. Distal centralizer must be used for the correct placement of the femoral component. Appropriate anteversion, valgus, and varus position of the femoral component must be provided in the period of cement polymerization. Modular or cemented stem should be used for extreme anteversion. Cemented femoral components have good long-term follow-up. Femoral component revision rates are 3–10% according to the literature [42, 56]. Cemented femoral component revision rates are lower than the cemented acetabular component. A total of 28 patients (35 hips) who underwent a cemented THA for DDH had been reviewed retrospectively. The overall revision rate was found 20%, and femoral revision rate was found 9% [57].

Noncemented femoral components are more popular nowadays. There is a risk of femur fracture while rasping the femoral canal and implantation of the noncemented femoral components. If a fracture occurs in that period, fixation must be achieved with cerclage wires or with a long femoral stem. Noncemented femoral component survival seems good. In a study of 15 patients with 17 hips, 57% underwent revision of the acetabular component at a mean of 14.6 years because of osteolysis. But no patient underwent revision because of femoral component loosening [46]. In another study with 106 patients with DDH, 18 acetabular revisions had been performed but there was no femoral component revision for any reason with mean follow-up period of 13.5 years [58]. Short-stem implants can be used for the reconstruction of the hip. Results of the hip arthroplasty with the short-stem implants in patients with DDH have good clinical outcome like primary osteoarthritis [59]. This type of implants can be used for lower grades of DDH.

Fixation of the subtrochanteric osteotomy with noncemented femoral components has favorable results. After the osteotomy and resection of the femoral segment, there can be inequality between proximal part cross-sectional area of the femoral canal and distal part cross-sectional area of the femoral canal. Long femoral stems improve stability. In some cases, modular femoral stems can be useful. Resected portion of femur can be used as auto graft over the osteotomy line. Also, this auto graft with cerclage wires has an additional support for stability (**Figure 3**). Crowe IV hips treated with subtrochanteric osteotomy using noncemented components show excellent healing rates [11, 60, 61]. But Park et al. reported three femoral nonunions on 24 hip arthroplasties with subtrochanteric shortening osteotomy [62].

There are several studies that compare THA outcomes in dysplastic and nondysplastic patients. As a result of a study which compares the dysplastic and nondysplastic hips, no significant difference was detected in Oxford Hip Score and revision rates between the two groups [63]. However, revision rates are more in dysplastic hips than in non-dysplastic hips in long-term follow-up [64]. Hip arthroplasty for DDH is complex surgery, and the cost of this procedure is more than a hip arthroplasty for primary osteoarthritis. Increased degree of dysplasia according to Crowe classification has been associated with higher costs [65].

10. Complications

Infection is an important complication that can occur after hip arthroplasty. The possibility of infection is increased in DDH. Surgical procedure time, exposure length, and use of more implants can be among the reasons. Nerve palsy, dislocation, and mechanical failure can be seen as a result of improper surgical technique and implant selection. Early loosening of the acetabular component, limping, and limb-length discrepancy can be seen in the high hip center type of reconstruction. Fracture and dislocation of the cup inside the pelvis are the most important complications for medialization technique. Nonunion of greater trochanter is an important complication after trochanteric osteotomy. Nonunion of the osteotomy site after femoral shortening procedures can be seen.

Author details

Özgür Korkmaz* and Melih Malkoç

*Address all correspondence to: ozkorkmaz00@yahoo.com

Department of Orthopedic and Traumatology, School of Medicine, Istanbul Medipol University, Turkey

References

[1] Argenson JN, Flecher X, Parratte S, Aubaniac JM: Anatomy of the dysplastic hip and consequences for total hip arthroplasty. Clin Orthop Relat Res. 2007;465:40–45. DOI: 10.1097/BLO.0b013e3181576052.

[2] Ito H, Matsuno T, Hirayama T, Tanino H, Yamanaka Y, Minami A: Three-dimensional computed tomography analysis of non-osteoarthritic adult acetabular dysplasia. Skeletal Radiol. 2009;38:131–139. DOI: 10.1007/s00256-008-0601-x.

[3] Sanchez-Sotelo J, Trousdale RT, Berry DJ, Cabanela ME: Surgical treatment of developmental dysplasia of the hip in adults: I. Nonarthroplasty options. J Am Acad Orthop Surg. 2002;10(5):321–333.

[4] Liu S, Zuo J, Li Z, Yang Y, Liu T, Xiao J, Gao Z: Study of three-dimensional morphology of the proximal femur in developmental adult dysplasia of the hip suggests that the on-shelf modular prosthesis may not be an ideal choice for patients with Crowe type IV hips. Int Orthop. 2016;14:1–7. DOI: 10.1007/s00264-016-3248-6.

[5] Liu R, Liang J, Wang K, Dang X, Bai C: Sciatic nerve course in adult patients with unilateral developmental dysplasia of the hip: implications for hip surgery. BMC Surg. 2015;31;15(1):1. DOI: 10.1186/1471-2482-15-14.

[6] Crowe JF, Mani VJ, Ranawat CS: Total hip replacement in congenital dislocation and dysplasia of the hip. J Bone Joint Surg Am. 1979;61(1):15–23.

[7] Hartofilakidis G, Stamos K, Karachalios T, Ioannidis TT, Zacharakis N: Congenital hip disease in adults. Classification of acetabular deficiencies and operative treatment with acetabuloplasty combined with total hip arthroplasty. J Bone Joint Surg Am. 1996;78(5):683–692.

[8] Kim JS, Park TS, Park SB, Kim JS, Kim IY, Kim SI: Measurement of femoral neck anteversion in 3D. Part 1: 3D imaging method. Med Biol Eng Comput. 2000;38:603–609.

[9] Dunn HK, Hess WE: Total hip reconstruction in chronically dislocated hips. J Bone Joint Surg Am. 1976;58:838–845.

[10] Kilicoglu OI, Turker M, Akgul T, Yazicioglu O: Cementless total hip arthroplasty with modified oblique femoral shortening osteotomy in Crowe type IV congenital hip dislocation. J Arthroplasty. 2013;28:117–125 DOI: 10.1016/j.arth.2012.06.014.

[11] Krych AJ, Howard JL, Trousdale RT, Cabanela ME, Berry DJ: Total hip arthroplasty with shortening subtrochanteric osteotomy in Crowe type-IV developmental dysplasia. J Bone Joint Surg Am. 2009;91:2213–2221. DOI: 10.2106/JBJS. H.01024.

[12] Bożek M, Bielecki T, Nowak R, Żelawski M: Arthroplasty in patients with congenital hip dysplasia—early evaluation of a treatment method. Ortop Traumatol Rehabil. 2013;15(1):49–59. DOI: 10.5604/15093492.1032794.

[13] Yalcin N, Kilicarslan K, Cicek H, Kayaalp C, Yildirim H: Crowe type I and II DDH managed by large diameter metal-on-metal total hip arthroplasty. Hip Int. 2011;21(2):168–175. DOI: 10.5301/HIP.2011.7418.

[14] Amstutz HC, Antoniades JT, Le Duff MJ: Results of metal-on-metal hybrid hip resurfacing for Crowe type-I and II developmental dysplasia. J Bone Joint Surg Am. 2007;89(2):339–346. DOI: 10.2106/JBJS.F.00576.

[15] Dapuzzo MR, Sierra RJ: Acetabular considerations during total hip arthroplasty for hip dysplasia. Orthop Clin North Am. 2012;43(3):369–375. DOI: 10.1016/j.ocl.2012.05.012.

[16] Paavilainen T, Hoikka V, Solonen KA: Cementless total replacement for severely dysplastic or dislocated hips. J Bone Joint Surg Br. 1990;72:205–211.

[17] Shen B, Yang J, Wang L, Zhou ZK, Kang PD, Pei FX: Midterm results of hybrid total hip arthroplasty for treatment of osteoarthritis secondary to developmental dysplasia of the hip-Chinese experience. J Arthroplasty. 2009;24:1157–1163. DOI: 10.1016/j.arth.2009.07.002.

[18] Farrell CM, Berry DJ, Cabanela ME: Autogenous femoral head bone grafts for acetabular deficiency in total-hip arthroplasty for developmental dysplasia of the hip: long-term effect on pelvic bone stock. J Arthroplasty. 2005;20(6):698–702. DOI: 10.1016/j.arth.2004.11.004.

[19] Mulroy RD, Harris WH: Failure of acetabular autogenous grafts in total hip arthroplasty. Increasing incidence: a follow-up note. J Bone Joint Surg Am. 1990;72(10):1536–1540.

[20] Komiyama K, Nakashima Y, Hirata M, Hara D, Kohno Y, Iwamoto Y: Does high hip center decrease range of motion in total hip arthroplasty? A computer simulation study. J Arthroplasty. 2016;15. DOI: 10.1016/j.arth.2016.03.014.

[21] Chen M, Luo ZL, Wu KR, Zhang XQ, Ling XD, Shang XF: Cementless total hip arthroplasty with a high hip center for hartofilakidis type B developmental dysplasia of the hip: results of midterm follow-up. J Arthroplasty. 2016;31(5):1027–1034. DOI: 10.1016/j.arth.2015.11.009.

[22] Terrier A, Levrero Florencio F, Rüdiger HA: Benefit of cup medialization in total hip arthroplasty is associated with femoral anatomy. Clin Orthop Relat Res. 2014;472(10):3159–3165. DOI: 10.1007/s11999-014-3787-3.

[23] Zha GC, Sun JY, Guo KJ, Zhao FC, Pang Y, Zheng X: Medial protrusio technique in cementless total hip arthroplasty for developmental dysplasia of the hip: a prospective 6- to 9-year follow-up of 43 consecutive patients. J Arthroplasty. 2016;31. DOI: 10.1016/j.arth.2016.01.052.

[24] Ewers A, Spross C, Ebneter L, Külling F, Giesinger K, Zdravkovic V, Erhardt J: 10-year survival of acetabular reinforcement rings/cages for complex hip arthroplasty. Open Orthop J. 2015;159:163–167. DOI: 10.2174/1874325001509010163.

[25] Sadri H, Pfander G, Siebenrock KA, Tannast M, Koch P, Fujita H, Ballmer P, Ganz R: Acetabular reinforcement ring in primary total hip arthroplasty: a minimum 10-year follow-up. Arch Orthop Trauma Surg. 2008;128(8):869–877. DOI: 10.1007/s00402-008-0612-z.

[26] Li W, Zhang W, Bai G, Huang Z, Shen R: Total hip arthroplasty for treatment of Crowe type IV congenital dysplasia of hip with dislocation in adults. Zhongguo Xiu Fu Chong Jian Wai Ke Za Zhi. 2013;27(10):1153–1156.

[27] Farrell CM, Springer BD, Haidukewych GJ, Morrey BF: Motor nerve palsy following primary total hip arthroplasty. J Bone Joint Surg Am. 2005;87:2619–2625. DOI: 10.2106/JBJS.C.01564.

[28] Eggli S, Hankemayer S, Müller ME: Nerve palsy after leg lengthening in total replacement arthroplasty for developmental dysplasia of the hip. J Bone Joint Surg Br. 1999;81:843–845.

[29] Kerboull L, Hamadouche M, Kerboull M: Transtrochanteric approach to the hip. Interact Surg. 2007;2:149–154.

[30] Menon PC, Griffiths WE, Hook WE, Higgins B: Trochanteric osteotomy in total hip arthroplasty: comparison of 2 techniques. J Arthroplasty. 1998;13:92–96.

[31] Kerboull M, Hamadouche M, Kerboull L: Total hip arthroplasty for Crowe type IV developmental hip dysplasia: a long-term follow-up study. J Arthroplasty. 2001;16:170–176.

[32] Chareancholvanich K, Becker DA, Gustilo RB: Treatment of congenital dislocated hip by arthroplasty with femoral shortening. Clin Orthop Relat Res. 1999;360:127–135.

[33] Yasgur DJ, Stuchin SA, Adler EM, DiCesare PE: Subtrochanteric femoral shortening osteotomy in total hip arthroplasty for high-riding developmental dislocation of the hip. J Arthroplasty. 1997;12(8):880–888.

[34] Becker DA, Gustilo RB: Double-chevron subtrochanteric shortening derotational femoral osteotomy combined with total hip arthroplasty for the treatment of complete congenital dislocation of the hip in the adult. Preliminary report and description of a new surgical technique. J Arthroplasty. 1995;10(3):313–318.

[35] Schmalzried TP, Peters PC, Maurer BT, Bragdon CR, Harris WH: Long duration metal-on-metal total hip arthroplasties with low wear of the articulating surfaces. J Arthroplasty. 1996;11:322.

[36] Sieber HP, Rieker CB, Kottig P. Analysis of 118 second-generation metal-on-metal retrieved hip implants: J Bone Joint Surg Br. 1999;81(1):46–50.

[37] Willert HG, Buchhorn GH, Fayyazi A, Flury R, Windler M, Köster G, Lohmann CH: Metal-on-metal bearings and hypersensitivity in patients with artificial hip joints. A clinical and histomorphological study. J Bone Joint Surg Am. 2005;87:280. DOI: 10.2106/JBJS.A.02039pp.

[38] Akiyama H, Kawanabe K, Iida H, Haile P, Goto K, Nakamura T: Long-term results of cemented total hip arthroplasty in developmental dysplasia with acetabular bulk bone grafts after improving operative techniques. J Arthroplasty. 2010;25(5):716–720. DOI: 10.1016/j.arth.2009.05.017.

[39] Chougle A, Hemmady MV, Hodgkinson JP: Severity of hip dysplasia and loosening of the socket in cemented total hip replacement. A long-term follow-up. J Bone Joint Surg Br. 2005;87(1):16–20.

[40] Stans AA, Pagnano MW, Shaughnessy WJ, Hanssen AD: Results of total hip arthroplasty for Crowe type III developmental hip dysplasia. Clin Orthop Relat Res. 1998;348:149–157.

[41] MacKenzie JR, Kelley SS, Johnston RC: Total hip replacement for coxarthrosis secondary to congenital dysplasia and dislocation of the hip. Long-term results. J Bone Joint Surg Am. 1996;78:55–61.

[42] Numair J, Joshi AB, Murphy JC, Porter ML, Hardinge K: Total hip arthroplasty for congenital dysplasia or dislocation of the hip. survivorship analysis and long-term results. J Bone Joint Surg Am. 1997;79:1352–1360.

[43] Morsi E, Garbuz D, Gross AE: Total hip arthroplasty with shelf grafts using noncemented cups. A long-term follow-up. J Arthroplasty. 1996;11(1):81–85.

[44] Silber DA, Engh CA: Cementless total hip arthroplasty with femoral head bone grafting for hip dysplasia. J Arthroplasty. 1990;5:231–240.

[45] Abdel MP, Stryker LS, Trousdale RT, Berry DJ, Cabanela ME: Noncemented acetabular components with femoral head autograft for acetabular reconstruction in developmental dysplasia of the hip: a concise follow-up report at a mean of twenty years. J Bone Joint Surg Am. 2014;96(22):1878–1882. DOI: 10.2106/JBJS.N.00061.

[46] Imbuldeniya AM, Walter WL, Zicat BA, Walter WK: Cementless total hip replacement without femoral osteotomy in patients with severe developmental dysplasia of the hip: minimum 15-year clinical and radiological results. Bone Joint J. 2014;96–B(11):1449–1454. DOI: 10.1302/0301-620X.96B11.33698.

[47] Garvin KL, Bowen MK, Salvati EA, Ranawat CS: Long-term results of total hip arthroplasty in congenital dislocation and dysplasia of the hip. A follow-up note. J Bone Joint Surg Am. 1991;73:1348–1354.

[48] Li H, Mao Y, Oni JK, Dai K, Zhu Z: Total hip replacement for developmental dysplasia of the hip with more than 30% lateral uncoverage of noncemented acetabular components. Bone Joint J. 2013;95–B(9):1178–1183. DOI: 10.1302/0301-620X.95B9.31398.

[49] Tikhilov R, Shubnyakov I, Burns S, Shabrov N, Kuzin A, Mazurenko A, Denisov A: Experimental study of the installation acetabular component with uncoverage in arthroplasty patients with severe developmental hip dysplasia. Int Orthop. 2015;40:1–5. DOI: 10.1007/s00264-015-2951-z.

[50] Russotti GM, Harris WH: Proximal placement of the acetabular component in total hip arthroplasty. A long-term follow-up study. J Bone Joint Surg Am. 1991;73(4):587–592.

[51] Schutzer SF, Harris WH: High placement of porous-coated acetabular components in complex total hip arthroplasty. J Arthroplasty. 1994;9(4):359–367.

[52] Murayama T, Ohnishi H, Okabe S, Tsurukami H, Mori T, Nakura N, Uchida S, Sakai A, Nakamura T: 15-year comparison of cementless total hip arthroplasty with anatomical or high cup placement for Crowe I to III hip dysplasia. Orthopedics. 2012;35(3):e313–e318. DOI: 10.3928/01477447-20120222-28.

[53] Pagnano W, Hanssen AD, Lewallen DG, Shaughnessy WJ: The effect of superior placement of the acetabular component on the rate of loosening after total hip arthroplasty. J Bone Joint Surg Am. 1996;78(7):1004–1014.

[54] Dorr LD, Tawakkol S, Moorthy M, Long W, Wan Z: Medial protrusio technique for placement of a porous-coated, hemispherical acetabular component withoutcement in a total hip arthroplasty in patients who have acetabular dysplasia. J Bone Joint Surg Am. 1999;81(1):83–92.

[55] Hartofilakidis G, Georgiades G, Babis GC, Yiannakopoulos CK: Evaluation of two surgical techniques for acetabular reconstruction in total hip replacement for congenital hip disease: results after a minimum 10-year follow-up. J Bone Joint Surg Br. 2008;90(6):724–730. DOI: 10.1302/0301-620X.90B6.20490.

[56] Sochart DH, Porter ML: The long-term results of Charnley low-friction arthroplasty in young patients who have congenital dislocation, degenerative osteoarthrosis, or rheumatoid arthritis. J Bone Joint Surg Am. 1997;79(11):1599–1617.

[57] Howie CR, Ohly NE, Miller B: Cemented total hip arthroplasty with subtrochanteric osteotomy in dysplastic hips. Clin Orthop Relat Res. 2010;468(12):3240–3247. DOI: 10.1007/s11999-010-1367-8.

[58] Kaneuji A, Sugimori T, Ichiseki T, Fukui K, Takahashi E, Matsumoto T: Cementless anatomic total hip femoral component with circumferential porous coating for hips with developmental dysplasia: a minimum 10-year follow-up period. J Arthroplasty. 2013;28(10):1746–1750. DOI: 10.1016/j.arth.2013.06.030.

[59] Budde S, Floerkemeier T, Thorey F, Ezechieli M, Claassen L, Ettinger M, Bredow J, Windhagen H, Lewinski GV: A short-stem hip implant with metaphyseal anchorage in patients with developmental dysplasia of the hip. Technol Health Care. 2016;59: 559–569. DOI: 10.3233/THC-161151.

[60] Bernasek TL, Haidukewych GJ, Gustke KA, Hill O, Levering M: Total hip arthroplasty requiring subtrochanteric osteotomy for developmental hip dysplasia: 5- to 14-year results. J Arthroplasty. 2007;22:145–150. DOI: 10.1016/j.arth.2007.05.014.

[61] Ollivier M, Abdel MP, Krych AJ, Trousdale RT, Berry DJ: Long-term results of total hip arthroplasty with shortening subtrochanteric osteotomy in Crowe IV developmental dysplasia. J Arthroplasty. 31. DOI: 10.1016/j.arth.2016.01.049.

[62] Park MS, Kim KH, Jeong WC: Transverse subtrochanteric shortening osteotomy in primary total hip arthroplasty for patients with severe hip developmental dysplasia. J Arthroplasty. 2007;22(7):1031–1036. DOI: 10.1016/j.arth.2007.05.011.

[63] Boyle MJ, Frampton CM, Crawford HA: Early results of total hip arthroplasty in patients with developmental dysplasia of the hip compared with patients with osteoarthritis. J Arthroplasty. 2012;27(3):386–390. DOI: 10.1016/j.arth.2011.06.024.

[64] Engesaeter LB, Furnes O, Havelin LI: Developmental dysplasia of the hip—good results of later total hip arthroplasty: 7135 primary total hip arthroplasties after developmental dysplasia of the hip compared with 59774 total hip arthroplasties in idiopathic coxarthrosis followed for 0 to 15 years in the Norwegian Arthroplasty Register. J Arthroplasty. 2008;23(2):235–240. DOI: 10.1016/j.arth.2007.03.023.

[65] Ashraf A, Larson AN, Maradit-Kremers H, Kremers WK, Lewallen DG: Hospital costs of total hip arthroplasty for developmental dysplasia of the hip. Clin Orthop Relat Res. 2014;472(7):2237–2244. DOI: 10.1007/s11999-014-3587-9.

5

Classifications Used in Total Hip Arthroplasty

Munis Ashraf

Abstract

Total hip arthroplasty is one of the most successful operation to be done and is definitely a rewarding procedure for both the surgeon and the patient. Ever since 3 days of low friction arthroplasty by Sir John Charnley, there has been considerable interest in improvement in the knowledge of surgical techniques and hip biomechanics. Over the past two decades there has been an exponential increase in total hip replacements. Therefore strategies to simplify the procedure and classifications to encounter difficulties in treatment plans were devised. It is imperative for consultants and trainees to be aware of these classifications systems which are helpful in pre op, intra op and postop planning.

Keywords: Vancouver, Paprosky, Brooker

1. Paprosky classification of acetabular deficiencies for revision hip arthroplasty

1.1. Introduction

Wayne Paprosky (Illinois, USA) proposed this classification in 1994 based on his experience with revision of 134 acetabular cups [1] (**Figure 1**).

1.2. Classification

Type I: Defect with undistorted rim.

Type II: Defect with distorted rim but adequate to support a hemispherical cup.

- **IIA:** Superior and medial with intact superior rim.

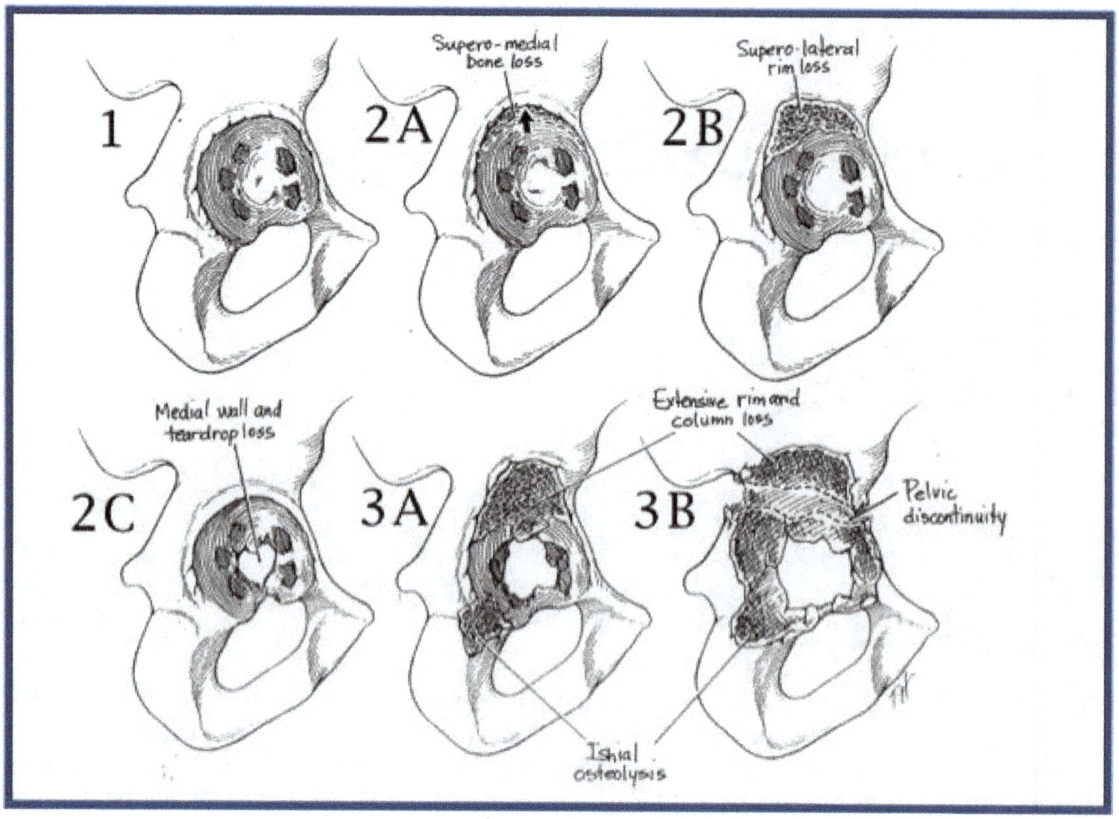

Figure 1. Paprosky classification of acetabular deficiencies.

- **IIB**: Superior with less than one-third superior rim deficient.
- **IIC:** Medial wall defect.

Type III: Defect with non-supportive rim.

- **III A:** Superior and lateral with 40 to 60% of the host bone intact and partial inherent mechanical stability.
- **III B:** Superior and medial with host bone less than 40% and possibility of occult discontinuity.

1.3. Clinical applications

Bone grafting techniques depends on the type of acetabular bone defect. Superior dome defect will need structural distal femoral allografts or trabecular metal wedges. Medial wall and ischial defect will need particulate bone grafts. Pelvic discontinuity needs ORIF versus triflanged custom cage. Unsupportive bone stock will need cup and cage construct.

1.4. Reliability

Gozzard et al. had performed a study to assess the reliability and validity of classification systems used for defects in acetabulum during revision arthroplasty [2]. It was found that there was poor to good intra observer agreement with the consultants (0.24) and moderate to good intra observer agreement with the registrars (0.36). Interobserver agreement was noted to be moderate with consultant and registrars scoring 0.56 and 0.27, respectively. Validity was deemed to be good (κ = 0.65). Overall, the authors found the system to be unreliable.

2. Saleh classification of acetabular deficiencies for revision hip arthroplasty

2.1. Introduction

This system of classification was proposed by Saleh et al. in 1999. The study had included 21 expert arthroplasty surgeons and was proposed based on estimation of anticipated bone stock following implant removal [3] (**Figure 2**).

2.2. Classification

Type I No significant bone loss.

Type II Contained loss of bone stock where there is cavitary enlargement of the acetabular cavity but no wall deficiency.

Type III Uncontained loss of bone stock where there is <50% segmental loss of the acetabulum involving anterior or posterior column.

Type IV Uncontained loss of bone stock where there is >50% segmental loss of the acetabulum affecting both anterior or posterior columns (if there is >50% loss of the acetabulum, involving

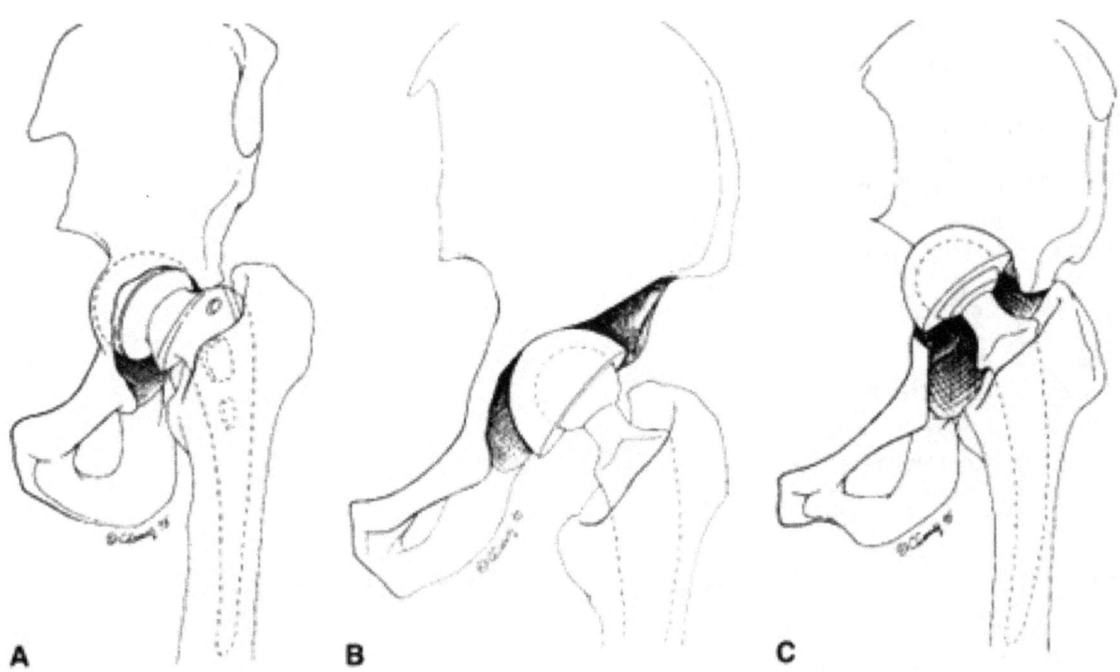

Figure 2. Saleh classification. (A) Type uncontained cavitary loss of bone stock. (B) Type III, uncontained (segmental) loss of bone stock involving <50% of acetabulum. (C) Type IV, uncontained (segmental) loss of bone stock involving >50% of the acetabulum.

mostly the medial wall but the columns are intact, then this type of defect is considered type II because of the availability of the columns for reconstruction).

Type V Acetabular defect with uncontained loss of bone stock in association with pelvic discontinuity.

2.3. Reliability

Gozzard et al. had observed an Inter-observer reliability testing revealed kappa values of 0.89 for the acetabulum. Average validation value was kappa = 0.86 for the acetabulum [2]. To put things into perspective: clinical epidemiologists consider correlation values of 0.6–0.8 to be "substantial" and between 0.8 and 1.0 to be "perfect association".

3. Hodgkinson classification of radiographic demarcation of the socket following total hip arthroplasty

3.1. Introduction

This classification was proposed by Hodgkinson et al. from Wrightington, UK in 1988. He reviewed 200 patients undergoing revision arthroplasty and found out strong correlation between the extent of radiographic demarcation at bone-cement interface and intraoperative loosening of cemented acetabular components [4].

3.2. Classification

Type 0: No demarcation.

Type 1: Demarcation of outer one-third.

Type 2: Demarcation of outer and middle thirds.

Type 3: Complete demarcation.

Type 4: Socket migration.

3.3. Clinical significance

This classification helps surgeon help decide between partial or complete revision preoperatively.

4. Paprosky classification of femoral bone deficiencies

4.1. Introduction

This classification was described by Wayne Paprosky et al. from Illinois, USA. He emphasized that his classification will help the surgeon determine the most appropriate option for

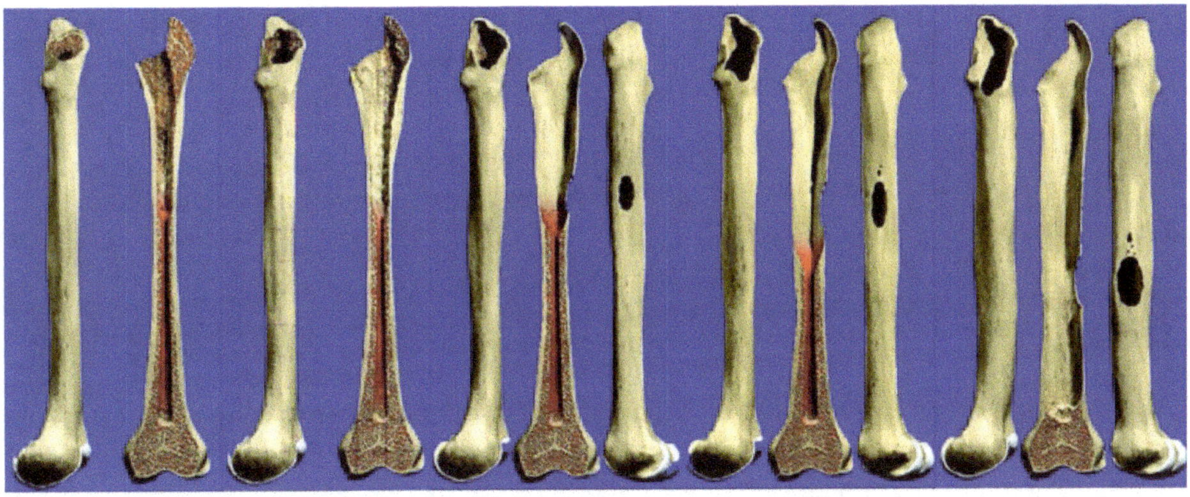

Figure 3. Paprosky classification.

reconstruction and thereby assists with ensuring that the appropriate implants and instruments are available at the time of surgery [5]. Gozzard et al. found moderate agreement between the preoperative and intraoperative validity; but the reliability of the classification was found to be fair (**Figure 3**).

4.2. Classification

Type 1: Minimal metaphyseal and diaphyseal bone loss.

Type 2A: Absent calcar extend just below the inter-trochanteric region.

Type 2B: Anterolateral metaphyseal bone loss wit absent calcar.

Type 2C: Posteromedial metaphyseal bone loss.

Type 3A: 2A plus diaphyseal bone loss but at least 4 cm of diaphyseal support possible.

Type 3B: 2B plus diaphyseal bone loss with less than 4 cm of diaphyseal support available.

Type 3C: 2C plus complete diaphyseal bone loss.

4.3. Clinical applications

Type 1: Cemented or proximally porous coated cementless implant can be used.

Type 2A, 2B, 2C: Extensively porous coated cementless stem is preferred. Cemented stem should be avoided because of loss of metaphyseal endosteal bone.

Type 3A: Extensively porous coated stems or modular distal fitting tapered stems can be used.

Type 3B: Modular tapered cementless stems are used if adequate bone stock.

Impaction bone grafting is also an option.

Type 4: Impaction bone grafting with tapered cemented stem if intact cortex. Composite prosthesis allograft if no proximal cortex. Long cemented stem is an option in elderly.

5. AAOS classification of femoral bone deficiencies for revision hip arthroplasty

5.1. Introduction

This classification was first proposed by D'Antonio et al. (Pennsylvania, USA) in 1989 and later adopted by American Academy of Orthopedic Surgeons (AAOS) [6] (**Figure 4**).

5.2. Classification

Type I: Segmental deficiencies.

  1a: Proximal either partial or complete.

  1b: Intercalary.

  1c: Greater trochanteric.

Type II: Cavitary deficiencies (cancellous, cortical or ectasia).

Type III: Combined.

Type IV: Rotational or angular malalignment.

Type V: Femoral stenosis.

Type VI: Femoral discontinuity.

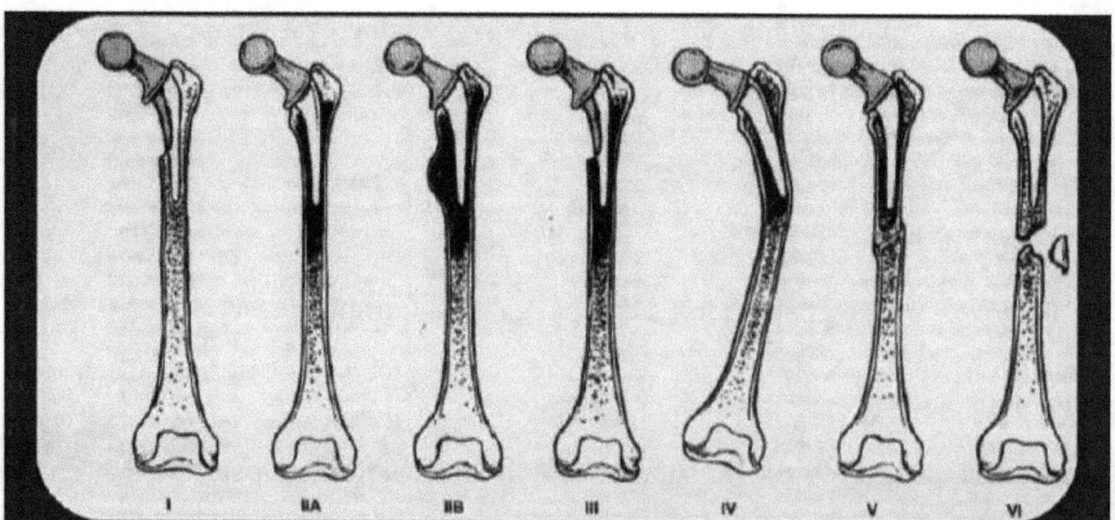

Figure 4. AAOS classification.

5.3. Clinical applications

This classification is very useful in describing the bone defect accurately but has less role in guiding the surgeon determine the reconstructive option.

5.4. Reliability

Gozzard et al. in their study observed the inter observer agreement among consultants and registrars. They noted a fair agreement (k value of 0.28) among consultants and a poor agreement (k value of −1.0) among the registrars.

6. Saleh classification of femoral bone deficiencies

6.1. Introduction

This system of classification was proposed by Saleh et al. in 1999. The study had included 21 expert arthroplasty surgeons and was proposed based on estimation of anticipated bone stock following implant removal [3].

6.2. Classification

Type	Defect	Treatment
I	No significant loss of bone stock.	Conventional cemented Uncemented components
II	Contained loss of bone stock, cortical sleeve intact	Proximal fixation Impaction grafting Porous coated implant Modular implant
III	Non-circumferential loss of bone stock uncontained Proximal circumferential loss of bone stock less than 5 cm in length	Cortical strut allograft Calcar replacing prosthesis
IV	Circumferential loss of bone stock more than 5 cm in length (distal to lesser trochanter)	Custom implant, proximal femoral allograft
V	Periprosthetic fracture with proximal circumferential loss of bone stock.	Restoration of bone stock plus long stem femoral component custom implant proximal femoral allograft.

6.3. Reliability

In the study by Saleh et al., they noted an inter observer reliability of k value 0.88 and average validity, k value of 0.88; indicating perfect association. The classification also provides probable treatment options for each type.

7. Dossick and Dorr classification of proximal femoral geometry

7.1. Introduction

Based on the calcar-to-canal ratio which is defined as the diameter of the femur at the midportion of the lesser trochanter divided by the diameter at a point 10 cm distal [7].

7.2. Classification

Type A: Calcar-to-canal ratio < 0.5.

No thinning of cortices on AP or lateral radiographs.

Type B: Calcar-to-canal ratio 0.5–0.75.

Thinning of the posterior cortex on the lateral view.

Type C: Calcar-to-canal ratio > 0.75.

Thinning of cortices on both views (Stovepipe femur) (**Figure 5**).

7.3. Clinical significance

Type A suitable for cementless femoral stem, type C requires use of cemented stem and type B is intermediate.

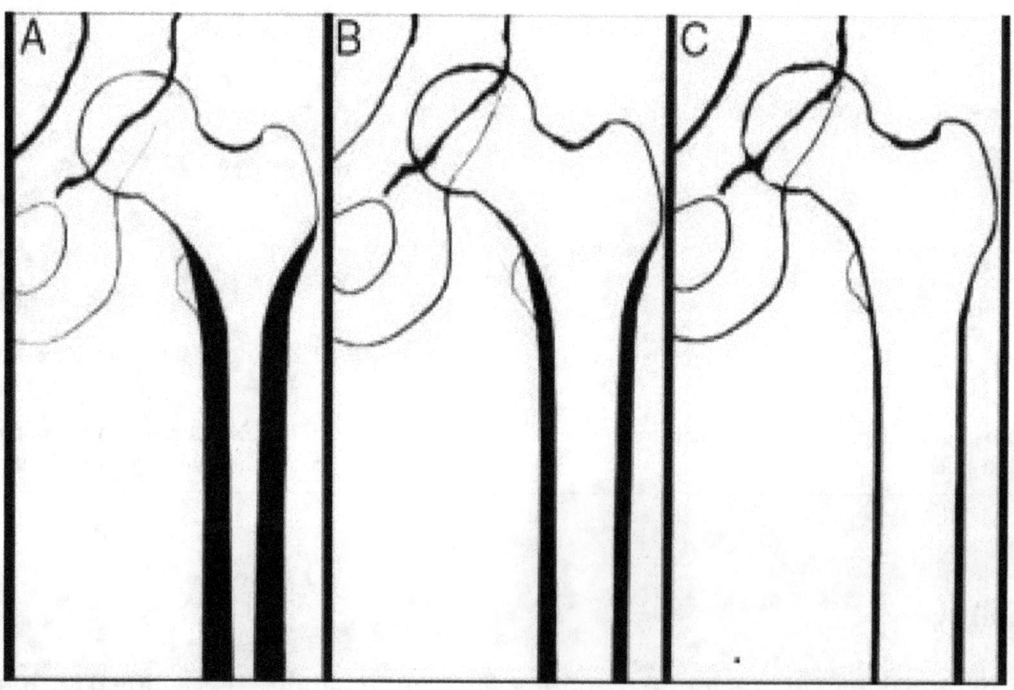

Figure 5. Dossick and Dorr classification.

8. Vancouver classification of intraoperative periprosthetic femur fractures around total hip arthroplasty

8.1. Classifications

Type A: Proximal metaphyseal.

A1: Cortical perforation.

A2: Undisplaced linear crack.

A3: Displaced or unstable fractures.

Type B: Proximal diaphyseal.

B1: Cortical perforation.

B2: Undisplaced linear crack.

B3: Displaced or unstable fractures.

Type C: Distal diaphyseal fractures.

C1: Cortical perforation.

C2: Undisplaced linear crack.

C3: Displaced or unstable fracture [8].

8.2. Clinical applications

Type A1: Bone graft alone.

Type A2: Circelage wire if using proximally porous coated stem and can be ignored if using fully porous coated stem and there is no distal extension into diaphysis.

Type A3: Needs fixation.

Type B1: Bypassing stem ± cortical allograft fixation.

Type B2: Circelage wire ± cortical allograft fixation.

Type B3: Long stem with cortical allograft fixation.

Type C1: Morselized bone graft ± bypass stem and cortical allograft.

Type C2: Circelage wire ± bypass stem and cortical allograft.

Type C3: ORIF (**Figure 6**).

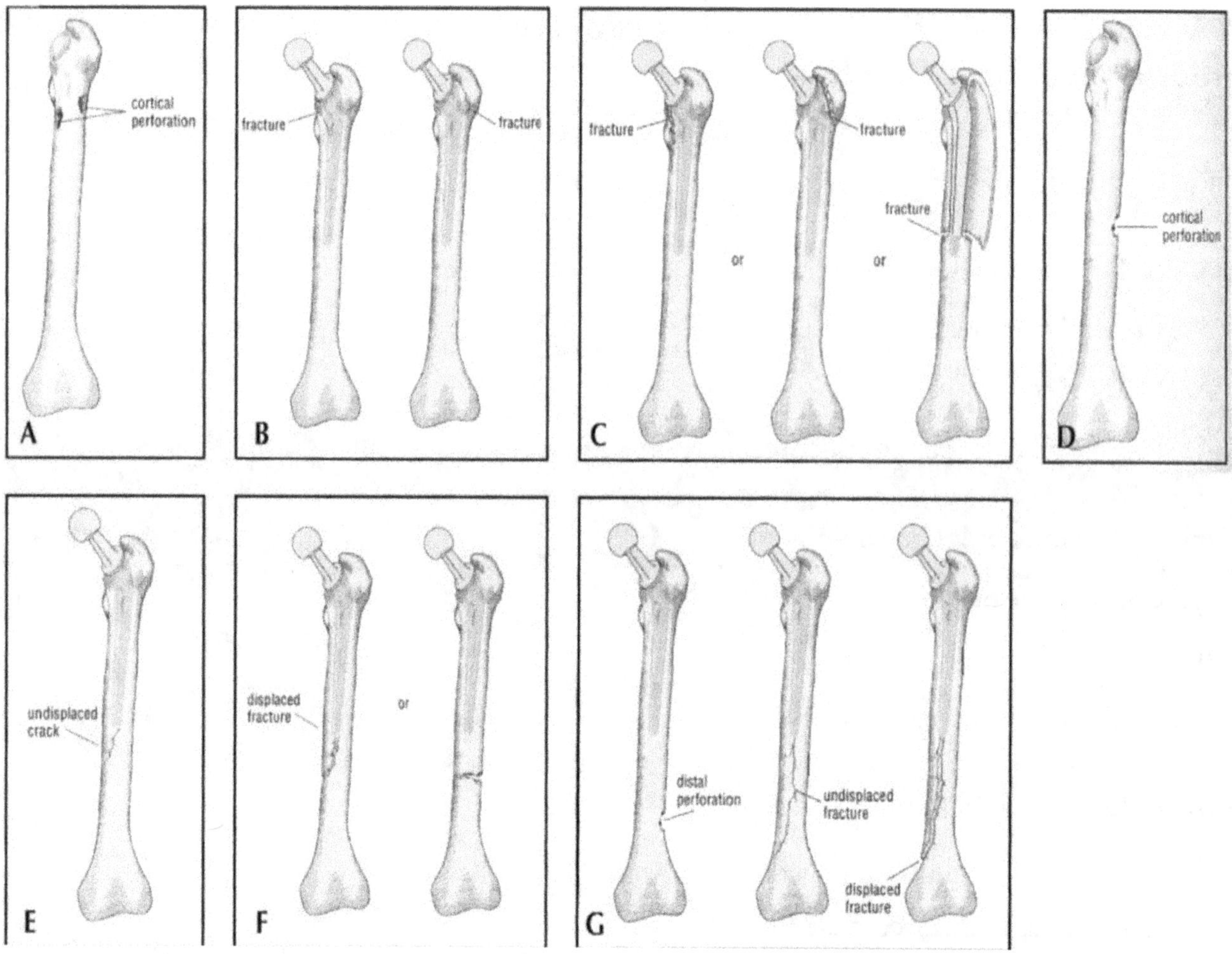

Figure 6. Intraoperative Vancouver classification.

9. Vancouver classification of postoperative periprosthetic femur fractures around total hip arthroplasty

9.1. Classification

Type A: Peritrochanteric.

AG: Greater trochanter.

AL: Lesser trochanter.

Type B: Around or just distal to the tip of the stem.

B1: Well-fixed femoral component.

B2: Loose femoral component.

B3: Loose femoral component and poor bone stock.

Type C: Well distal to the stem.

9.2. Clinical application

This classification guides the surgeon with treatment decision.

AG and AL: Usually stable and can be treated non-operatively.

B1: ORIF if displaced.

B2: Revision to long stem.

B3: Revision with struct grafting.

C: ORIF.

9.3. Reliability

A European validation for this classification was performed by Rayan et al. The study had included consultants, trainees and medical students. It was noted to have an inter observer reliability of substantial agreement among consultants (k value of 0.72–0.74) orthopedic trainees (k value of 0.68–0.70) and medical students (k value of 0.61). The validity within B type fractures revealed an agreement of 77% with a k value of 0.67 [9, 10] (**Figure 7**).

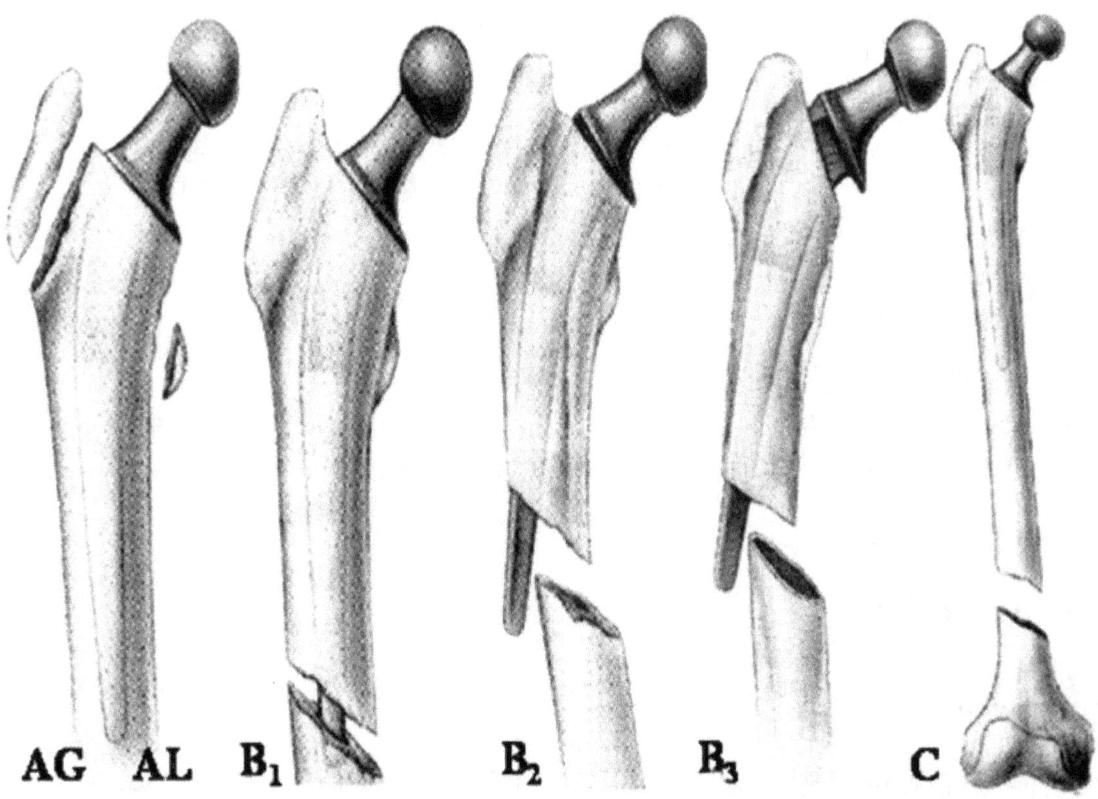

Figure 7. Postoperative Vancouver classification.

10. Tsukayama classification of infected hip joint prosthesis

10.1. Introduction

Tsukayama et al. proposed the classification based on the study of 97 patients with infected hip joint prosthesis [11].

10.2. Classification

Positive intraoperative cultures: Two out of five intraoperative specimens positive on culture in a patient undergoing revision hip arthroplasty with no clinical evidence of infection at the time of revision.

Early postoperative infection: Wound infection developed less than 1 month after the operation.

Late chronic infection: Wound infection developed 1 month or more after the index operation and with insidious course.

Acute hematogenous infection: Associated with a documented or suspected antecedent bacteremia and characterized by an acute onset of symptoms in the affected joint with the prosthesis.

10.3. Clinical implication (treatment guidelines)

Positive intraoperative cultures: Intravenous administration of antibiotics for 6 weeks without operative intervention.

Early postoperative infection: Debridement, replacement of the polyethylene inserts of the acetabular component, retention of the prosthesis, and intravenous administration of antibiotics for 4 weeks.

Late chronic infection: Debridement; removal of all prosthetic components and bone cement; and placement of antibiotic beads. Intravenous antibiotics for 6 weeks. Revision arthroplasty 2 weeks after cessation of antibiotic therapy.

Acute hematogenous infection: Debridement, replacement of the polyethylene insert, retention of the prosthesis if it was not loose, and intravenous administration of antibiotics for 6 weeks [11].

11. Brooker's classification

11.1. Introduction

This system was proposed by Brooker et al. from John Hopkins Hospital in 1973 on a series of 100 consecutive patients undergoing Total hip arthroplasty. Since then it has been in widespread use and has stood the test of time [12].

11.2. Classification

Class I: Isolated islands of bone.

Class II: Gap between bones at least 1 cm.

Class III: Gap between bones less than 1 cm.

Class IV: Apparent ankylosis.

11.3. Clinical application

This classification is useful in the follow up of the high-risk patients and in patients with post HO resection.

11.4. Reliability

Vasileiadis et al. from mayo clinic in their study noted a moderate to substantial agreement (k value 0.49–0.71) in the inter observer reliability. Grade IV had best inter observer reliability [13, 14] (**Figure 8**).

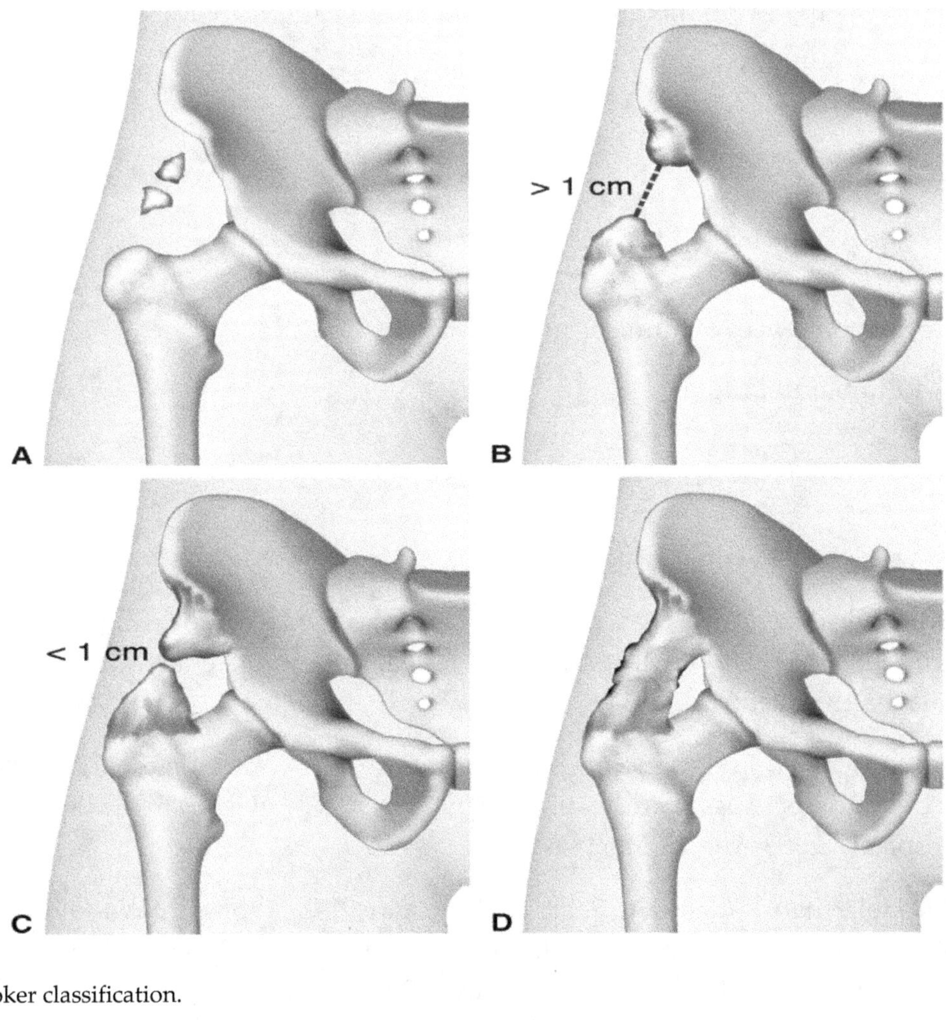

Figure 8. Brooker classification.

12. Barrack grading of cementing

12.1. Introduction

This classification was proposed by Barrack et al. based-on review of 50 second generation cemented femoral stems [15].

12.2. Classification

Grade A: White-out with complete filling.

Grade B: Slight defects at the cement-bone interface.

Grade C: Defective cement mantle or radiolucency involving 50 to 99% of the cement-bone interface.

Grade D: 100% lucency or failure to cover the tip of the stem.

12.3. Clinical applications

This classification helps in predicting the survivability of the implant based on the grade of cementing.

Author details

Munis Ashraf

Address all correspondence to: munis6@gmail.com

KG Hospital, Coimbatore, India

References

[1] Paprosky WG, Perona PG, Lawrence JM. Acetabular defect classification and surgical reconstruction in revision arthroplasty. A 6-year follow-up evaluation. The Journal of Arthroplasty. 1994 Feb;**9**(1):33-44

[2] Gozzard C, Blom A, Taylor A, Smith E, Learmonth I. A comparison of the reliability and validity of bone stock loss classification systems used for revision hip surgery. The Journal of Arthroplasty. 2003 Aug;**18**(5):638-642

[3] Saleh KJ, Holtzman J, Gafni A, Saleh L, Jaroszynski G, Wong P, Woodgate I, Davis A, Gross AE. Development, test reliability and validation of a classification for revision hip arthroplasty. Journal of Orthopaedic Research. 2001 Jan 1;**19**(1):50-56

[4] Hodgkinson JP, Shelley P, Wroblewski BM. The correlation between the roentgenographic appearance and operative findings at the bone-cement junction of the socket in Charnley low friction arthroplasties. Clinical Orthopaedics and Related Research. 1988 Mar;**228**: 105-109

[5] Valle CJ, Paprosky WG. Classification and an algorithmic approach to the reconstruction of femoral deficiency in revision total hip arthroplasty. The Journal of Bone and Joint Surgery. American Volume. 2003;**85-A**(Suppl 4):1-6

[6] D'Antonio J, McCarthy JC, Bargar WL, Borden LS, Cappelo WN, Collis DK, Steinberg ME, Wedge JH. Classification of femoral abnormalities in total hip arthroplasty. Clinical Orthopaedics and Related Research. 1993 Nov;**296**:133-139

[7] Dossick PH, Dorr LD, Gruen T, Saberi MT. Techniques for preoperative planning and postoperative evaluation of noncemented hip arthroplasty. Techniques in orthopaedics. 1991 Sep 1;**6**(3):1-6

[8] Greidanus NV, Mitchell PA, Masri BA, Garbuz DS, Duncan CP. Principles of management and results of treating the fractured femur during and after total hip arthroplasty. Instructional Course Lectures. 2003;**52**:309-322

[9] Brady OH, Garbuz DS, Masri BA, Duncan CP. The reliability and validity of the Vancouver classification of femoral fractures after hip replacement. The Journal of Arthroplasty. 2000 Jan;**15**(1):59-62

[10] Rayan F, Dodd M, Haddad FS. European validation of the Vancouver classification of periprosthetic proximal femoral fractures. Journal of Bone and Joint Surgery. British Volume (London). 2008 Dec;**90**(12):1576-1579

[11] Tsukayama DT, Estrada R, Gustilo RB. Infection after total hip arthroplasty. A study of one hundred and six infections. The Journal of Bone and Joint Surgery. American Volume. 1996;**78**:512-523

[12] Brooker AF, Bowerman JW, Robinson RA, Riley LH Jr. Ectopic ossification following total hip replacement. Incidence and a method of classification. The Journal of Bone and Joint Surgery. American Volume. 1973 Dec;**55**(8):1629-1632

[13] Toom A, Fischer K, Märtson A, Rips L, Haviko T. Inter-observer reliability in the assessment of heterotopic ossification: Proposal of a combined classification. International Orthopaedics. 2005 Jun;**29**(3):156-159

[14] Vasileiadis GI, Itoigawa Y, Amanatullah DF, Pulido-Sierra L, Crenshaw JR, Huyber C, Taunton MJ, Kaufman KR. Intraobserver reliability and interobserver agreement in radiographic classification of heterotopic ossification. Orthopedics. 2017 Jan 24;**40**(1):e54-e58

[15] Barrack RL, Mulroy RD Jr, Harris WH. Improved cementing techniques and femoral component loosening in young patients with hip arthroplasty. A 12-year radiographic review. Journal of Bone and Joint Surgery. British Volume (London). 1992 May;**74**(3):38

6

Total Hip Replacement in Developmental Dysplasia

Maximilian F. Kasparek and Friedrich Boettner

Abstract

Total hip arthroplasty (THA) for osteoarthritis secondary to development dysplasia of the hip (DDH) is facing increasing levels of complexity with increasing grade of deformity. The dysplastic acetabulum is characterized by diminished bone stock with decreased lateral coverage. Therefore, it is challenging to restore the anatomic center of rotation and ensure adequate acetabular component fixation. Surgical strategies include a medialization of the acetabular component, a higher hip center, lateral structural bone grafting and the selection of smaller component sizes to improve native bone coverage. Excessive femoral anteversion is commonly encountered in patients with developmental dysplasia. Moreover, the intramedullary canal is narrow and the neck often aligned in valgus. Modular implants are helpful to address the altered femoral anatomy and also facilitate femoral shortening osteotomies in patients with high hip dislocation. Although clinical results are comparable to primary total hip replacement in primary osteoarthritis, the risk for revision surgery due to dislocation and loosening is increased. The current chapter reviews classification, preoperative planning, and surgical strategies for patients undergoing THA for osteoarthritis secondary to developmental dysplasia.

Keywords: developmental dysplasia, secondary osteoarthritis, primary total hip arthroplasty, bone grafting, femoral shortening osteotomy, complication

1. Introduction

Development dysplasia of the hip (DDH) is a common reason for primary total hip arthroplasty (THA) in young female adults. Surgical treatment is complicated by subluxation or dislocation of the femoral head out of the dysplastic acetabulum [1]. Complications occur more frequently due to the increased surgical complexity compared to THA in primary osteoarthritis. Understanding the underlying anatomical abnormalities in patients with DDH is of paramount importance for successful surgical treatment. The complexity is related to a dysplastic acetabulum with decreased lateral bone stock and coverage. Femoral anteversion is common especially in patients with lower levels of dysplasia [2]. In addition, most patients have a valgus neck alignment and a narrow medullary canal [3, 4].

2. Classification

The etiology of DDH is multifactorial and DDH is associated with positive family history and female gender [5]. Classification systems are based on the amount of displacement of the femoral head in relationship to the teardrop and predict the complexity of surgery. With increasing grade of deformity the acetabular bone stock is diminished. The most commonly used classification system was described by Crowe et al. [6] and Hartofilakidis et al. [7].

2.1. Crowe classification

Crowe et al. [6] classified DDH based on the grade of proximal subluxation of the femoral head (**Table 1**). The subluxation is calculated on anterior-posterior radiographs by measuring the proximal subluxation distance between the inter-teardrop line and the transition point of the femoral head to the femoral neck (**Figures 1** and **2**). The grade of subluxation is defined as the proximal subluxation in relation to the undeformed femoral head diameter.

In Crowe grade I, the proximal subluxation of the transition point is under <50% of the vertical femoral head diameter and in Crowe grade II between 50 and 74%. In grade III, proximal migration is about 75–100% and in grade IV more than 100% (**Table 1**).

If the femoral head is deformed, the vertical diameter of the femoral head is calculated as 20% of the height of the pelvis (distance between the iliac crest and the inferior margin of the ischial tuberosity).

The Crowe classification predicts the complexity of surgery and with increasing Crowe grade complications are more common [8]. Furthermore, it was reported that the Crowe classification correlates with grade of acetabular and femoral anteversion [2].

Grade	Crowe classification	Acetabular anteversion	Femoral anteversion
I	<50% subluxation	15°	42°
II	50–74% subluxation	10°	30°
III	75–100% subluxation	7°	43°
IV	>100% subluxation	4°	27°

Table 1. Crowe classification and relationship with acetabular and femoral anteversion [2, 6].

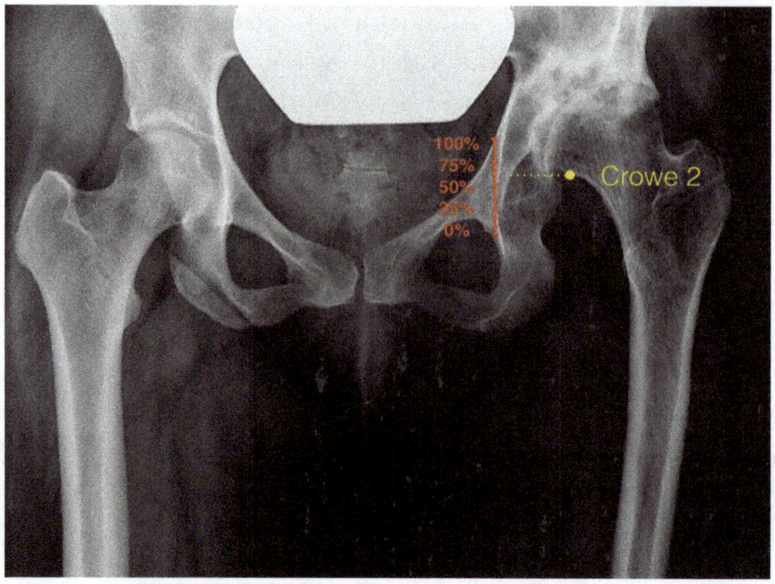

Figure 1. On the radiographs a Crowe grade II deformity is shown (50–74% subluxation). The subluxation is calculated by measuring the proximal migration between the teardrop line and the transition point of femoral head-neck.

2.2. Hartofilakidis classification

Hartofilakidis et al. [7] classified dysplastic hips in three overall categories based on radiographic appearance of the hip: in Type A the femoral head is articulating with the true acetabulum; in Type B the femoral head articulate with a false acetabulum and the false and true acetabulum are still connected; finally in a Type C the femoral head has migrated further proximal (**Table 2**) and therefore true and actual acetabulum are separated. This classification

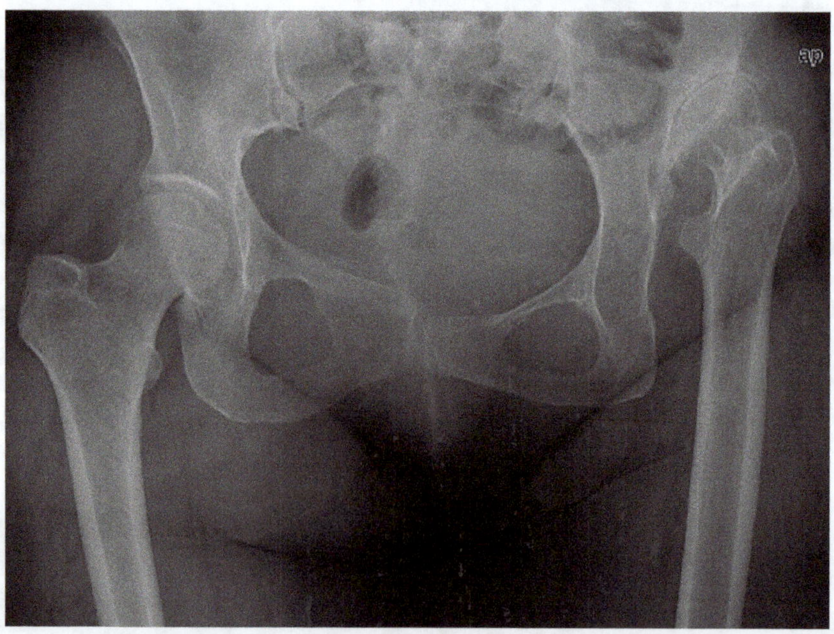

Figure 2. Radiograph of a Crowe grade IV deformity.

Hartofilakidis		Acetabular deficiency
Type A	The femoral head is contained within the original acetabulum despite some degree of subluxation	1. Superior segmental deficiency
		2. Secondary shallowing due to fossa-covering osteophyte
Type B	The femoral head articulates with a false acetabulum that partially covers the true acetabulum	1. Anterior and posterior segmental deficiency
		2. Narrow opening
		3. Inadequate depth
		4. Increased anteversion
Type C	With high dislocation, the femoral head has migrated superiorly and posteriorly. The true acetabulum is inferior and anterior to the false acetabulum along the iliac wing	1. Segmental deficiency of the entire acetabular rim
		2. Narrow opening
		3. Inadequate depth
		4. Excessive anteversion
		5. Abnormal distribution of bone stock, mainly superoposteriorly

Table 2. Hartofilakidis classification [7].

system describes the anatomical deformity and predicts the complexity of acetabular reconstruction.

3. Preoperative planning

Standardized radiographs including calibrated anterior-posterior (AP) pelvis radiographs at the level of the anterior superior iliac spine and lateral hip views are required for templating. Standard AP pelvis radiographs including the iliac crest are necessary to grade the DDH using the Crowe classification. Computer tomography is useful for determining: (1) acetabular component position and bone stock, (2) the amount of femoral anteversion, and (3) the size of the femoral canal in order to determine if standard implants are feasible. Preoperative planning should incorporate planning of the center of rotation before and after surgery as well as the need for femoral shortening osteotomies. This is essential to restore adequate leg lengths. In addition, overall amount of lengthening should be determined to anticipate the risk of sciatic nerve palsy. Adequate sizing of the femoral canal is important in patients at risk for a shortening osteotomy (Crowe type 3 and 4) to assure adequate distal press fit.

4. Surgical approaches

Surgeons should use the surgical approach they are most comfortable with. Standard surgical approaches include the direct anterior, anterolateral, direct lateral, and posterior approach. Advantages of the lateral and posterior approaches are a good view of the acetabulum. The posterior approach also facilitates the access to the femur for shortening osteotomies. While the posterior approach has advantages for patients with more deficient lateral bone stock and high hip dislocations, the direct anterior approach facilitates acetabular component reaming and placement due to intraoperative C-Arm imaging [9]. In addition, operating in a supine position facilitates restoration of leg length. Moreover, in cases with prior periacetabular osteotomies the surgeon can often utilize the same incision [10].

In patients with severe DDH that require shortening osteotomy, it is advantageous to start with femoral preparation since the shortening osteotomy itself often greatly facilitates acetabular exposure. Occasionally, a sliding trochanteric osteotomy can be required to improve abductor muscle tension [11]. Also the posterior capsule and external rotators should be preserved and repaired to reduce the risk of postoperative dislocation [12]. Postoperative weight bearing status is influenced by the type of surgical reconstruction and implant rather than the surgical approach. More advanced postoperative precautions are usually applied to patients undergoing a posterior and direct lateral approach.

5. Acetabular component implantation

In DDH, the acetabulum is often shallow and oval. This results in altered anatomic landmarks and it can be challenging to identify the true acetabulum. Identifying the teardrop (junction of the ischium and pubis) either clinically or using intraoperative fluoroscopy is of absolute importance to locate the true acetabulum [13].

Finding the balance between restoration of the center of rotation and adequate lateral bone coverage requires careful preoperative templating and surgical experience. Lateral coverage can be improved by medialization of the cup and decreasing its size to improve coverage in case of lateral bone deficiency.

In most cases the center of rotation is slightly elevated to improve lateral coverage. This does impact on postoperative leg length and needs to be carefully considered when restoring postoperative leg lengths. Finding the right compromise is also important to avoid a high hip center that can affect postoperative function [1, 14, 15]. In addition, a high hip center increases the forces on the acetabulum and can increase the risk for cup loosening [16, 17]. Therefore, in general it is recommended to restore the center of rotation within 15 mm of the center of the true acetabulum or <35 mm superior to the interteardrop line [18].

A modern porous coated spherical cup, including smaller sizes (40–46 mm) should be available with maximal head size to improve stability. During acetabular reaming, the anterior wall should be protected, as it is often very thin and most of the bone stock is available posterior (**Figure 3**). Therefore, the authors recommend to ream preferentially

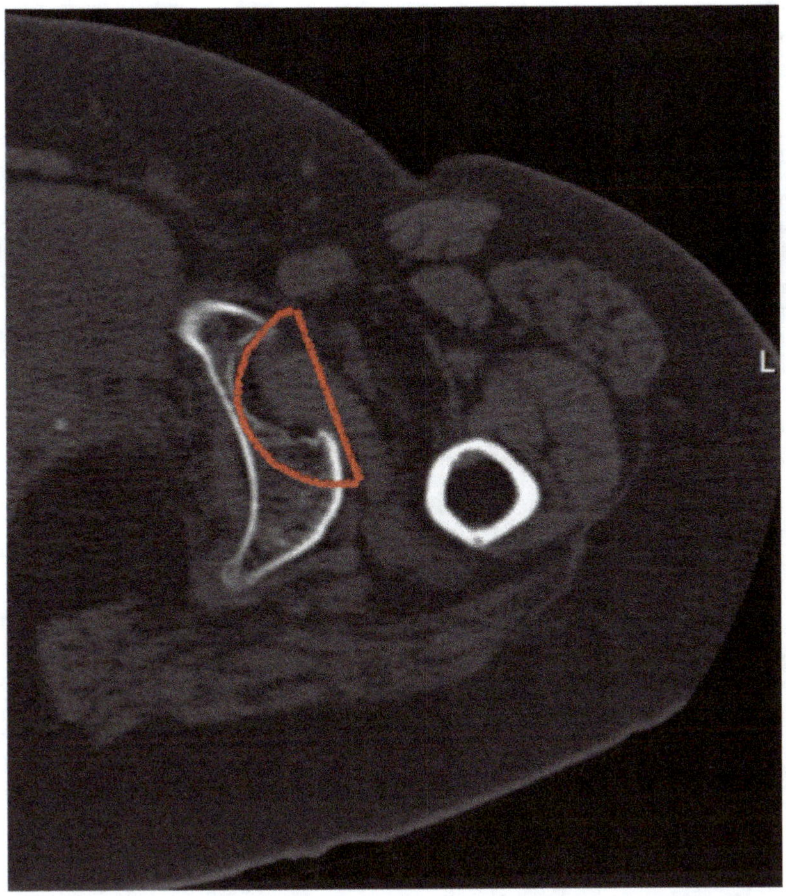

Figure 3. Computer tomography reveals that in the posterior part of the acetabulum there is more bone stock available. Reaming should be done more posteriorly to protect the anterior wall of the acetabulum.

posterior. While medialization is important, care should be taken to avoid over medialization with loss of medial bone fixation. The authors prefer reaching the inner table without penetrating it completely. Whenever the cup extends medially beyond Kohler's line medial bone grafting with graft from the reamer can help later restoration of the medial wall.

Lack of lateral coverage up to 17 mm of uncovered implant arc is acceptable for all implant sizes [19]. For larger acetabular components (52 and up) with less than 45 degree of cup inclination up to 25 mm of the cup can remain uncovered. If preoperative templating suggests that a larger area of the cup is not covered by bone than lateral bone grafting, utilizing the femoral head fixed with two screws (Harris plastic) is recommended [20] (**Figure 4**). Good long-term results with incorporation of the graft were reported for this technique [21, 22]. Metal augments can alternatively be utilized to improve lateral fixation [23], however, the authors prefer a biological restoration of bone stock using the Harris plastic. To facilitate the graft fixation and reaming, it is usually advised to make the decision to proceed with bone grafting early during the acetabular reaming. Modern robotic cup implantation using the Mako® system (Stryker, Kalamazoo, MI) allows for perfect reaming of the acetabulum

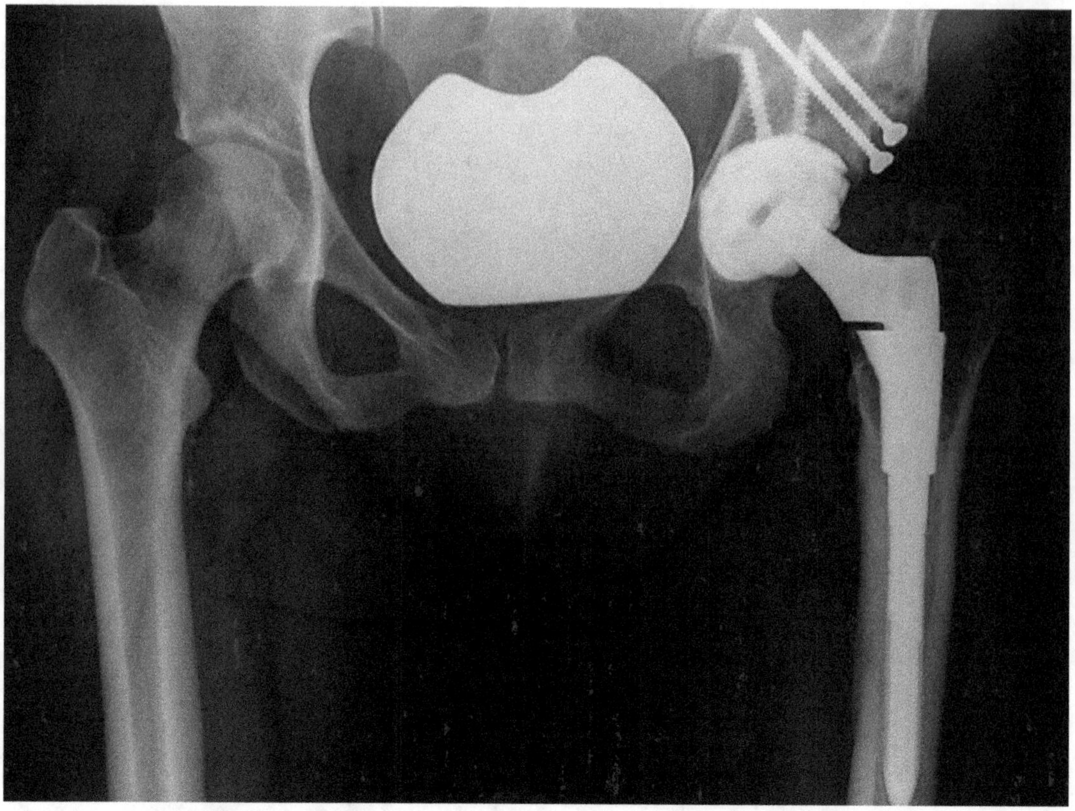

Figure 4. Postoperative radiographs after restoration of a Crowe grade III deformity. The anatomical hip center is restored with a femoral bone graft (Harris plastic).

according to the preoperative plan and is an appealing treatment option for patients undergoing THA for DDH.

5.1. Crowe classification: how it impacts acetabular fixation

In Crowe grade 1 deformities acetabular component fixation is often not too difficult, because in most cases adequate bone stock is available. Therefore, good implant-bone coverage can be achieved almost always without bone grafting or excessive medialization.

Crowe grade II and III deformities are the most difficult defects to restore. In these deformities the femoral head is more subluxated, and significant parts of the lateral bone stock are missing. However, while most Crowe 2 and 3 can be managed similar to grade I by placing the cup proximal-medial and by using a smaller cup size, occasionally a Harris plastic is indicated.

Crowe grade IV deformities are easier to manage because the femoral head was dislocated from the acetabulum without continuous pressure on the lateral bone stock. In most cases the hip center can be restored with a smaller acetabular component in anatomic position. In these cases care should be taken not to over ream since the bone is often soft due to the lack of weight bearing. Restoration of the center of rotation in Crowe grade IV might require a femoral shortening osteotomy to facilitate reduction of the hip.

6. Femoral reconstruction

In comparison to patients with primary osteoarthritis, the dysplastic femur has a narrower and straighter intramedullary canal [24, 25]. In mildly dysplastic hips standard femoral stems can often be used. However, the proximal bone is often osteopenic and its valgus alignment can increase the risk of calcar fractures if broached implants are used. A femoral wire-cerclage of the proximal femur just above the lesser trochanter can be used prophylactically.

Modular implants (for instance S-Rom® system, DePuy, Warsaw, IN) allow the surgeon to use a standard implant for patients with small canal diameter and excessive anteversion while preserving the option to do a femoral shortening osteotomy [26]. The proximal modular sleeve can be selected according to the proximal metaphysis shape and size.

Modular implants also allow to correct excessive anteversion and adjusts the medial spout according to the amount of valgus present [12]. Surgeons should be aware that excessive femoral anteversion is more common in patients with lower Crowe grades. Excessive femoral anteversion can also be corrected using derotation of the proximal fragment during a femoral shortening osteotomy [13].

In grade Crowe III and especially IV, subtrochanteric shortening osteotomies are often indicated [27]. Limb lengthening is generally possible between 2.5 and 4.5 cm [28]. If more lengthening is required, femoral shortening is recommended to avoid sciatic nerve palsy [29, 30]. Especially patients with prior surgeries are at increased risk for sciatic nerve palsy and less lengthening might be possible in these patients.

Preoperative planning is crucial to assess the location of the osteotomy, diameter of the stem as well as extend of lengthening. While a shortening osteotomy can be performed using a cemented stem, today, usually a modular uncemented femoral component is preferred. The removed bone segment can be split in coronal plane and utilized as bone graft by wiring the bone shells on each side of the osteotomy to improve rotational stability. Theoretically, an oblique osteotomy can improve rotational stability; today transverse osteotomies are usually preferred to facilitate derotation of the proximal fragment.

Alternatives to shortening osteotomies are swan neck prosthesis or two stage skeletal traction followed by THA [31–33].

To facilitate intraoperative reduction soft tissue releases including release of the gluteus maximus insertion on the proximal femur, elevation of the gluteus medius of its insertion on the ilium, release of the psoas off the lesser trochanter as well as releases of the anterior and posterior capsule might be necessary. In case of a severe adduction contracture, a postoperative percutaneous release of the adductor tendons can be considered. It is crucial to carefully balance the need for soft tissue releases to facilitate reduction and the need for stability of the hip to minimize postoperative dislocations.

Recommended bearing options in THA for DDH are metal or ceramic on highly crosslinked polyethylene-bearing combinations.

7. Hip resurfacing

In young male patients with Crowe grade I or II deformity, hip resurfacing can be a valuable treatment option with satisfactory results [34, 35]. However, hip resurfacing can face a number of challenges in patients with DDH: because of the valgus neck alignment restoration of hip offset is usually challenging; excessive femoral anteversion and leg shortening cannot be corrected using a hip resurfacing; finally, acetabular components rely on primary press fit and screw augmentation is not possible for most resurfacing components. If a limb-length discrepancy of more than 2 cm or a Crowe grade III or IV deformity is present, hip resurfacing is not recommended [36]. Advantages of hip resurfacing include preservation of bone stock, better range of motion, and stability as well as increased ability to participate in sport compared to conventional THA.

8. Postoperative mobilization

While early mobilization is encouraged in patients undergoing THA for DDH, patients requiring modular implants or more advanced bone grafting and shortening osteotomies often need to observe toe touch weight bearing on crutches for 4–6 weeks. Standard postoperative antithrombotic prophylaxis is recommended.

Shortening osteotomies might require additional abductor precautions during the first 4–6 weeks. Hip precautions are usually enforced for patients undergoing a posterior approach.

9. Complications

Complications are more common in patients undergoing THA for DDH [37]. A higher incidence of proximal femoral fractures is encountered due to the dysplastic narrow femoral canal.

The incidence of dislocations in dysplastic hips is increased and postoperative dislocation is the most common reason for revision surgeries within the first 6 months [38]. Dislocations are commonly anterior as a result of extensive combined anteversion and are not influenced by Crowe grade or the need for shortening osteotomies [39]. Moreover, smaller head diameters due to smaller acetabular component sizes and a decreased femoral offset are additional risk factors for dislocation. The medialization of the cup can result in a decreased femoral offset and bony impingement.

Increased polyethylene wear can occur because of the smaller component sizes with thinner polyethylene inserts, resulting in osteolysis and acetabular component loosening [40].

Also the risk for sciatic nerve palsy is increased and its risk is associated with surgical complexity and history of prior surgeries [41]. Nonunion or delayed union can be encountered in patients with femoral shortening osteotomies [42, 43].

A higher incidence of infections was reported for patients undergoing THA for DDH compared to osteoarthritis. This might be secondary to the increased surgical complexity, increased surgical time, as well as the need for extensive soft tissue releases and utilization of bone grafts [13].

10. Outcome

The functional outcome of THA in DDH is comparable to primary THA in osteoarthritis [44, 45]. However, the revision rate is higher compared to patients with osteoarthritis and increases with severity of the deformity [8, 37]. Increased revision rates in cemented components due to loosening and increased wear were reported in the past, but modern implants and surgical techniques have remarkably improved the long-term survival rates [46]. Even in cases with shortening osteotomies modern implants provide satisfactory mid- and long-term functional results [47, 48].

A proper restoration of hip mechanics and soft tissue balance is important to provide the best functional results after THA. An anatomical restoration of the hip center improves function and decreases acetabular component loosening [18]. Functional results in severe DDH are poor compared to primary osteoarthritis [42], which might be related to the accompanying soft tissue contractures and preoperative functional status. Patients may also have a limb after surgery due to muscle weakness of the abductors. However, in general THA in DDH provides significant increase in function and quality of life in the long-term follow up [49]. Prior pelvis osteotomies can increase the surgical complexity, but do not influence the complication rate or outcome [50, 51].

11. Conclusion

Preoperative planning is crucial in developmental dysplasia. With increasing grade of deformity, the surgeon should have special modular implants available and should be prepared to perform femoral shortening osteotomies as well as lateral acetabular bone grafting. Modern THA provides good long-term results, however, complication rates are increased compared to THA in primary osteoarthritis. It is important to communicate realistic expectations, discuss the increased risk of complications and alert the patient to the possible need for protected weight-bearing.

Contribution statement

I attest to the fact that all authors have participated in the research, read the manuscript, attest to the validity and legitimacy of the data and its interpretation, and agree to its submission.

Conflict of interest statement

We certify that we have not signed any agreement with commercial interest related to this book chapter, which would in any way limit publication of any and all data generated for the study or to delay publication for any reason.

Dr. Boettner reports personal fees from Smith & Nephew, personal fees from Ortho Development Corporation and personal fees form DePuy, outside the submitted work.

Author details

Maximilian F. Kasparek and Friedrich Boettner*

*Address all correspondence to: boettnerf@hss.edu

Adult Reconstruction and Joint Replacement Division, Hospital for Special Surgery, New York, NY, USA

References

[1] Hartofilakidis G, Karachalios T. Total hip arthroplasty for congenital hip disease. J Bone Joint Surg Am 2004;86-a(2):242–50.

[2] Bernasek TL, Haidukewych GJ, Gustke KA, Hill O, Levering M. Total hip arthroplasty requiring subtrochanteric osteotomy for developmental hip dysplasia: 5- to 14-year results. J Arthroplasty 2007;22(6 Suppl 2):145–50. doi:10.1016/j.arth.2007.05.014.

[3] Argenson JN, Flecher X, Parratte S, Aubaniac JM. Anatomy of the dysplastic hip and consequences for total hip arthroplasty. Clin Orthop Relat Res 2007;465:40–5. doi:10.1097/BLO.0b013e3181576052.

[4] Argenson JN, Ryembault E, Flecher X, Brassart N, Parratte S, Aubaniac JM. Three-dimensional anatomy of the hip in osteoarthritis after developmental dysplasia. J Bone Joint Surg Br 2005;87(9):1192–6. doi:10.1302/0301-620x.87b9.15928.

[5] Hoaglund FT, Shiba R, Newberg AH, Leung KY. Diseases of the hip. A comparative study of Japanese Oriental and American white patients. J Bone Joint Surg Am 1985;67(9):1376–83.

[6] Crowe JF, Mani VJ, Ranawat CS. Total hip replacement in congenital dislocation and dysplasia of the hip. J Bone Joint Surg Am 1979;61(1):15–23.

[7] Hartofilakidis G, Stamos K, Karachalios T, Ioannidis TT, Zacharakis N. Congenital hip disease in adults. Classification of acetabular deficiencies and operative treat-

ment with acetabuloplasty combined with total hip arthroplasty. J Bone Joint Surg Am 1996;78(5):683–92.

[8] Cameron HU, Botsford DJ, Park YS. Influence of the Crowe rating on the outcome of total hip arthroplasty in congenital hip dysplasia. J Arthroplasty 1996;11(5):582–7.

[9] Gromov K, Greene ME, Huddleston JI, Emerson R, Gebuhr P, Malchau H et al. Acetabular dysplasia and surgical approaches other than direct anterior increases risk for malpositioning of the acetabular component in total hip arthroplasty. J Arthroplasty 2016;31(4):835–41. doi:10.1016/j.arth.2015.10.045.

[10] Baque F, Brown A, Matta J. Total hip arthroplasty after periacetabular osteotomy. Orthopedics 2009;32(6):399. doi:10.3928/01477447-20090511-04.

[11] Lakstein D, Backstein DJ, Safir O, Kosashvili Y, Gross AE. Modified trochanteric slide for complex hip arthroplasty: clinical outcomes and complication rates. J Arthroplasty 2010;25(3):363–8. doi:10.1016/j.arth.2009.02.017.

[12] Sanchez-Sotelo J, Berry DJ, Trousdale RT, Cabanela ME. Surgical treatment of developmental dysplasia of the hip in adults: II. Arthroplasty options. J Am Acad Orthop Surg 2002;10(5):334–44.

[13] Rogers BA, Garbedian S, Kuchinad RA, Backstein D, Safir O, Gross AE. Total hip arthroplasty for adult hip dysplasia. J Bone Joint Surg Am 2012;94(19):1809–21. doi:10.2106/jbjs.k.00779.

[14] Doehring TC, Rubash HE, Shelley FJ, Schwendeman LJ, Donaldson TK, Navalgund YA. Effect of superior and superolateral relocations of the hip center on hip joint forces. An experimental and analytical analysis. J Arthroplasty 1996;11(6):693–703.

[15] Delp SL, Wixson RL, Komattu AV, Kocmond JH. How superior placement of the joint center in hip arthroplasty affects the abductor muscles. Clin Orthop Relat Res 1996;(328):137–46.

[16] Bicanic G, Delimar D, Delimar M, Pecina M. Influence of the acetabular cup position on hip load during arthroplasty in hip dysplasia. Int Orthop 2009;33(2):397–402. doi:10.1007/s00264-008-0683-z.

[17] Stans AA, Pagnano MW, Shaughnessy WJ, Hanssen AD. Results of total hip arthroplasty for Crowe Type III developmental hip dysplasia. Clin Orthop Relat Res 1998;(348): 149–57.

[18] Watts CD, Abdel MP, Hanssen AD, Pagnano MW. Anatomic hip center decreases aseptic loosening rates after total hip arthroplasty with cement in patients with Crowe type-II dysplasia: a concise follow-up report at a mean of thirty-six years. J Bone Joint Surg Am 2016;98(11):910–5. doi:10.2106/jbjs.15.00902.

[19] Li H, Mao Y, Oni JK, Dai K, Zhu Z. Total hip replacement for developmental dysplasia of the hip with more than 30% lateral uncoverage of uncemented acetabular components. Bone Joint J 2013;95-b(9):1178–83. doi:10.1302/0301-620x.95b9.31398.

[20] Harris WH, Crothers O, Oh I. Total hip replacement and femoral-head bone-grafting for severe acetabular deficiency in adults. J Bone Joint Surg Am 1977;59(6):752–9.

[21] Spangehl MJ, Berry DJ, Trousdale RT, Cabanela ME. Uncemented acetabular components with bulk femoral head autograft for acetabular reconstruction in developmental dysplasia of the hip: results at five to twelve years. J Bone Joint Surg Am 2001;83-a(10):1484–9.

[22] Abdel MP, Stryker LS, Trousdale RT, Berry DJ, Cabanela ME. Uncemented acetabular components with femoral head autograft for acetabular reconstruction in developmental dysplasia of the hip: a concise follow-up report at a mean of twenty years. J Bone Joint Surg Am 2014;96(22):1878–82. doi:10.2106/jbjs.n.00061.

[23] Bicanic G, Barbaric K, Bohacek I, Aljinovic A, Delimar D. Current concept in dysplastic hip arthroplasty: techniques for acetabular and femoral reconstruction. World J Orthop 2014;5(4):412–24. doi:10.5312/wjo.v5.i4.412.

[24] Noble PC, Kamaric E, Sugano N, Matsubara M, Harada Y, Ohzono K et al. Three-dimensional shape of the dysplastic femur: implications for THR. Clin Orthop Relat Res 2003;(417):27–40. doi:30.3097/01.blo.0000096819.67494.32.

[25] Robertson DD, Essinger JR, Imura S, Kuroki Y, Sakamaki T, Shimizu T et al. Femoral deformity in adults with developmental hip dysplasia. Clin Orthop Relat Res 1996;(327):196–206.

[26] Tamegai H, Otani T, Fujii H, Kawaguchi Y, Hayama T, Marumo K. A modified S-ROM stem in primary total hip arthroplasty for developmental dysplasia of the hip. J Arthroplasty 2013;28(10):1741–5. doi:10.1016/j.arth.2013.04.041.

[27] Gustke K. The dysplastic hip: not for the shallow surgeon. Bone Joint J 2013;95-b(11 Suppl A):31–6. doi:10.1302/0301-620x.95b11.32899.

[28] Lewallen DG. Neurovascular injury associated with hip arthroplasty. Instr Course Lect 1998;47:275–83.

[29] Sener N, Tozun IR, Asik M. Femoral shortening and cementless arthroplasty in high congenital dislocation of the hip. J Arthroplasty 2002;17(1):41–8.

[30] Reikeraas O, Lereim P, Gabor I, Gunderson R, Bjerkreim I. Femoral shortening in total arthroplasty for completely dislocated hips: 3–7 year results in 25 cases. Acta Orthop Scand 1996;67(1):33–6.

[31] Huo MH, Salvati EA, Lieberman JR, Burstein AH, Wilson PD, Jr. Custom-designed femoral prostheses in total hip arthroplasty done with cement for severe dysplasia of the hip. J Bone Joint Surg Am 1993;75(10):1497–504.

[32] DiFazio F, Shon WY, Salvati EA, Wilson PD, Jr. Long-term results of total hip arthroplasty with a cemented custom-designed swan-neck femoral component for congenital dislocation or severe dysplasia: a follow-up note. J Bone Joint Surg Am 2002;84-a(2):204–7.

[33] Yoon PW, Kim JI, Kim DO, Yu CH, Yoo JJ, Kim HJ et al. Cementless total hip arthroplasty for patients with Crowe type III or IV developmental dysplasia of the hip: two-stage total hip arthroplasty following skeletal traction after soft tissue release for irreducible hips. Clin Orthop Surg 2013;5(3):167–73. doi:10.4055/cios.2013.5.3.167.

[34] Wang Q, Zhang XL, Chen YS, Shen H, Shao JJ. Resurfacing arthroplasty for hip dysplasia: a prospective randomised study. J Bone Joint Surg Br 2012;94(6):768–73. doi:10.1302/0301-620x.94b6.28522.

[35] Amstutz HC, Le Duff MJ, Harvey N, Hoberg M. Improved survivorship of hybrid metal-on-metal hip resurfacing with second-generation techniques for Crowe-I and II developmental dysplasia of the hip. J Bone Joint Surg Am 2008;90 Suppl 3:12–20. doi:10.2106/jbjs.h.00711.

[36] Amstutz HC, Beaule PE, Dorey FJ, Le Duff MJ, Campbell PA, Gruen TA. Metal-on-metal hybrid surface arthroplasty. Surgical Technique. J Bone Joint Surg Am 2006;88 Suppl 1 Pt 2:234–49. doi:10.2106/jbjs.f.00273.

[37] Krych AJ, Howard JL, Trousdale RT, Cabanela ME, Berry DJ. Total hip arthroplasty with shortening subtrochanteric osteotomy in Crowe type-IV developmental dysplasia. J Bone Joint Surg Am 2009;91(9):2213–21. doi:10.2106/jbjs.h.01024.

[38] Thillemann TM, Pedersen AB, Johnsen SP, Soballe K. Implant survival after primary total hip arthroplasty due to childhood hip disorders: results from the Danish Hip Arthroplasty Registry. Acta Orthop 2008;79(6):769–76. doi:10.1080/17453670810016830.

[39] Wang L, Trousdale RT, Ai S, An KN, Dai K, Morrey BF. Dislocation after total hip arthroplasty among patients with developmental dysplasia of the hip. J Arthroplasty 2012;27(5):764–9. doi:10.1016/j.arth.2011.08.021.

[40] Murray PJ, Hwang KL, Imrie SN, Huddleston JI, 3rd, Goodman SB. Polyethylene wear and osteolysis is associated with high revision rate of a small sized porous coated THA in patients with hip dysplasia. J Arthroplasty 2014;29(7):1373–7. doi:10.1016/j.arth.2014.02.027.

[41] Eggli S, Hankemayer S, Muller ME. Nerve palsy after leg lengthening in total replacement arthroplasty for developmental dysplasia of the hip. J Bone Joint Surg Br 1999;81(5):843–5.

[42] Yalcin N, Kilicarslan K, Karatas F, Mutlu T, Yildirim H. Cementless total hip arthroplasty with subtrochanteric transverse shortening osteotomy for severely dysplastic or dislocated hips. Hip Int 2010;20(1):87–93.

[43] Hartofilakidis G, Babis GC, Georgiades G, Kourlaba G. Trochanteric osteotomy in total hip replacement for congenital hip disease. J Bone Joint Surg Br 2011;93(5):601–7. doi:10.1302/0301-620x.93b5.24780.

[44] Boyle MJ, Frampton CM, Crawford HA. Early results of total hip arthroplasty in patients with developmental dysplasia of the hip compared with patients with osteoarthritis. J Arthroplasty 2012;27(3):386–90. doi:10.1016/j.arth.2011.06.024.

[45] Engesaeter LB, Furnes O, Havelin LI. Developmental dysplasia of the hip—good results of later total hip arthroplasty: 7135 primary total hip arthroplasties after developmental dysplasia of the hip compared with 59774 total hip arthroplasties in idiopathic coxarthrosis followed for 0 to 15 years in the Norwegian Arthroplasty Register. J Arthroplasty 2008;23(2):235–40. doi:10.1016/j.arth.2007.03.023.

[46] Perka C, Fischer U, Taylor WR, Matziolis G. Developmental hip dysplasia treated with total hip arthroplasty with a straight stem and a threaded cup. J Bone Joint Surg Am 2004;86-a(2):312–9.

[47] Takao M, Ohzono K, Nishii T, Miki H, Nakamura N, Sugano N. Cementless modular total hip arthroplasty with subtrochanteric shortening osteotomy for hips with developmental dysplasia. J Bone Joint Surg Am 2011;93(6):548–55. doi:10.2106/jbjs.i.01619.

[48] Park MS, Kim KH, Jeong WC. Transverse subtrochanteric shortening osteotomy in primary total hip arthroplasty for patients with severe hip developmental dysplasia. J Arthroplasty 2007;22(7):1031–6. doi:10.1016/j.arth.2007.05.011.

[49] Roidis NT, Pollalis AP, Hartofilakidis GC. Total hip arthroplasty in young females with congenital dislocation of the hip, radically improves their long-term quality of life. J Arthroplasty 2013;28(7):1206–11. doi:10.1016/j.arth.2012.09.025.

[50] Tokunaga K, Aslam N, Zdero R, Schemitsch EH, Waddell JP. Effect of prior Salter or Chiari osteotomy on THA with developmental hip dysplasia. Clin Orthop Relat Res 2011;469(1):237–43. doi:10.1007/s11999-010-1375-8.

[51] Duncan S, Wingerter S, Keith A, Fowler SA, Clohisy J. Does previous osteotomy compromise total hip arthroplasty? A systematic review. J Arthroplasty 2015;30(1):79–85. doi:10.1016/j.arth.2014.08.030.

7

Preoperative Planning of Total Hip Arthroplasty

Aamir H. Shaikh

Abstract

Preoperative planning is a crucial step towards a successful hip replacement. It is approached in five easy steps that includes a comprehensive history and examination, ordering weight bearing standardized radiographs, assessment of patients for fitness in the pre-assessment clinic, choosing the best implants as per individual case basis along with choosing method of implantation and templating the radiographs before starting the procedure to replicate the patient joint anatomy for the best patient outcome and to restore hip joint biomechanics. This further allows anticipating difficulties and pitfalls prior to surgery and thereby reducing the risk of complications associated with the hip replacement surgery.

Keywords: preoperative, planning, hip arthroplasty, results, templating

1. Introduction

Total hip arthroplasty (THA) provides an excellent pain relief and improvement in functional capacity along with improvement in the objective performance scores in patients with established debilitating arthritis of the hip joint. The success of the above treatment is multifactorial including proper patient selection, preoperative procedure planning and surgeons ability to perform a satisfactory procedure that restores the biomechanics of the hip joint [1, 2]. The outcome is limited by the fact that no single prosthesis is suitable for all patients due to personal patient factors including variation in bone quality, bone anatomy, patient activity level and the postoperative expectations of the patient. However, with thorough preoperative planning, these goals are achievable while minimizing perioperative risks and complications.

A famous quote of an American polymath, a scientist Benjamin Franklin is, "By failing to prepare, you are preparing to fail." This is why preoperative planning is a vital step in the actual total hip arthroplasty.

2. Preoperative planning

Preoperative planning is presented here as a five step process that begins with the introduction of surgeon to the patient. These steps include:

- Obtaining meticulous history and examination.
- Ordering appropriate investigations including weight-bearing X-ray.
- Assessment of the patients for fitness in the pre assessment clinics.
- Selection of the most appropriate implants as per patient's need and anatomy along with the method of implantation of prosthesis.
- Templating procedure to help accurately size the implants before start of the procedure.

2.1. Obtaining meticulous history and examination

There is no substitute of a thorough history and examination, which will make a clinician to arrive at a working diagnosis of arthritis of the hip joint. Bear in mind radiculopathy pain can also present as pain surrounding gluteal region and thigh and has to be excluded by examination. It is a good practice to both subjectively and objectively determine patient's loss of function on Harris Hip score [3] and its impact on the quality of life using SF36 [4] or other acceptable scores of reporting system.

Patient past medical history should be obtained including significant comorbidities of other body systems as this will help clinician to obtain further assessment of patient body reserve prior to major surgery and in obtaining risk assessment which will help the clinician to optimize these risk beforehand and on occasion to book a special care bed post-surgery in a high dependency unit (HDU) to facilitate proper patient care.

Further, it is vital to obtain from patient history of medical comorbidities, which could have a serious bearing on response to healing after surgery like diabetes and immune deficiency states e.g. steroid use and liver or kidney disorders.

Medication history with any known allergies has to be documented and assessed carefully. This include allergy to any metal type or latex material. Antiplatelet medication like clopidogrel need to be assessed by cardiologist to consider holding it a week before planned surgery, as this would otherwise increase the risk for perioperative bleeding with increased incidence of transfusion. Likewise anticoagulant medication will all need to be assessed for their indication of use and consideration given for holding them if possible otherwise bridging them with a low molecular weight heparin.

Past surgical history with anesthesia given in the past helps to identify additional knowledge of patient's response to prior anesthetic medication and their tolerance. Further, any issues with spinal problems or previous spinal surgeries will require evaluating safety of the spinal anesthesia. Likewise any prior incisions at the operative area will require surgeon to carefully plan their surgical site incision, as this will create a flap with its healing problem if not selected properly. Any past surgical procedure with its effect should be determined that could possibly increase the risk of prosthetic joint infection as colostomy, ileostomy or urinary conduit close to the operating site.

During robust clinical examination attention is paid to findings like fixed flexion deformity (FFD), leg length discrepancy (LLD), gait assessment including Trendelenburg or antalgic gait. Skin condition of the leg been operated is of paramount importance and any signs suggestive of severe eczema or infection should need to be addressed before the surgery itself. Likewise vascular status should be properly assessed and documented.

Patient's body mass index (BMI) is an important assessment parameter as obese population is at higher risk for prosthetic joint infection (PJI) and other wound problems post-surgery.

2.2. Ordering appropriate investigations including weight-bearing X-ray

It is prudent to obtain weight-bearing radiographs of the patient that accurately assess patient's anatomy with measurable dimensions of the bone. If there are concerns with alignment or limb length discrepancy then obtain long leg radiographs. Consider putting blocks under short leg, as this will correct pelvic obliquity from the effect of limb shortening.

In essence good quality radiographs that will show square pelvis with standardized magnification are essential for preoperative planning. The typical views include an anteroposterior (AP) pelvis along with AP views and Lowenstein lateral views of the affected hip. The AP views are obtained with legs internally rotated by 15–20° (**Figure 1**). This allows assessment of the neck shaft angle; the lateral hip offset and helps in comparison with the opposite unaffected hip.

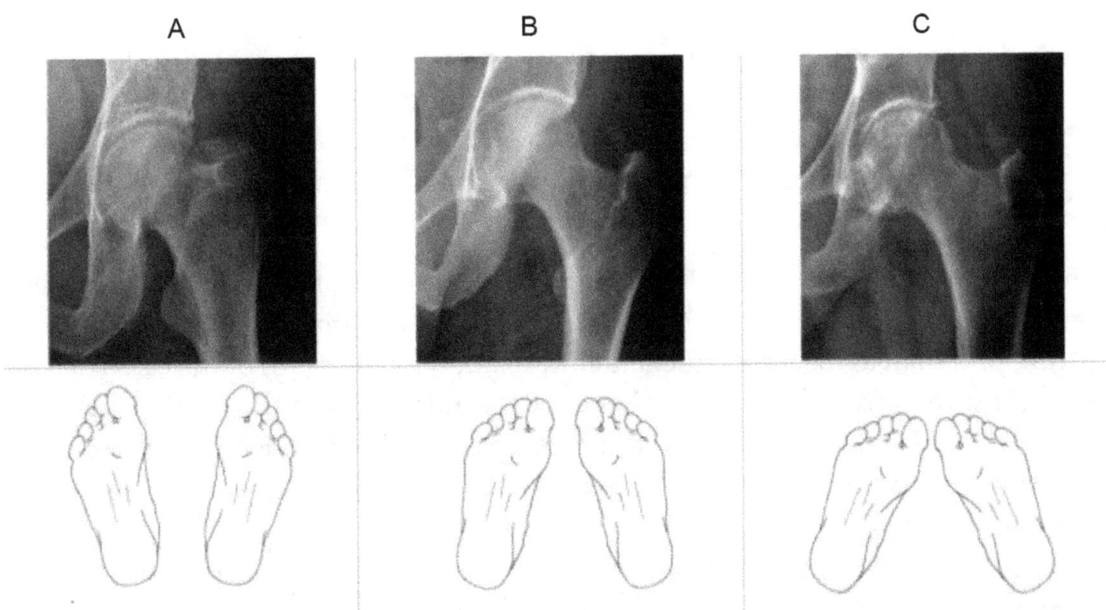

Figure 1. Hip X-ray taken with leg in (A) External rotation, (B) Internal rotation (C) extra internal rotation over 15–20°. (B) is considered optimum image.

2.3. Assessment of patients for fitness in the pre assessment clinics

The investigations obtained for determining anesthetic suitability starts with the blood work up. These include full blood count (FBC), renal function test (U&E), fasting blood glucose, coagulation profile, liver function test (LFT) if required. Other tests if needed in special circumstances will be ordered as per need like sickle cell test for certain African population, C-reactive protein (CRP) in infection cases. Blood group and hold is valid for few weeks and should be ordered if pre assessment of patient will lead to surgery promptly within acceptable time frame. Recently, there has been increased use of Tranexamic acid to prevent per operative bleeding and also the use of autologous blood transfusion by using cell saver preoperatively for long and complex primary and revision hip replacement cases.

Patient electro cardio graph (ECG) should be obtained with a recording of 12 lead ECG in this clinic appointment.

If patient is over 60 years of age and those under 60 years but smokers and those with respiratory conditions, obtain a base line chest X-ray. Consider repeating weight bearing joint X-ray if the earlier X-rays are over 12 months old for looking into any interim progress in the arthritic pattern.

2.4. Selection of the most appropriate implants as per patient's need and anatomy along with the method of implantation of prosthesis

Several factors are considered in selecting an appropriate implant. The patient's age and activity level are important. Other factors most important in consideration for choosing implants are national joint registry 10 years implant survival results published annually [5] and orthopedic data evaluation panel (ODEP) level rating [6], which depends on the revision rate in 10 years follow up.

Generally speaking the younger and more active patients are considered to have the highest physical demand; for them cement-less implants and some of the new bearing surface like ceramic head should be considered. On the contrary for older subjects with less activity profile or low demand patients treatment with hybrid THA along with the use of traditional bearing surface like metal on poly should be preferred.

The quality of bone is another factor that influences the method of implant fixation. Medullary canal configuration, as described by Noble et al. [7] by calculating the ratio of femoral canal width 20 mm proximal to the lesser trochanter in relation to the width of the canal at the femoral isthmus (**Figure 2**). This ratio is called canal flare index (CFI). If this ratio is less than 3.0, the canal has stovepipe configuration and the best implant fixation is by utilizing cementing technique. If this ratio is greater than 4.7, the femoral canal then has a champagne flute configuration and will require meticulous reaming to safeguard risk of periprosthetic fracture. Wider population has a ratio of 3.0–4.7, which is considered normal and may benefit from cement less implants if the cortex is simultaneously thick.

Next, the extent of arthritic involvement in the joint itself can influence the type of implant selection. Example, isolated femoral head wear with various stages of avascular necrosis (AVN) of the femur head, some surgeon will prefer a resurfacing hemiarthroplasty (**Figure 3**).

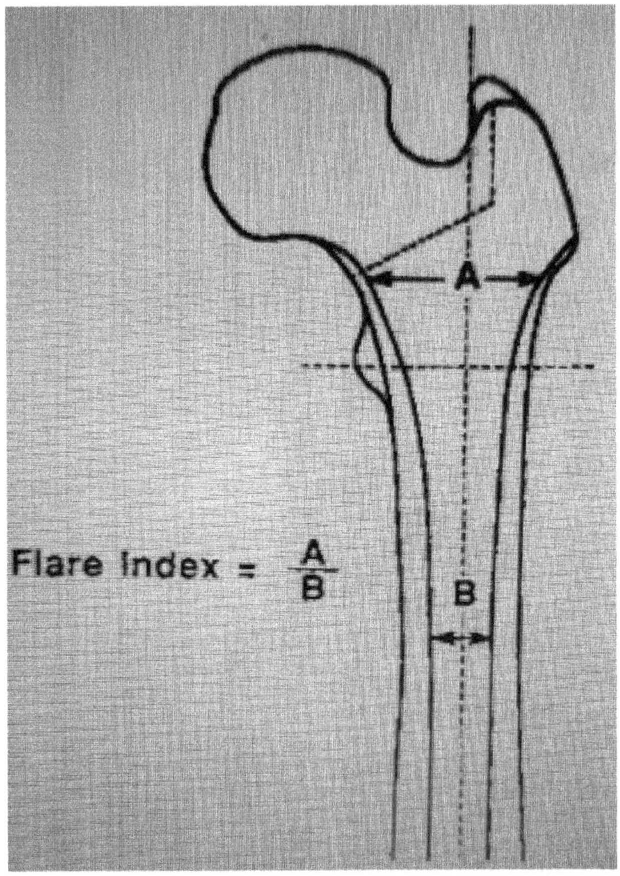

Figure 2. Canal flare index as described by Noble et al. [7].

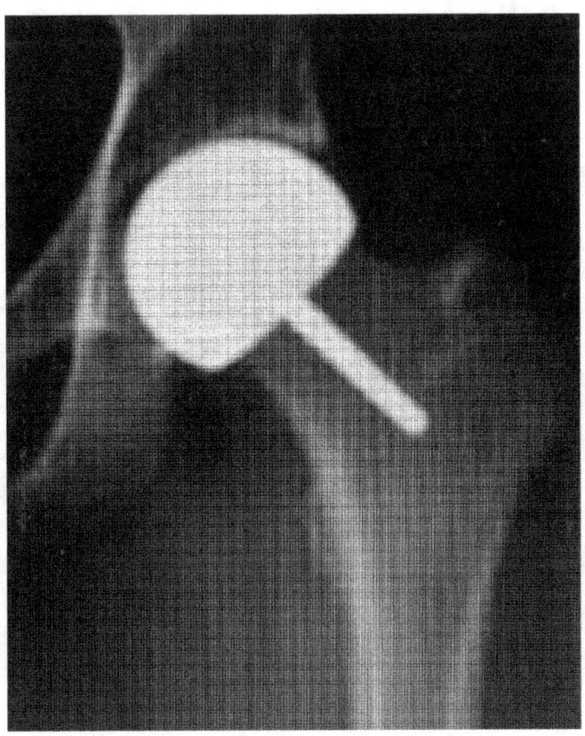

Figure 3. Resurfacing hemiarthroplasty for selected patients with isolated femoral head involvement from AVN.

In cases where proximal femur is excessively anteverted like development dysplasia of hip (DDH) population, the surgeon may prefer to use modular (**Figure 4**) or custom made prosthesis that will allow to adjust for extra anteversion when cement less implant system is used.

Further, on the acetabular side a protrusio configuration (**Figure 5**) can be accommodated with a deeper profile acetabular component. Acetabular protrusion is an anatomical finding encountered in cases of rheumatoid arthritis, ankylosing spondylitis, Paget's disease and in patients with severe osteoporosis with bone stock deficiency. Radiographic assessment of protrusio acetabulum is established by finding the extent of femoral head displacement medially relative to Kohler's line (ilioischial line) or can be defined by a center edge angle (CEA) of Wiberg exceeding 35°. This deformity is corrected by restoring the center of acetabular rotation to the correct anatomical position. During surgery any medial side reaming of the acetabular floor should be avoided. Acetabular component fixation is then achieved by good peripheral rim contact with the acetabular bone. Any associated medial wall defect can then be filled with autologous bone graft or by utilizing deeper profile acetabular cup that should be arranged preoperatively.

In nutshell it is prudent to define any anatomical distortion, whether on the femoral or acetabular side.

2.5. Templating procedure to help accurately size the implants before start of the procedure

Hip joint templating requires anticipating the size and position of the implants before the actual hip surgery is undertaken. Both Charnley [8] and Müller [9] emphasized the importance of preoperative templating utilizing radiographs in determining the type and size of prosthesis.

Preoperative planning for THA is performed by superposing acetate template drawings on the standardized AP radiographs of the hip using hard copies X-rays [10, 11], while other surgeons have favored using digital templating [12]. An old misconception, which some surgeons

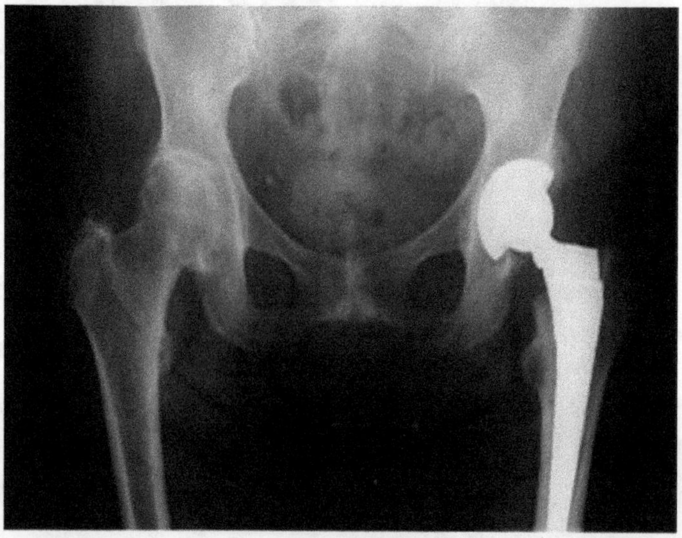

Figure 4. Modular THR for adjusting extra anteversion of the femur.

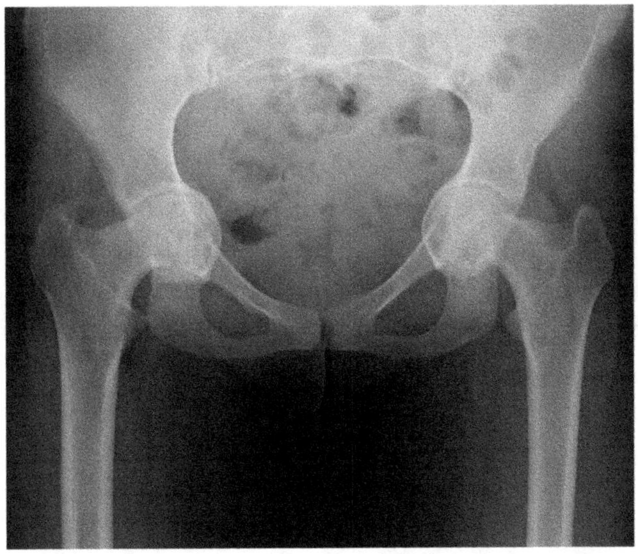

Figure 5. Protrusio acetabulum requiring marginal reaming with bone grafting on the floor of the acetabulum together with fitting a deeper profile cup.

hold about templating process, is that it only helps to guess about the size of the acetabular and femoral components. In reality this becomes difficult and inaccurate, as radiographs are a projection of three-dimensional structure. Many other factors like image magnification [13, 14] and distortion due from projection has also likely to play its role.

It is important to remember from literature that accurate prediction for a cup size is found in between 16 and 62% [11, 14, 15] while stem size accurate prediction is found in between 30 and 69% [11, 15] those accounting for cemented stem up to 78% [14] while cement less stem up to 42% [14]. More importantly, templating is more accurate in predicting within a range of +/− one size, for cup and stem size 52–98% [11, 15]. While its accuracy to predict hip offset is reasonably better in between 58 and 91% [11, 15].

Templating process does not only help to predict the implant size but its major benefit lies in helping an operating surgeon to estimate the position and insertion depth of both components to reproduce hip biomechanics. This also helps surgeon to anticipate any potential difficulties with the available implants.

To begin with this process, standardization of the magnification of hip and pelvis X-rays are of paramount importance. This can be achieved by calibration object of known magnification. Ideally a metal sphere of known dimension is placed at the level of the hip joint in the AP plane, in order to achieve same magnification. The best place is considered to be close to the pubis between the patient's legs and in the plane of greater trochanter [16].

A systematic five-step approach is recommended to proceed for smooth planning during templating process of the hip joints before surgery.

A. Anatomical landmarks identification.

B. Analyzing quality of the radiograph.

C. Choosing mechanical references.

D. Implant selection and positioning.

E. The templating task.

2.5.1. *Anatomical landmarks identification*

To qualify as an anatomical landmark, it must be simple to identify them both on X-rays and simultaneously, while looking at the surgical specimen. At the acetabular side, the roof and the teardrop are adequate landmarks. Importantly acetabular roof is easy to identify at its supero-lateral corner during procedure. The teardrop is radiographic marker formed by superposition of the most medial part of acetabulum distally along with anterior and posterior horn of the acetabulum [17]. The main anatomical concept, which applies for the teardrop, is that it actually corresponds to the most distal and medial part of the acetabulum, that sits behind the transverse acetabular ligament (TAL) and at the superior border of the obturator foramen (OF) (**Figure 6**).

While on the femoral side, recognition of the anatomical reference landmarks include identifying greater trochanter (GT), Lesser trochanter (LT), the medullary canal (MC) and the sloppy saddle (SS) where distally the lower aspect of the neck meets greater trochanter (**Figure 6**).

2.5.2. *Analyzing quality of the radiographs*

Properly exposed, high quality standardized AP radiographs with set magnification are prerequisite for hip joint templating (**Figure 6**). Although this looks simple but it is a real challenging

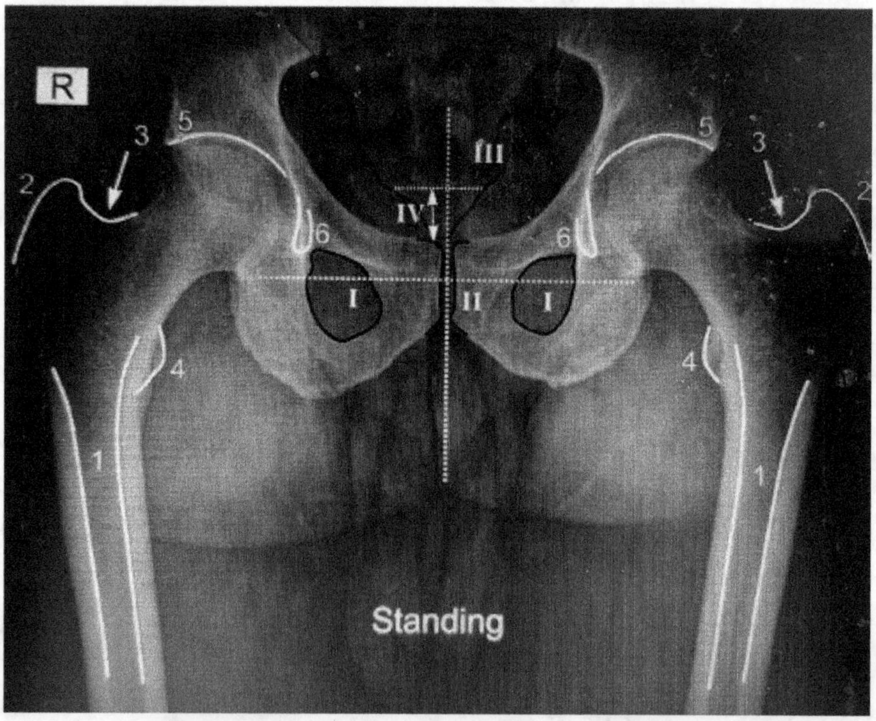

Figure 6. Standing AP hip X-rays suitable for templating. Anatomical Landmarks: (1) femoral medullary canal; (2) greater trochanter; (3) saddle; (4) lesser trochanter; (5) acetabular roof; (6) teardrop; (I) obturator foramina; (II) symphysis pubis; (III) sacrococcygeal joint; (IV) distance to measure for pelvic tilt observation.

task in our modern day practice for acquiring proper exposure. A low pelvis radiographs centered over pubis is preferred for hip templating. With this approach the entire proximal third of the femur is obtained. Pelvis should be kept square in an ideal radiograph. To gain insight into leg length discrepancy, pelvic tilt in both frontal and sagittal plane should be observed. To exclude this effect, keep the AP radiographs in standing position with iliac spines at the same distance bilaterally. This will be confirmed when the symphysis pubis is passing right through the middle of sacrum (**Figure 6**). To calculate sagittal tilt, distance between sacrococcygeal joint and the upper aspect of symphysis pubis is calculated. In neutral alignment it reflects a distance of 32 mm (range: 8–50 mm) in women and 47 mm (range: 15–72 mm) in men. This distance increases when pelvis is tilted forward and the reciprocal is true as well [18].

Another task is to determine femoral neck length (femur offset). To obtain real measurements both femurs should be kept about 15–20° of internal rotation (IR) corresponding to the femoral anteversion. This will highlight actual neck length and thus help in obtaining correct femoral offset (**Figure 7**) while radiographs obtained of femur with more or less IR will underestimate the true femoral neck length and thus femoral offset. Hananouchi et al. [19] highlighted that femoral rotation can be estimated by measuring lesser trochanter projection. By keeping femoral neck parallel to the film, the lesser trochanter is on the average 2.3 ± 3.1 mm broad. This means in most cases around 5 mm of lesser trochanter should be visible medially before attempting to calculate neck length and femoral offset.

2.5.3. Choosing mechanical references

Important mechanical references to determine include:

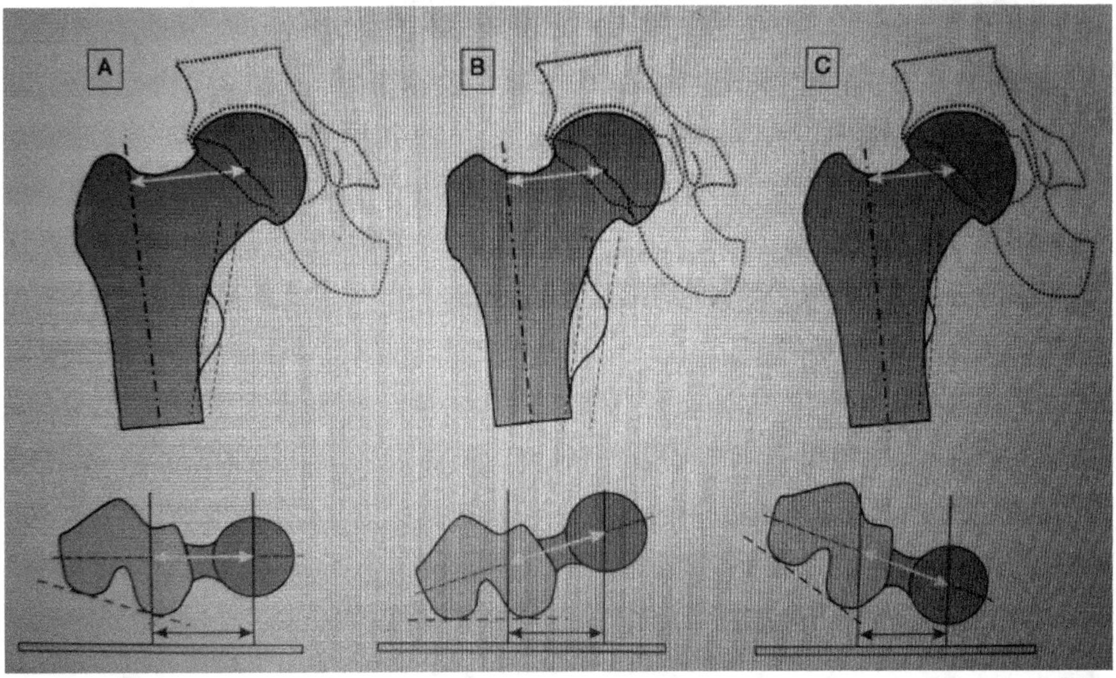

Figure 7. Femoral rotation influence on neck length. (A) IR corresponding to 15–20° with measuring neck length and femoral offset. (B) Femur kept in neutral position underestimating neck length and offset. (C) Femur kept in excessive IR also has same effect in underestimating neck length and femoral offset.

2.5.3.1. *Hip, femoral and acetabular rotation Center*

The hip joint rotation center is the central point around which all hip joint movement occurs. If the acetabulum and femoral head are concentric, then realistically their center of rotation projects on the hip joint center of rotation. As such, the hip rotation center can be easily found as the center of a circle fitted to the projection of the femoral head (**Figure 8**).

On the other hand, if the hip joint is deformed due from dysplastic cup or femoral head dysplasia then it makes very difficult to find hip joint center as its position may vary during hip joint movements. To make such situation easier we will define the "original rotation center" where the native femoral head and acetabulum rotates on the centers before the deformity occurs. This can be usually identified on the preserved inferior one-third of the femoral head and the preserved part of the acetabulum (generally the teardrop and the medial wall). Applying both rotation centers on each other, will likely give a good idea of the native hip joint center of rotation before appearance of the secondary changes.

2.5.3.2. *Femoral, acetabular and combined offset*

The femoral offset is defined as the least distance between the femoral head center of rotation and the longitudinal axis of the femur [20]. The longitudinal axis of femur is drawn as a line in the middle of projected femoral canal. In cases of dysplastic femoral head, the original

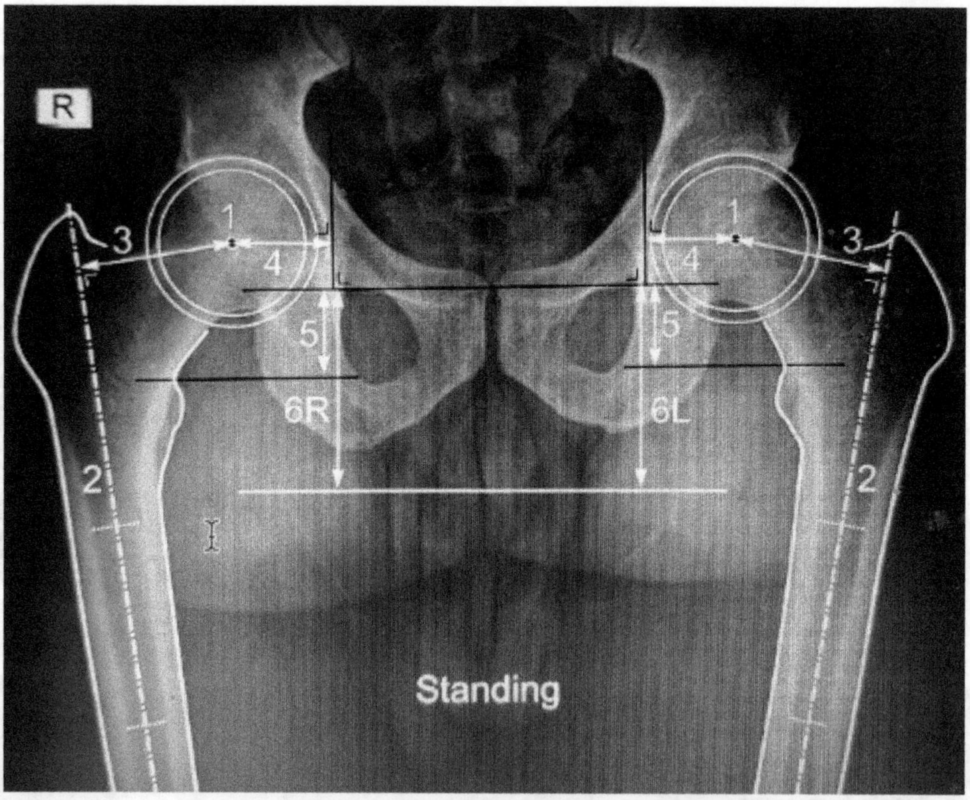

Figure 8. Mechanical landmarks: (1) hip rotation center; (2) longitudinal axis of proximal femur; (3) femoral offset; (4) acetabular offset; (5) hip length; (6) LLD is calculated as difference between distances 6R and 6L.

femoral offset can be estimated between original femoral center of rotation and the longitudinal axis of the proximal femur. Remember femoral offset calculation depends on leg rotation and inevitably it will under estimate femoral offset if the neck is not kept parallel to the radiographic film (**Figure 7**).

Acetabular offset is defined as the distance between acetabular center of rotation and a vertical line drawn through the teardrop. If acetabulum is dysplastic then the original acetabular offset can be found in the same way except replacing hip center of rotation with the original acetabular center of rotation by considering tear drop segment of acetabulum reflecting true acetabular landmark.

The combined hip offset is defined as the cumulative sum of the femoral and acetabular offset. This parameter is important as it bears the tension in hip abductor muscles along with the soft tissues as it controls relative position of greater trochanter with respect to the pelvis.

2.5.3.3. Leg length versus hip length

The "leg length" is defined by measuring distance between a fixed reference point on the pelvis, ideally teardrop inferior edge and the floor where heel lies on the ground. In real sense this measurement is not possible as the floor is not visible on any single radiographic image.

The "hip length" is defined by measuring distance between teardrop inferior edge and a horizontal line through a fixed point on the proximal femur like upper part of the lesser trochanter (**Figure 8**). Remember hip length is influenced by position of the hip in flexion/extension or abduction/adduction therefore, both hips should be kept in a similar position to determine hip lengths and simultaneously to help determine in "hip length discrepancy."

2.5.4. Implant selection and positioning

After labeling of the anatomical landmarks on standardized radiograph and choosing the mechanical reference points, an ideal fitting implant size is chosen for both the acetabular and the femoral component. Our aim is to restore the original hip anatomy and biomechanics. However in certain cases it is not feasible and compromise has to be considered.

2.5.5. The templating task

If the pathological hip undergoing surgery for arthritis is anatomically acceptable then it is preferred to have templating performed on it otherwise it will be technically difficult and a substitute choice should be to template contralateral hip to determine the implant sizes for the operative hip.

2.5.5.1. Positioning: aim to restore the native hip anatomy and biomechanics

First, acetabular cup is selected to fit the acetabular cavity based on line to line reaming or press fit technique to restore the native acetabular center of rotation. Acetabular component should be templated with an abduction angle of 40–45° between longitudinal axis of the cup and the teardrop [21], while template still kept in its position, cup insertion depth compared to the medial acetabular wall, the insertion height compared to the inferior border of the teardrop and the cup margins sitting on the superolateral border of the acetabular roof is noted. These anatomical reference marks are easily identifiable during surgery and will help in restoring original hip anatomy. In cases of protrusio acetabuli, planning is made for lateralizing the acetabular component while grafting the medial acetabular wall will help restoring the acetabular center of rotation thereby avoiding impingement [1]. In dysplastic hips, our goal again is to restore acetabular center of rotation. However, as the acetabulum is often secondarily deformed and shallow, obtaining superolateral roof coverage is a challenging task. This may require consideration for bone grafting or at times will require an additional use of shell and mesh to reconstruct the superolateral defect [1].

Secondly, a femoral implant is selected to fit the medullary canal based on the trial implant size. The longitudinal axis of the implant should be following the longitudinal axis of the femur, while approximate insertion depth is chosen to correctly restore the leg or the hip length. Three techniques are available to achieve the native femoral center of rotation and the femur offset.

i. Lateralizing or medializing the femur by choosing standard versus high offset stem.

ii. Modifying the size of the femoral head component.

iii. Choosing a stem with different neck shaft angle.

Opting between a standard or high offset stem is an easy option as it has no effect on the leg and hip length while the other options does influences on the hip length. By opting to use a stem with less neck shaft angle, compromise is made on the hip length, which can be adjusted by the use of increase in head size or by keeping the stem proud. Using a large size femoral head component will increase both femur offset and hip length and thus will require a more distal stem insertion to control hip length.

More importantly, if a radiograph is obtained with leg in altered rotation. This will impact in determining adequate hip offset and should always be born in mind while decision is made on choosing right offset for the involved hip.

With templating, an appropriate neck cut and its orientation can be planned along with the insertion depth of the stem prosthesis.

2.5.5.2. Equating a balance when failure to restore the native hip anatomy

When it becomes impossible to restore adequate native hip anatomy in that scenario it becomes ideal to restore the combined femoro-acetabular offset and the hip length. When acetabular offset is decreased and hip rotation center is medialized then it becomes prudent to increase the femoral offset. Likewise, increasing the acetabular offset can compensate loss of the femoral offset. This will maintain the soft tissue tension between pelvis and the proximal femur and thus hip abductor function will be optimized.

Similarly, keeping stem more or less proud can compensate for a low or high set hip center of rotation.

Soft tissue balancing is of paramount importance when our goal is to increase or decrease in the leg length. When considering lengthening it is vital to consider for decreasing combined femoro-acetabular offset by medializing the cup or reducing femoral offset by using low offset stem. On the contrary, when planning shortening of the leg, it would be best to consider increasing combined hip offset to minimize the risk of dislocation and gluteal muscle weakness due from lack in the soft tissue tension.

2.5.5.3. Challenges in tackling extreme varus and valgus hips

In a varus hip, with its excessive femoral offset, surgeon can help restore the native anatomy by using high offset stem combined with a large head. To avoid with increase in the leg length with these choice of implants, surgeon may plan a distal neck osteotomy together with low stem insertion. Rarely, this may be benefited further if required with the use of large cup positioned laterally as possible or by using a lateral cup insert thereby helping in increasing acetabular offset. This will restore correct soft tissue tension. However, this increase in the acetabular center of rotation should be opted as the last resort as it increases the acetabular loading [20].

In a valgus hip, with its associated reduced combined hip offset should be respected as over stretching the soft tissues by increase the hip offset could lead to trochanteric bursa pain. This can be maintained by an attempt in medializing the cup. This further helps in reducing the mechanical load at the acetabular component and optimizing abductor function by improving femoral offset [20]. If femoral offset needs to be reduced further, a low offset stem combined with short head should be considered. However, this will require leaving the stem proud if it shortens the leg length.

3. Newer innovation in preoperative planning

Complex primary hip cases involving dysplasia at either side of the joint, trauma cases with fractures requiring arthroplasty, ankylosing spondylitis, protrusio cup and revision hip cases are a big challenge for arthroplasty surgeons. Rapid prototyping (RP) is a new concept adopted from industrial designing. This involves laying down series of additional layers of a material to regenerate a 3D model. Computer aided designing (CAD) program enables rapid production of a component with super accuracy [22]. This model is adopted in medical specialties including orthopedics to develop accurate replica of a body part in cross-section using CT scan as an input source. They are further printed using layered material to generate a 3D-printing model. This rapid prototype model provides a unique opportunity in preoperative planning, in terms of understanding deformity pattern, providing intraoperative referencing and surgical simulation. This further helps an arthroplasty surgeon for inventory planning as they can order necessary implants to make their availability on the day of surgery. This will save time during surgery and minimize on table bleeding, infection rate and thereby patient morbidity.

3.1. Customized instruments and implants

With advancement in the modern day technology, patient specific instruments can be obtained by using rapid prototyping [23]. This will aid in complex cases and will aid in improvement in operative results. In future more customized implants will be developed to use for the individual case demand that will fit for the purpose and will have better survival outcome for our patients by improving joint kinematics.

4. Conclusion

Preoperative planning is an important step in the actual delivery of joint replacement as it allows the patient to go through a comprehensive assessment and preparation for undertaking joint replacement in a schematic fashion. This begins with a thorough clinical assessment by their operating surgeon and a series of investigations followed by actual planning of their hip joint replacement, utilizing template on their standardized radiographs. Templating process allows assessment of their anatomical landmarks to mark as reference points while implanting prosthesis with correct depth. This will allow the surgeons to restore hip biomechanics and thereby improving post-surgical outcomes. This will further allow anticipating difficulties and pitfalls prior to surgery.

Some surgeons do not like to proceed with this important step of templating prior to their joint replacement surgeries. However, unless it is done systematically, it might be difficult, even for the experience hip surgeons to identify those hips, which will definitely benefit from a proper anatomical and mechanical assessment. Moreover, these less planed cases without templating are at increase risk to suffer inadequate hip biomechanics and higher complication rates including trendelenburg gait, joint dislocation, significant leg length discrepancy, peri prosthetic fracture and trochanteric pain. It has been proven to have similar efficacy of preoperative templating by the junior surgeons in training as their senior counter parts [11]. Thus it makes it a legitimate cause for carrying out this vital process of templating of the hip joint prior to actual implantation of the prosthesis. In crux this will improve the long-term outcome and patient satisfaction in both subjective and objective manner [3, 4].

Author details

Aamir H. Shaikh

Address all correspondence to: draamir@mail.com

North Middlesex University Hospital, London, United Kingdom

References

[1] Blackley HRL, Howell GED, Rorabeck CH. Planning and management of the difficult primary hip replacement: Preoperative planning and technical considerations. Instructional Course Lectures. 2000;**49**:3-11

[2] Capello WN. Preoperative planning of total hip arthroplasty. Instructional Course Lectures. 1994;**43**:323-327

[3] Harris WH. Traumatic arthritis of the hip after dislocation and acetabular fractures: Treatment by mold arthroplasty. An end-result study using a new method of result evaluation. The Journal of Bone and Joint Surgery. American Volume. 1969 Jun;**51**(4):737-755

[4] 36-Item Short Form Survey from the RAND Medical Outcomes Study. RANDHealth. Available from: http://www.rand.org/health/surveys_tools/mos/mos_core_36item.html. [Accessed Nov 5, 2014]

[5] Available from: https://www.hqip.org.uk/media/NJR%2014th%20Annual%20Report%20 2017.pdf

[6] Available from: www.odep.org.uk/.../0/ODEPStatements/ODEP%20Benchmarks%20 2017_rev.6.pdf

[7] Noble PC, Alexander JW, Lindahl LJ, et al. The anatomic basis of femoral component design. Clinical Orthopaedics. 1988;**235**:25-34

[8] Charnley J. Low friction arthroplasty of the hip. Vol. 246. Berlin: Springer Verlag; 1979

[9] Müller ME. Lessons of 30 years of total hip arthroplasty. Clinical Orthopaedics. 1992; **274**:12-21

[10] Iorio R, Siegel J, Specht LM, et al. A comparison of acetate vs. digital templating for preoperative planning of total hip arthroplasty is digital templating accurate and safe? The Journal of Arthroplasty. 2009;**24**:180

[11] Kearney R, Shaikh AH, O'Byrne JM. The accuracy and inter-observer reliability of acetate templating in total hip arthroplasty. Irish Journal of Medical Science. 2013 Sep;**182**(3):409-414

[12] Gamble P, Beer JD, Petruccelli D, et al. The accuracy of digital templating in uncemented total hip arthroplasty. The Journal of Arthroplasty. 2010;**25**:529-532

[13] Conn KS, Clarke MT, Hallett JP. A simple guide to determine the magnification of radiographs and to improve the accuracy of preoperative templating. Journal of Bone and Joint Surgery. 2002;**84-B**:269-272

[14] Knight JL, Atwater RD. Preoperative planning for total hip arthroplasty. Quantitating its utility and precision. The Journal of Arthroplasty. 1992;**7**:403-409

[15] Della VAG, Comba F, Taveras N, et al. The utility and precision of analogue and digital preoperative planning for total hip arthroplasty. International Orthopaedics. 2008;**32**: 289-294

[16] Wimsey S, Pickard R, Shaw G. Accurate scaling of digital radiographs of the pelvis. A prospective trial of two methods. The Journal of Bone and Joint Surgery. 2006;**88**:1508-1512

[17] Bowerman JW, Sena JM, Chang R. The teardrop shadow of the pelvis; anatomy and clinical significance. Radiology. 1982;**143**:659-662

[18] Siebenrock KA, Kalbermatten DF, Ganz R. Effect of pelvic tilt on acetabular retroversion: A study of pelvis from cadavers. Clinical Orthopaedics and Related Research. 2003; **407**:241-248

[19] Hananouchi T, Sugano N, Nakamura N, et al. Preoperative templating of femoral components on plain X-rays. Archives of Orthopaedic and Trauma Surgery. 2007;**127**:381-385

[20] Charles MN, Bourne RB, Davey JR, et al. Soft tissue balancing of the hip. The role of femoral offset restoration. Journal of Bone and Joint Surgery. 2004;**86-A**:1078-1088

[21] Wan Z, Boutary M, Dorr LD. The influence of acetabular component position on wear in total hip arthroplasty. The Journal of Arthroplasty. 2008;**23**:51-56

[22] Torabi K, Farjood E, Hamedani S. Rapid prototyping technologies and their applications in prosthodontics, a review of literature. Journal of Dentistry. 2015 Mar;**16**(1):1-9

[23] Basalah A, Shanjani Y, Esmaeili S, Toyserkani E. Characterizations of additive manufactured porous titanium implants. Journal of Biomedical Materials Research. Part B, Applied Biomaterials. 2012 Oct;**100**(7):1970-1979

8

Evaluation of Adaptive Bone Remodeling after Total Hip Arthroplasty Using Finite Element Analysis

Yutaka Inaba, Hiroyuki Ike, Masatoshi Oba and Tomoyuki Saito

Abstract

We compared equivalent stress and strain energy density (SED) to bone mineral density (BMD) in the femur after total hip arthroplasty (THA) using subject-specific finite element analysis (FEA). Equivalent stress and BMD were maintained in the distal femur after THA, whereas both decreased in the proximal femur. A significant correlation was observed between the rates of changes in BMD and equivalent stress before and after THA. Therefore, FEA can predict adaptive bone remodeling after mechanical loading changes. Additionally, we evaluated the effects of two different types of stem geometries (Zweymüller-type stem and fit-and-fill-type stem) on load distribution and BMD using the same method. Equivalent stress and BMD in the medial side of the proximal femur were significantly lower with the Zweymüller-type stem than with the fit-and-fill-type stem. Therefore, FEA can assess the effects of stem geometry on bone remodeling after THA. Moreover, we evaluated the effects of bone geometry on load distribution and BMD after THA. Equivalent stress in the medial side of the proximal femur was significantly lower in the stovepipe model implanted with large tapered wedge-type stems than in the champagne flute and intermediate models, and there was a significant loss of BMD in the stovepipe model. Therefore, a large tapered wedge-type stem and stovepipe femur may be associated with significant proximal BMD loss.

Keywords: finite element analysis, dual-energy X-ray absorptiometry, bone remodeling, hip, arthroplasty

1. Introduction

Periprosthetic bone loss, i.e., a decrease in bone mineral density (BMD) around an implant, is a major concern following total hip arthroplasty (THA) [1, 2]. Severe periprosthetic bone loss may contribute to aseptic loosening of the prosthesis or the risk of periprosthetic fracture [3] and presents serious problems if revision surgery becomes necessary [4]. Several studies have reported that BMD decreases following THA, particularly in the proximal femur [5, 6]. Most changes in BMD occur during the first postoperative year, and subsequently, BMD is maintained [7–9]. This phenomenon is considered to be an adaptive remodeling response of the bone structure to alter its stress environment owing to the presence of an implant. Therefore, mechanical stress may be associated with the patterns of BMD changes. In particular, in cementless THA, an optimal fit of the stem into the metaphyseal region of the femur has been reported to lead to a reduction in periprosthetic bone loss [10].

Wolff [11] proposed that trabecular bone in the proximal femur adapts to external mechanical loads. This structural change is caused by bone remodeling, which couples bone resorption by osteoclasts and bone formation by osteoblasts [12]. It is generally accepted that bone tissue can detect and respond to its mechanical environment, but the exact mechanical signal that drives remodeling remains controversial [13]. Various biomechanical parameters have been investigated to determine the remodeling stimulus. Huiskes et al. [14] examined whether strain energy density (SED) controls bone remodeling. Carter et al. [15] examined stress, and Stulpner et al. [16] examined equivalent strain as signals for remodeling. Adachi et al. [17] proposed that the driving force of remodeling is the local nonuniformity of the scalar function of stress. The existence of various theories indicates that the mechanism of bone remodeling is not well understood.

Subject-specific finite element (FE) models based on geometry and mechanical properties derived from computed tomography (CT) scans have been described in several studies [18–20]. Furthermore, relationships between results of subject-specific finite element analysis (FEA) and bone density have been investigated previously. Cody et al. [21] performed subject-specific FEA and bone density measurements for predicting the fracture load of the femur. Tawara et al. [22] evaluated vertebral strength using subject-specific FEA and BMD. We previously examined the usefulness of subject-specific FEA, which was validated by BMD changes, after THA. We found that equivalent stress through subject-specific FEA correlated with BMD changes before and after THA [23]. The distribution of mechanical loads within the femur after THA might be influenced by the stem geometry and the femur structure. Our previous results suggest that subject-specific FEA could be used to evaluate the effects of stem and femoral geometry on adaptive bone remodeling after THA [24].

This chapter initially provides general information on subject-specific FEA and then presents a brief overview of our work regarding adaptive bone remodeling after THA.

2. Finite element analysis

2.1. Finite element analysis and bone mineral density

It is difficult to assess the stress and strain distributions throughout the entire bone using simplified mathematical models or implanted prostheses or through experiments with cadaveric tissue. An alternative approach to analyze bone mechanics is the FE method, which can accommodate large intersubject variations in bone geometry and material properties [25]. When the ability to perform three-dimensional FE contact analysis is available, subject-specific geometry should be analyzed. This provides the opportunity to examine normal populations of individuals and populations with specific injuries or other pathologies. Ultimately, patient-specific modeling might be used in surgical planning and large-scale studies of treatment efficacy [26]. As mentioned above, we investigated the relationships between the FEA results and BMD. Several previous studies have described the application of FEA for investigating bone-remodeling patterns around implants. However, most of these were not subject-specific models. Weinans et al. [27] reported that subject-specific FE models might be useful for explaining variations in bone adaptation responsiveness among different subjects.

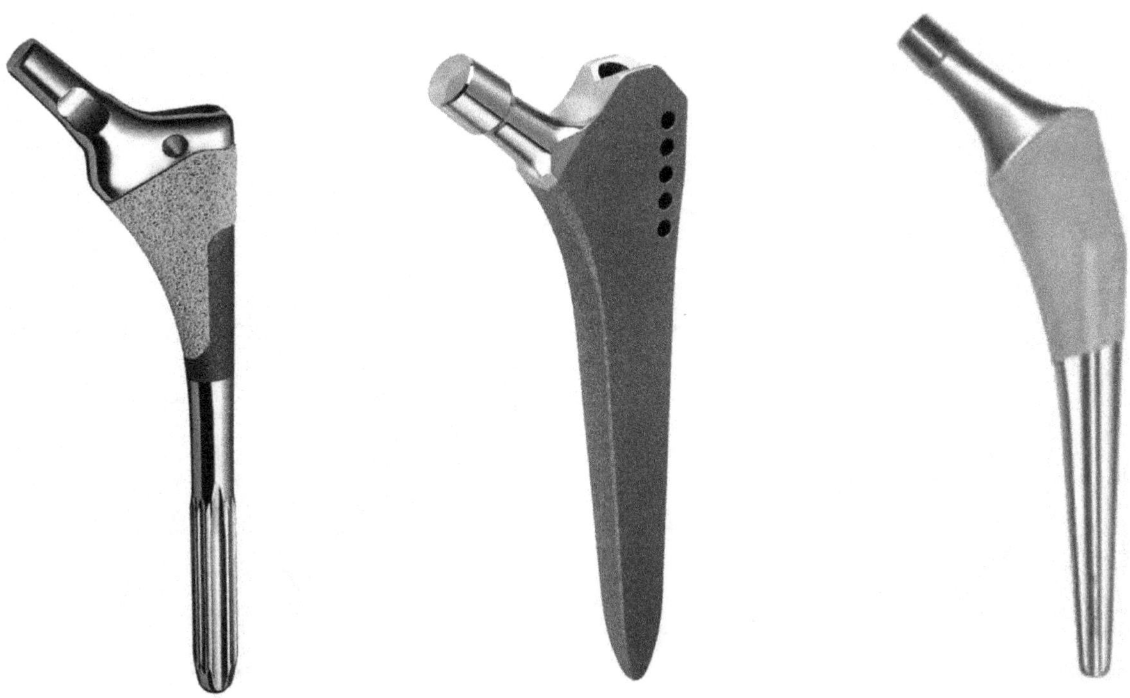

(a) (b) (c)

Figure 1. Diagrams of (a) collarless VerSys Fiber Metal MidCoat, (b) SL-PLUS, and (c) Accolade TMZF stems. (a) Collarless VerSys Fiber Metal MidCoat (Zimmer Inc., Warsaw, IN) is a fit-and-fill-type stem composed of titanium alloy with fiber-metal porous coating at the proximal region. (b) SL-PLUS (Smith & Nephew Inc., Memphis, TN) is a Zweymüller-type stem composed of titanium alloy with a dual taper, rectangular, and trochanteric wing design. (c) Accolade TMZF stem (Stryker Orthopaedics, Mahwah, NJ) is a cementless tapered wedge-type stem composed of beta titanium alloy with a proximal hydroxyapatite-coated porous surface and a distal smooth-finished surface.

We investigated 24 patients (16 women and 8 men) who underwent primary cementless THA using the same fit-and-fill type of prosthesis (collarless VerSys Fiber Metal MidCoat, Zimmer Inc., Warsaw, IN) (**Figure 1**). Collarless VerSys Fiber Metal MidCoat is a stem composed of titanium alloy with a fiber-metal porous coating at the proximal region. Patients were excluded from the study if they were receiving systemic estrogen, vitamin D, or bisphosphonate for osteoporosis. The mean patient age at surgery was 63 years (range, 44–82 years). After surgery, all patients were allowed to use a wheelchair, with full weight bearing, on postoperative day 1, and gait exercise was performed as soon as possible [23]. BMD was assessed with dual-energy X-ray absorptiometry (DEXA) using the Hologic Discovery system (Hologic Inc., Waltham, MA). Baseline DEXA measurements were performed 1 week after surgery as reference, and subsequent measurements were performed at 3, 6, and 12 months postoperatively. Patients were placed in the supine position, and the affected leg was maintained in 20 ° internal rotation to minimize measurement errors. DEXA measurements were performed using the "array prosthetic" mode, which excludes metal from analysis of the regions of interest (ROIs). ROIs were defined according to Gruen's system [28]. The pixel size was 1.1 × 0.56 mm.

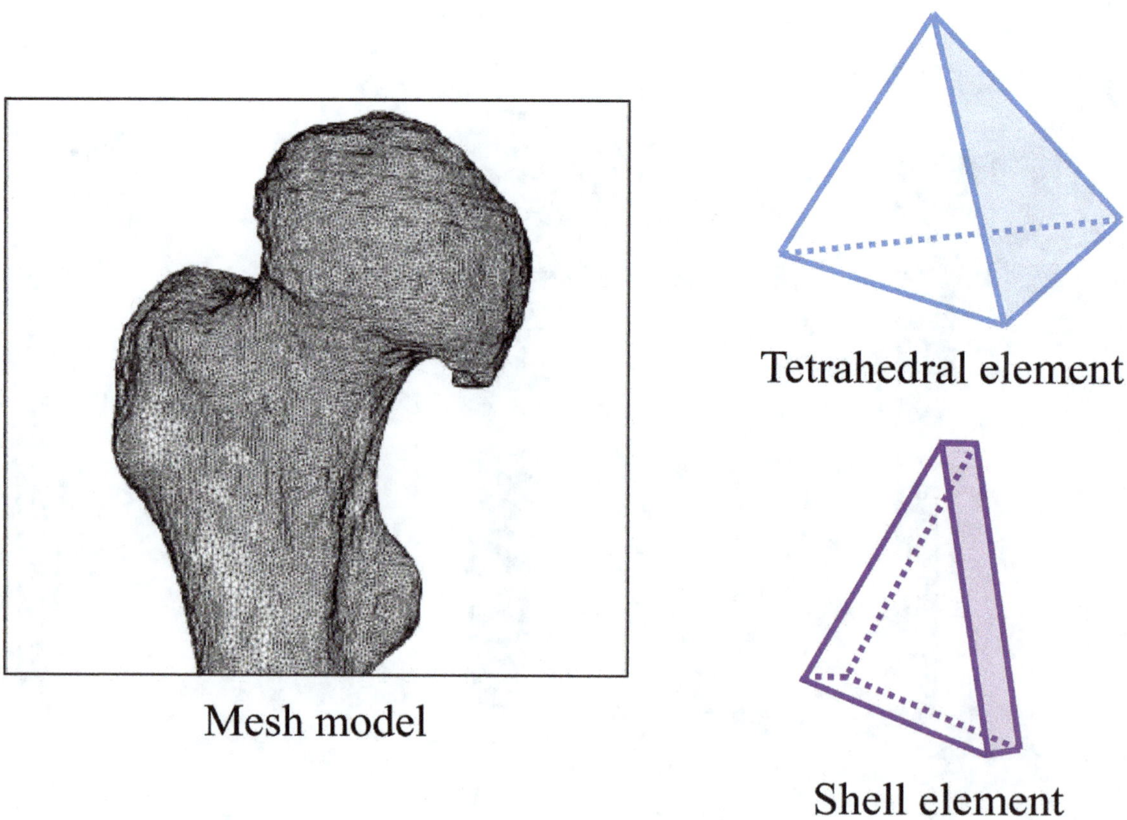

Figure 2. Finite element mesh of the femur. Three-dimensional FE models are constructed using 1- to 4-mm tetrahedral elements for the trabecular and inner cortical bone. The outer surface of the cortical bone is represented with three nodal-point shell elements having a thickness of 0.3 mm.

CT scans of the femurs of all patients were performed pre- and postoperatively (1 week after surgery). The scanner settings were approximately 140 kV and 300 mA, with a slice thickness of 2 mm, pixel resolution of 512 × 512, and voxel size of 0.70 × 0.70 × 2 mm. Three-dimensional FE models of the femur and stem were constructed according to pre- and postoperative CT data using the Mechanical Finder ver. 6.0 software (Research Center of Computational Mechanics Inc., Tokyo, Japan). This software creates FE models after considering individual bone shape and density distribution [29]. We used a global threshold algorithm for determining the bone area with a threshold of 200 mg/cm^3 and with manual correction if necessary. We applied a closing algorithm in addition to the global threshold algorithm for determining the bone area when the density was extremely low [29]. In addition, the global threshold algorithm was applied to determine the stem area with a threshold of 2,000 Hounsfield units. We used 1 to 4 mm tetrahedral elements to construct three-dimensional FE models for the trabecular and inner cortical bone. The outer surface of the cortical bone was represented with three nodal-point shell elements having a thickness of 0.3 mm (**Figure 2**). The FE models of the femur consisted of approximately 600,000 elements in addition to 200,000 elements for the stem. Bone density was determined according to CT density values, using a calibration equation (**Table 1**). Additionally, the elastic modulus of the bone was determined according to bone density values, using the equations proposed by Keyak et al. [18, 30] and Keller [31] (**Table 1**). Poisson's ratio of the bone was assumed to be 0.40. The stem was an isotropic titanium alloy, and it had an elastic modulus of 109.0 GPa and a Poisson's ratio of 0.28. The models assumed a completely bonded interface between the stem and bone. The models were restrained at the distal end of the femoral shaft, and loads were applied to the femoral head and greater trochanter. We applied a load of 2400 N to the surface of the femoral head at an angle of 15° to the femoral axis and applied a load of 1200 N to the greater trochanter at an angle of 20° [32, 33]. Linear FEA was performed. Equivalent stress and SED were analyzed in ROIs 1–7 and were compared with the DEXA data.

Bone density	Elastic modulus (MPa)
$\rho = 0$	0.001
$0 < \rho \leq 0.27$	$33{,}900\rho^{2.20}$
$0.27 < \rho < 0.6$	$5307\rho + 469$
$0.6 \leq \rho$	$10{,}200\rho^{2.01}$

$$\rho\left(\mathrm{g/cm^3}\right) = (\mathrm{H.U.} + 1.4246) \times 0.001 \big/ 1.508\ (\mathrm{H.U.} > -1)$$

$$= 0.0\ (\mathrm{H.U.} \leq -1)$$

H.U. represents CT density values in Hounsfield Units. The elastic modulus of the bone is determined according to computed tomography density values, using the equations proposed by Keyak et al. [18, 30] and Keller [31].

Table 1. Equations used for calculating the elastic modulus of the bone.

Changes in the BMD of the femur during the first postoperative year are shown in **Figure 3**. BMD was maintained in ROIs 3, 4, 5, and 6, whereas it significantly decreased in ROIs 1, 2, and 7 by 19, 11, and 27%, respectively, 12 months after THA. The changes in BMD noted in this study were similar to those reported in other studies [34, 35].

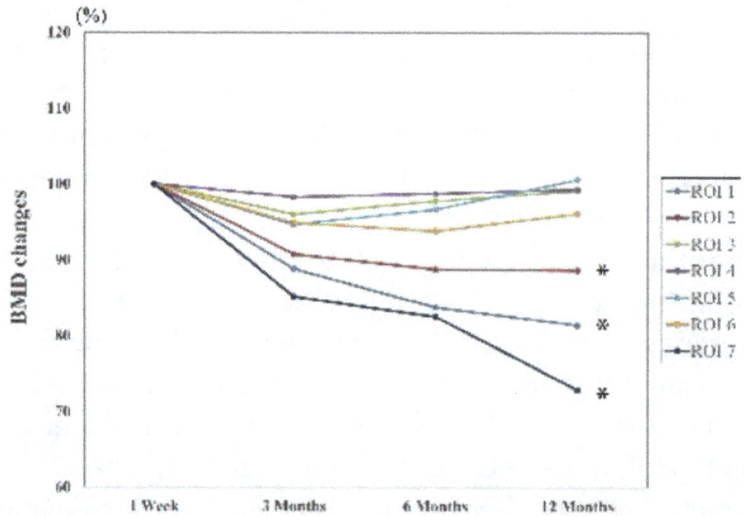

Figure 3. The median percentage change in bone mineral density (BMD) after surgery with the fit-and-fill-type stem. The periprosthetic BMDs at 3, 6, and 12 months after total hip arthroplasty (THA) are expressed as percentage changes from the baseline BMD measured at 1 week after surgery. BMD is maintained 12 months after THA in regions of interest (ROIs) 3, 4, 5, and 6, whereas it has significantly decreased by 19, 11, and 27% in ROIs 1, 2, and 7, respectively, 12 months after THA (*$p < 0.05$).

The pre- and postoperative equivalent stress and SED are shown in **Figure 4**. The equivalent stress and SED were maintained in ROIs 3, 4, and 5, whereas both decreased in ROIs 1, 2, 6, and 7 after THA (**Figure 5**). The lowest values of equivalent stress, SED, and relative BMD were observed in ROI 7 ($p < 0.05$). There was a relatively strong correlation between equivalent stress and BMD changes ($R = 0.426$, $p < 0.01$), whereas there was a weak correlation between SED and BMD changes ($R = 0.183$, $p = 0.053$) (**Figure 6**).

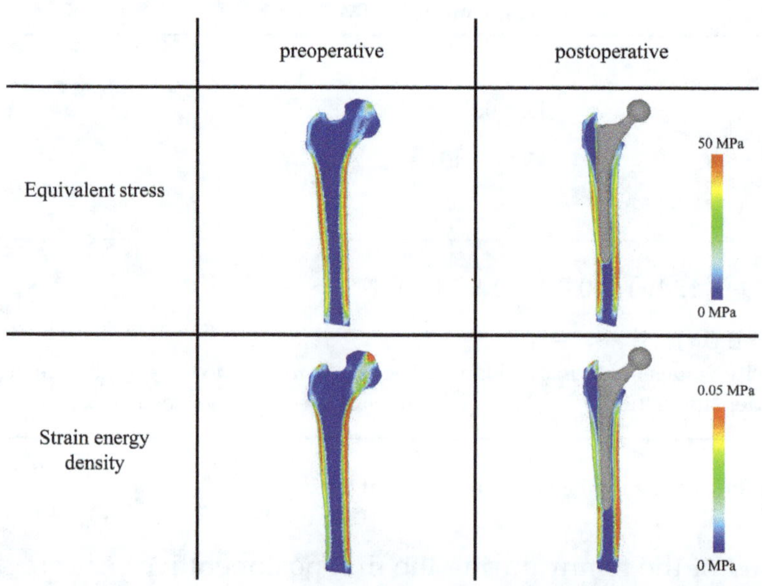

Figure 4. Distributions of equivalent stress and strain energy density (SED) in the femur. Equivalent stress and SED are maintained in the distal femur after total hip arthroplasty, whereas both decreased in the proximal femur.

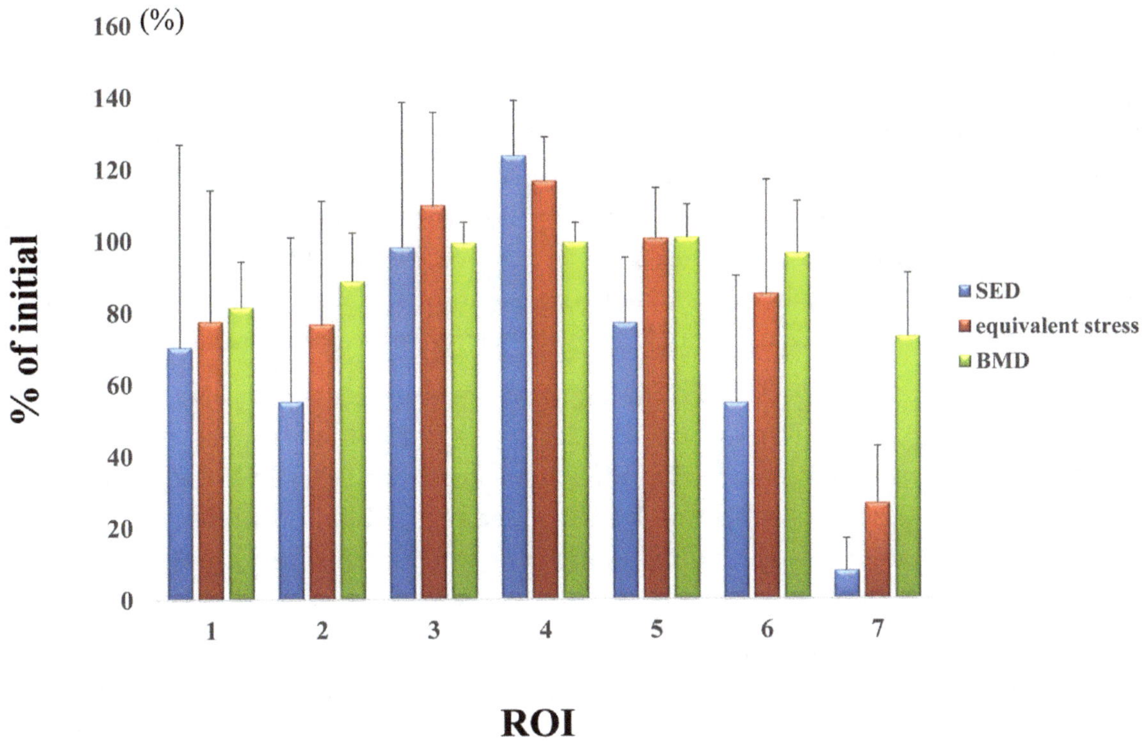

Figure 5. Strain energy density (SED), equivalent stress, and bone mineral density (BMD) 12 months after total hip arthroplasty. In ROI 7, equivalent stress, SED, and relative BMD show the lowest values of all regions examined.

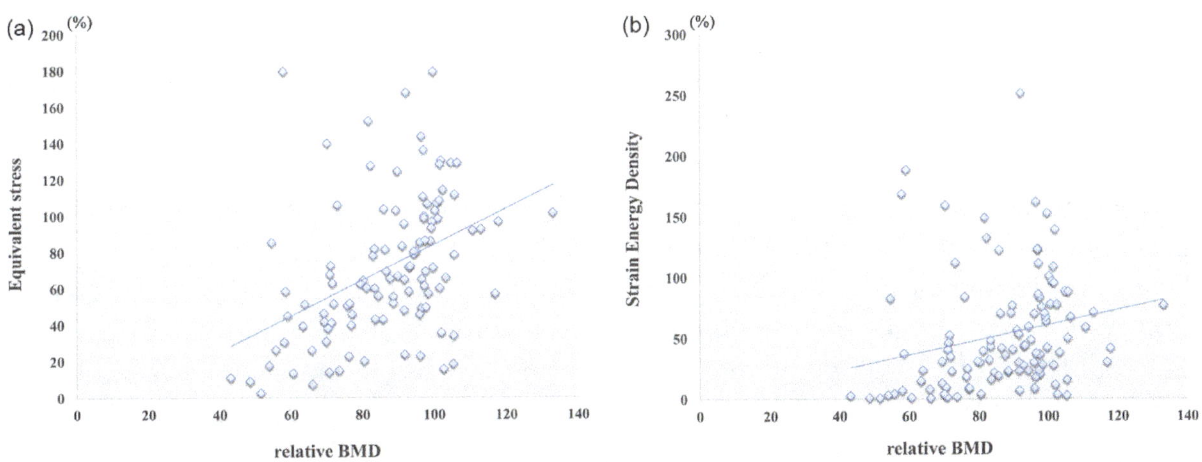

Figure 6. Scatter plots of the relationships (a) between bone mineral density (BMD) and equivalent stress and (b) between BMD and strain energy density (SED). The periprosthetic BMD at 12 months after total hip arthroplasty (THA) is expressed as the percentage change from the baseline BMD measured at 1 week after surgery. Postoperative equivalent stress and SED are expressed as percentage changes from the preoperative values. (a) Equivalent stress has a relatively strong correlation with the changes in BMD ($R = 0.426$, $p < 0.01$). (b) SED has a weak correlation with the changes in BMD ($R = 0.183$, $p = 0.053$).

Periprosthetic BMD loss may be related to changes in the mechanical loading environment. The purpose of this study was to investigate the relationships between periprosthetic BMD loss and changes in the mechanical loading environment after cementless THA according to subject-specific FEA. This subject-specific FEA exhibited a significant correlation between BMD changes and equivalent stress. After THA, the stress load is transferred to the distal femur through the stem rather than to the periprosthetic bone owing to the high elastic modulus of the stem [36, 37]. Therefore, equivalent stress in the proximal femur may decrease after stem implantation. These results are consistent with those of previous studies [20, 33]. We investigated the effect of a porous-coated titanium-alloy fit-and-fill-type stem on bone remodeling after THA. Although this implant is designed to achieve proximal fixation, equivalent stress and BMD decreased postoperatively at the proximal femur. These results indicate that load transmission to the proximal femur may not be sufficient for maintaining BMD.

The present study demonstrated that equivalent stress correlates with BMD changes in the femur 12 months after THA. In this study, CT scans were performed from all patients pre- and postoperatively, and subject-specific FE models were constructed to investigate bone heterogeneity by using the equations proposed by Keyak et al. [18, 30] and Keller [31]. Our results suggest that the rate of changes in equivalent stress could be an important factor for BMD changes.

The strain-adaptive bone-remodeling theory has been used to simulate BMD changes after THA; Huiskes et al. [14] reported that the SED distribution indicates the regions where resorption and apposition are expected. However, other studies have reported that bone remodeling can be better predicted with stress parameters than with strain parameters. Simulation results and clinical data have shown that there is a positive correlation between average equivalent stress and BMD [38, 39]. Therefore, controversy still exists with regard to whether equivalent stress or SED is an appropriate parameter for evaluating bone remodeling. Our results suggest that a decrease in equivalent stress caused a decrease in BMD in the proximal femur after THA.

2.2. Effects of stem geometry

A number of factors, such as geometry, roughness and coating of the stem, technique of preparation, and bone quality, influence initial stability or primary fixation. Femoral stems with various geometries are currently in use. The implant shape has been shown to determine cortical contact and initial stability [40]. Our recent study showed that differences in stem design could affect the postoperative BMD loss of the proximal femur [41]. We studied the effects of stem geometry on BMD changes and equivalent stress in the femur after THA.

We investigated 20 patients who underwent primary cementless THA for osteoarthritis or osteonecrosis of the hip. Of these patients, 10 underwent THA with a Zweymüller-type stem (SL-PLUS; Smith & Nephew Inc.), and the other 10 underwent THA with a fit-and-fill-type stem (collarless VerSys Fiber Metal MidCoat; Zimmer Inc.) (**Figure 1**). The mean age of the patients at the time of THA was 63 years (range, 54–72 years) in the Zweymüller-type stem group and 64 years (range, 57–69 years) in the fit-and-fill-type stem group. There was no significant difference in age between the two groups. In the Zweymüller-type stem group, all patients were diagnosed with osteoarthritis, while in the fit-and-fill-type stem group, eight patients were diagnosed with osteoarthritis, and two were diagnosed with osteonecrosis. We compared equivalent stress and BMD between the two groups.

In the preoperative models, no significant differences in equivalent stress were observed between the two groups. In the postoperative models, maximum equivalent stress was observed in ROI 4, and minimum equivalent stress was observed in ROI 1 in both groups. In ROI 4, equivalent stress was significantly higher in the Zweymüller-type stem group than in the fit-and-fill-type stem group ($p < 0.05$). On the other hand, in ROI 7, equivalent stress was significantly higher in the fit-and-fill-type stem group than in the Zweymüller-type stem group ($p < 0.05$) (**Figure 7**).

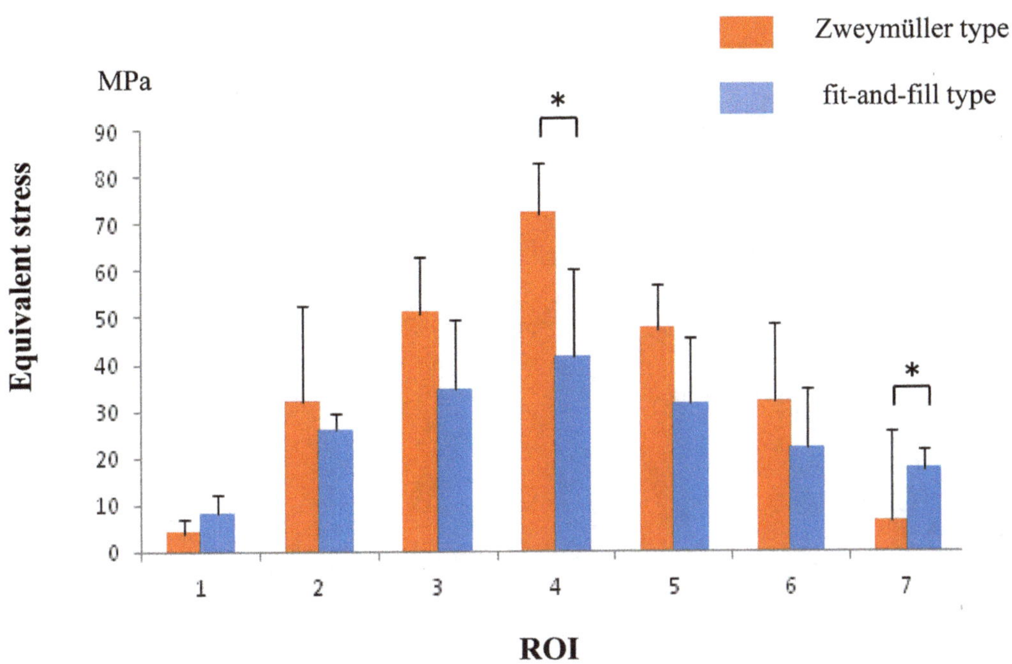

Figure 7. Comparison of equivalent stress between the fit-and-fill-type stem and Zweymüller-type stem groups. The equivalent stress in ROI 4 is higher, and the stress in ROI 7 is lower in the Zweymüller-type stem group than in the fit-and-fill-type stem group *$p < 0.05$.

Changes in the BMD of the femur during the first postoperative year are shown in **Figure 8**. In both the Zweymüller-type stem and fit-and-fill-type stem groups, BMD decreased in ROIs 2, 6, and 7, whereas BMD was maintained in ROIs 3, 4, and 5. In ROIs 6 and 7, BMD was significantly lower in the Zweymüller-type stem group than in the fit-and-fill-type stem group ($p < 0.05$). In ROI 1, the fit-and-fill-type stem group showed a continuous decrease in BMD for 12 months after surgery, while the Zweymüller-type stem group showed a decrease in BMD up to 6 months after surgery and then showed an increase 12 months after surgery. In ROI 4, BMD was significantly lower in the fit-and-fill-type stem group than in the Zweymüller-type stem group at 3 months after surgery ($p < 0.05$); however, there were no differences in BMD between the two groups at 6 months or 12 months after surgery [24].

Stress at the proximal femur was lower, and stress at the distal femur was higher in the Zweymüller-type stem group than in the fit-and-fill-type stem group. BMD at the proximal femur was significantly lower in the Zweymüller-type stem group than in the fit-and-fill-type stem group ($p < 0.05$). The FEA results and postoperative BMD changes in the femur suggest that implantation of the Zweymüller-type stem leads to insufficient load transmission to the proximal femur and may be associated with proximal BMD loss. These findings indicate that subject-specific FEA can assess the effects of stem geometry on adaptive bone remodeling after THA.

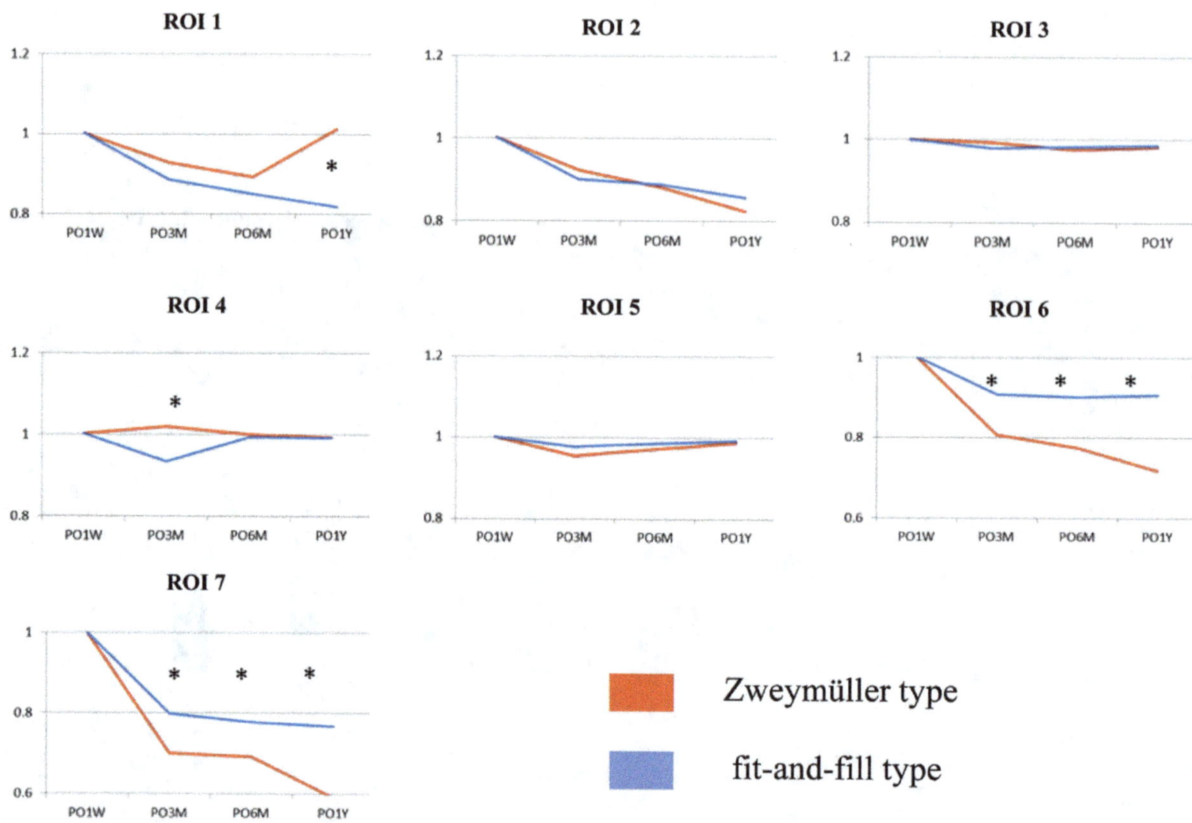

Figure 8. Median percentage change in bone mineral density (BMD) after surgery in the fit-and-fill-type stem and Zweymüller-type stem groups. The periprosthetic BMDs at 3, 6, and 12 months after surgery are expressed as percentage changes from the baseline BMD measured at 1 week after surgery (*$p < 0.05$).

2.3. Effects of bone geometry

Noble et al. [42] demonstrated the femoral anatomy variations in the mediolateral and anteroposterior dimensions and the need for multiple stem designs to achieve a close fit. Close adaptation of the prosthesis to the bone geometry is required to achieve optimal primary stability and secondary biologic fixation [43]. We studied the effects of bone geometry on BMD changes and equivalent stress in the femur after THA.

We investigated 20 patients who underwent THA using the Accolade TMZF stem (Stryker Orthopaedics) after reviewing the preoperative anterior-posterior hip radiographs of 90 consecutive patients who had undergone THA using the Accolade TMZF stem (**Figure 1**). The width of the proximal femoral canal on the operated side was measured from preoperative anterior-posterior hip radiographs, and Noble's canal flare index (CFI) was calculated for each patient [42]. Based on Noble's classification, the femurs were divided into the following three groups of femoral canal shapes: champagne flute (CFI ≥ 4.7), intermediate (CFI 3–4.7), and stovepipe (CFI < 3). Among the 20 study femurs, 7 had a champagne flute canal shape, 5 had a stovepipe shape, and 8 had an intermediate canal shape. The 8 femurs with an intermediate canal shape were randomly selected from among the remaining 78 hips with an intermediate canal shape to balance the groups for analysis.

The mean percentage changes in equivalent stress in each ROI between the pre- and postoperative femur models were calculated from the FEA results, and they are plotted in **Figure 9**. Between-group differences in the pattern of postoperative changes in equivalent stress were identified, and specific differences were observed in ROIs 6 ($p = 0.01$) and 7 ($p = 0.02$). Post hoc analysis indicated that the decrease in equivalent stress in ROI 6 was significantly greater in the stovepipe group (−63.8%) than in the champagne flute group (−38.8%) and intermediate group (−47.2%) ($p = 0.01$). Additionally, the decrease in equivalent stress in ROI 7 was significantly greater in the stovepipe group (−70.9%) than in the champagne flute group (−53.7%) and intermediate group (−51.4%) ($p = 0.03$).

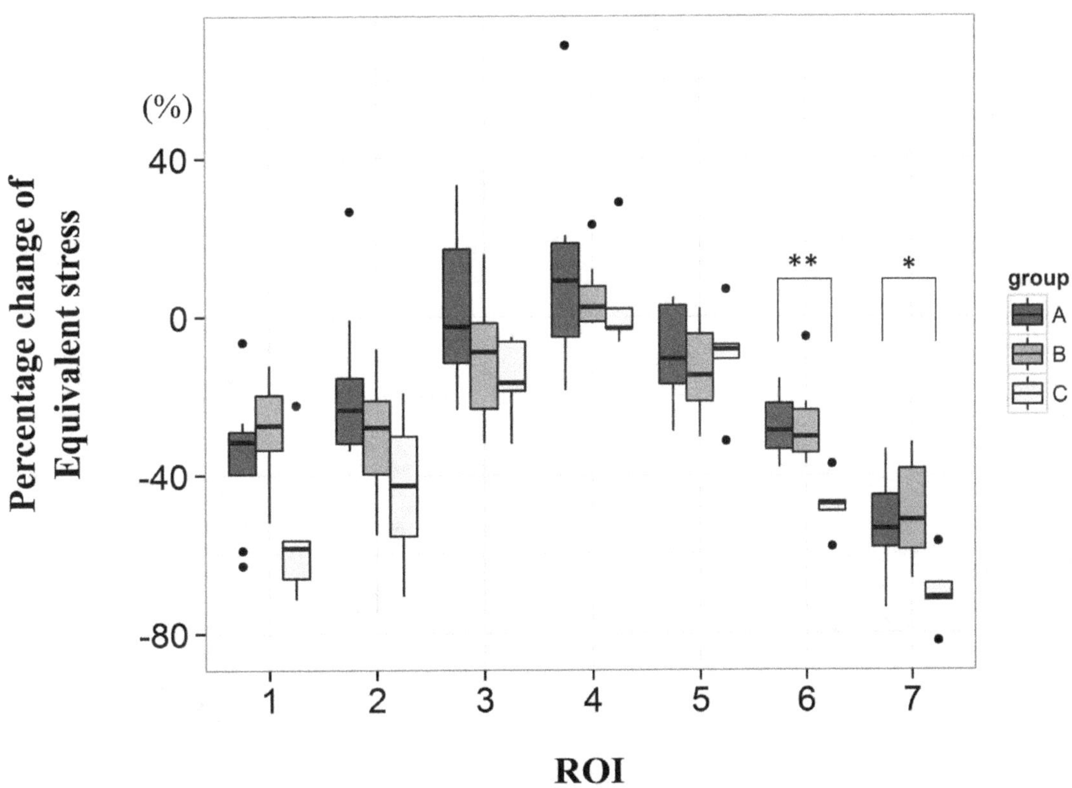

Figure 9. Comparison of the relative percentage changes in equivalent stress between the pre- and postoperative femur models for the three femoral canal shape groups. Postoperative relative percentage changes in equivalent stress in each region of interest compared to that of the preoperative models. Dots in the box plot show the outliers (*p = 0.02, **p = 0.01).

BMD changes in the femurs during the first postoperative year are shown in **Figure 10**. Significant between-group differences in BMD were evident in ROIs 6 ($p = 0.01$) and 7 ($p = 0.04$). In ROI 6, a marked decrease in BMD was identified only in the stovepipe group during the first postoperative year; the ROI 6 BMD showed a significantly higher decrease in the stovepipe group (−14.3%) than in the champagne flute group (−1.4%) and intermediate group (+3.6%) ($p = 0.01$). A postoperative decrease in ROI 7 BMD was evident in all the groups during the first postoperative year (champagne flute group, −23.1%; intermediate group, −22.7%; and stovepipe group, −36.5%). Additionally, the ROI 7 BMD showed a significantly higher decrease in the stovepipe group than in the other two groups ($p = 0.045$). BMDs in ROIs 1 and 2 were relatively lower in the stovepipe group than in the champagne flute and stovepipe groups during the first postoperative year; however, the differences were not significant.

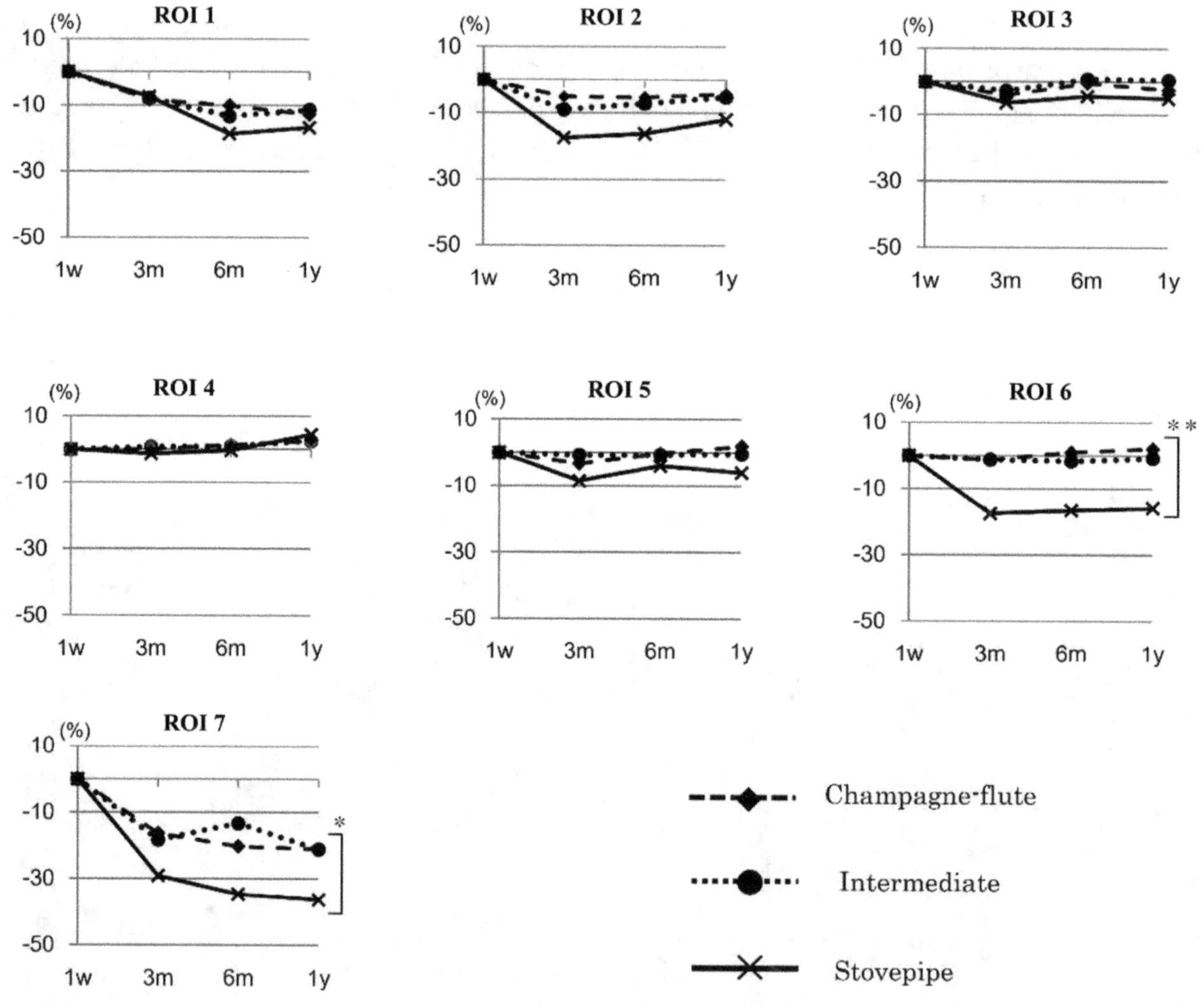

Figure 10. Comparison of bone mineral density (BMD) in the three femoral canal shape groups. The periprosthetic BMDs at 3, 6, and 12 months after surgery are expressed as percentage changes from the baseline BMD measured at 1 week after surgery (*$p = 0.04$, **$p = 0.01$).

The percentage changes in equivalent stress in each ROI were positively correlated with the postoperative BMD changes (**Figure 11**). A significant correlation was observed between equivalent stress and BMD changes ($p < 0.01$), and the adjusted R^2 value showed that the percentage changes in equivalent stress (adjusted $R^2 = 0.79$) could predict the postoperative BMD changes in our simulation model.

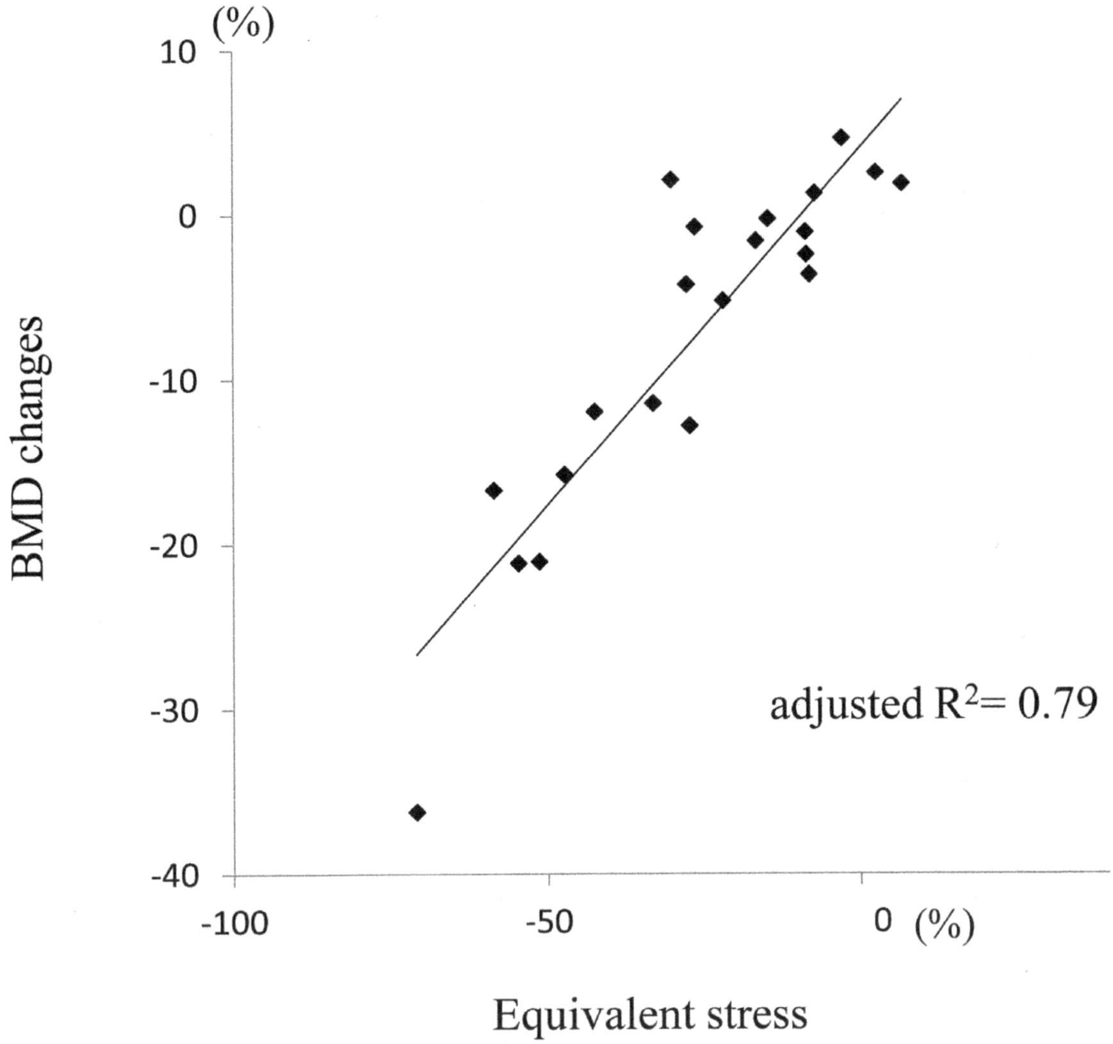

Figure 11. Scatter plot illustrating the relationship between the percentage changes in equivalent stress and postoperative bone mineral density (BMD). The 21 points plotted in this scatter plot display the average relative percentage changes in equivalent stress (finite element analysis results) and BMD for the three femoral canal shape groups. A significant correlation is observed between equivalent stress and BMD changes (adjusted $R^2 = 0.79$, $p < 0.01$).

The FEA results and postoperative BMD changes of the femur suggest that the combination of a large, tapered wedge-type stem and stovepipe femur may be associated with proximal BMD loss. Our simulation-based outcomes predicted a stronger stress-shielding effect in the stovepipe femur group than in the other groups. These results indicate that subject-specific FEA can assess the effects of bone geometry on adaptive bone remodeling after THA.

The present studies have limitations. First, the interface condition between the stem and the femur in the FEA model was assumed to be fully bonded. Consideration of the surface properties of the implant and degree of stem fixation would be useful for constructing realistic models. Second, the maximum length of the tetrahedral elements (4 mm) was relatively large, and therefore the elements might straddle the boundary between the cortical and cancellous area in the FE models. Therefore, the elastic modulus of the elements straddling the boundary would contain some errors.

3. Summary

We focused on equivalent stress as a mechanical parameter associated with adaptive bone remodeling and found that equivalent stress changes were positively correlated with postoperative BMD changes in the femur. BMD and equivalent stress were maintained in the distal femur and decreased in the proximal femur after THA. Thus, the proposed subject-specific FEA is useful for evaluating adaptive bone remodeling after THA and could predict BMD changes after THA. Furthermore, subject-specific FEA can be used to evaluate the effects of stem geometry and bone geometry on bone remodeling and can help in the understanding of the altered mechanical environment after THA.

Abbreviations

BMD, bone mineral density

CFI, canal flare index

CT, computed tomography

DEXA, dual-energy X-ray absorptiometry

FEA, finite element analysis

ROIs, regions of interest

SED, strain energy density

THA, total hip arthroplasty

Author details

Yutaka Inaba*, Hiroyuki Ike, Masatoshi Oba and Tomoyuki Saito

*Address all correspondence to: yute0131@med.yokohama-cu.ac.jp

Department of Orthopaedic Surgery, Yokohama City University, Yokohama, Japan

References

[1] Malchau H, Herberts P, Ahnfelt L. Prognosis of total hip replacement in Sweden. Follow-up of 92,675 operations performed 1978-1990. Acta Orthop Scand. 1993; 64:497–506.

[2] Dorr LD, Lewonowski K, Lucero M, Harris M, Wan Z. Failure mechanisms of anatomic porous replacement I cementless total hip replacement. Clin Orthop Relat Res. 1997; 334:157–167.

[3] Bougherara H, Bureau M, Campbell M, Vadean A, Yahia L. Design of a biomimetic polymer-composite hip prosthesis. J Biomed Mater Res. 2007; 82:27–40.

[4] Kerner J, Huiskes R, van Lenthe GH, Weinans H, van Rietbergen B, Engh CA, Amis AA. Correlation between pre-operative periprosthetic bone density and post-operative bone loss in THA can be explained by strain-adaptive remodelling. J Biomech. 1999; 32:695–703.

[5] Kroger H, Miettinen H, Arnala I, Koski E, Rushton N, Suomalainen O. Evaluation of periprosthetic bone using dual-energy X-ray absorptiometry: precision of the method and effect of operation on bone mineral density. J Bone Miner Res. 1996; 11:1526–1530.

[6] Kim YH, Yoon SH, Kim JS. Changes in the bone mineral density in the acetabulum and proximal femur after cementless total hip replacement: alumina-on-alumina versus alumina-on-polyethylene articulation. J Bone Joint Surg Br. 2007; 89:174–179.

[7] Nishii T, Sugano N, Masuhara K, Shibuya T, Ochi T, Tamura S. Longitudinal evaluation of time related bone remodeling after cementless total hip arthroplasty. Clin Orthop Relat Res. 1997; 339:121–131.

[8] Kroger H, Venesmaa P, Jurvelin J, Miettinen H, Suomalainen O, Alhava E. Bone density at the proximal femur after total hip arthroplasty. Clin Orthop Relat Res. 1998; 352:66–74.

[9] Rosenthall L, Bobyn JD, Brooks CE. Temporal changes of periprosthetic bone density in patients with a modular noncemented femoral prosthesis. J Arthroplasty. 1999; 14:71–76.

[10] Ostbyhaug PO, Klaksvik J, Romundstad P, Aamodt A. An in vitro study of the strain distribution in human femora with anatomical and customised femoral stems. J Bone Joint Surg Br. 2009; 91:676–682.

[11] Wolff J. Das Gesetz der Transformation der Knochen. Berlin, Germany: Verlag von August Hirschwald; 1892.

[12] Jaworski ZF. Coupling of bone formation to bone resorption: a broader view. Calcif Tissue Int. 1984; 36:531–535.

[13] Zadpoor AA. Open forward and inverse problems in theoretical modeling of bone tissue adaptation. J Mech Behav Biomed Mater. 2013; 27:249–261.

[14] Huiskes R, Weinans H, Grootenboer HJ, Dalstra M, Fudala B, Slooff TJ. Adaptive bone-remodeling theory applied to prosthetic-design analysis. J Biomech. 1987; 20:1135–1150.

[15] Carter DR, Van Der Meulen MC, Beaupre GS. Mechanical factors in bone growth and development. Bone. 1996; 18:5S–10S.

[16] Stulpner MA, Reddy BD, Starke GR, Spirakis A. A three-dimensional finite analysis of adaptive remodelling in the proximal femur. J Biomech. 1997; 30:1063–1066.

[17] Adachi T, Tomita Y, Sakaue H, Tanaka M. Simulation of trabecular surface remodeling based on local stress uniformity. Jpn Soc Mech Eng. 1997; 40:782–792.

[18] Keyak JH, Rossi SA, Jones KA, Skinner HB. Prediction of femoral fracture load using automated finite element modeling. J Biomech. 1998; 31:125–133.

[19] Taddei F, Schileo E, Helgason B, Cristofolini L, Viceconti M. The material mapping strategy influences the accuracy of CT-based finite element models of bones: an evaluation against experimental measurements. Med Eng Phys. 2007; 29:973–979.

[20] Pettersen SH, Wik TS, Skallerud B. Subject specific finite element analysis of stress shielding around a cementless femoral stem. Clin Biomech (Bristol, Avon). 2009; 24:196–202.

[21] Cody DD, Gross GJ, Hou FJ, Spencer HJ, Goldstein SA, Fyhrie DP. Femoral strength is better predicted by finite element models than QCT and DXA. J Biomech. 1999; 32:1013–1020.

[22] Tawara D, Sakamoto J, Murakami H, Kawahara N, Oda J, Tomita K. Mechanical evaluation by patient-specific finite element analyses demonstrates therapeutic effects for osteoporotic vertebrae. J Mech Behav Biomed Mater. 2010; 3:31–40.

[23] Ike H, Inaba Y, Kobayashi N, Hirata Y, Yukizawa Y, Aoki C, Choe H, Saito T. Comparison between mechanical stress and bone mineral density in the femur after total hip arthroplasty by using subject-specific finite element analyses. Comput Methods Biomech Biomed Engin. 2015; 18:1056–1065.

[24] Hirata Y, Inaba Y, Kobayashi N, Ike H, Fujimaki H, Saito T. Comparison of mechanical stress and change in bone mineral density between two types of femoral implant using finite element analysis. J Arthroplasty. 2013; 28:1731–1735.

[25] Anderson AE, Peters CL, Tuttle BD, Weiss JA. Subject-specific finite element model of the pelvis: development, validation and sensitivity studies. J Biomech Eng. 2005; 127:364–373.

[26] Ateshian GA, Henak CR, Weiss JA. Toward patient-specific articular contact mechanics. J Biomech. 2015; 48:779–786.

[27] Weinans H, Sumner DR, Igloria R, Natarajan RN. Sensitivity of periprosthetic stress-shielding to load and the bone density-modulus relationship in subject-specific finite element models. J Biomech. 2000; 33:809–817.

[28] Gruen TA, McNeice GM, Amstutz HC. "Modes of failure" of cemented stem-type femoral components: a radiographic analysis of loosening. Clin Orthop Relat Res. 1979; 141:17–27.

[29] Bessho M, Ohnishi I, Matsuyama J, Matsumoto T, Imai K, Nakamura K. Prediction of strength and strain of the proximal femur by a CT-based finite element method. J Biomech. 2007; 40:1745–1753.

[30] Keyak JH, Lee IY, Skinner HB. Correlations between orthogonal mechanical properties and density of trabecular bone: use of different densitometric measures. J Biomed Mater Res. 1994; 28:1329–1336.

[31] Keller TS. Predicting the compressive mechanical behavior of bone. J Biomech. 1994; 27:1159–1168.

[32] Bergmann G, Deuretzbacher G, Heller M, Graichen F, Rohlmann A, Strauss J, Duda GN. Hip contact forces and gait patterns from routine activities. J Biomech. 2001; 34:859–871.

[33] Herrera A, Panisello JJ, Ibarz E, Cegonino J, Puertolas JA, Gracia L. Comparison between DEXA and finite element studies in the long-term bone remodeling of an anatomical femoral stem. J Biomech Eng. 2009; 131:041013.

[34] Aldinger PR, Sabo D, Pritsch M, Thomsen M, Mau H, Ewerbeck V, Breusch SJ. Pattern of periprosthetic bone remodeling around stable uncemented tapered hip stems: a prospective 84-month follow-up study and a median 156-month cross-sectional study with DXA. Calcif Tissue Int. 2003; 73:115–121.

[35] Boden H, Adolphson P. No adverse effects of early weight bearing after uncemented total hip arthroplasty: a randomized study of 20 patients. Acta Orthop Scand. 2004; 75:21–29.

[36] Maistrelli GL, Fornasier V, Binnington A, McKenzie K, Sessa V, Harrington I. Effect of stem modulus in a total hip arthroplasty model. J Bone Joint Surg Br. 1991; 73:43–46.

[37] Decking R, Puhl W, Simon U, Claes LE. Changes in strain distribution of loaded proximal femora caused by different types of cementless femoral stems. Clin Biomech (Bristol, Avon). 2006; 21:495–501.

[38] Herrera A, Panisello JJ, Ibarz E, Cegonino J, Puertolas JA, Gracia L. Long-term study of bone remodelling after femoral stem: a comparison between dexa and finite element simulation. J Biomech. 2007; 40:3615–3625.

[39] Kwon JY, Naito H, Matsumoto T, Tanaka M. Estimation of change of bone structures after total hip replacement using bone remodeling simulation. Clin Biomech (Bristol, Avon). 2013; 28:514–518.

[40] Khanuja HS, Vakil JJ, Goddard MS, Mont MA. Cementless femoral fixation in total hip arthroplasty. J Bone Joint Surg Am. 2011; 93:500–509.

[41] Inaba Y, Kobayashi N, Oba M, Ike H, Kubota S, Saito T. Difference in postoperative periprosthetic bone mineral density changes between 3 major designs of uncemented stems: a 3-year follow-up study. J Arthroplasty. DOI: 10.1016/j.arth.2016.02.009.

[42] Noble PC, Alexander JW, Lindahl LJ, Yew DT, Granberry WM, Tullos HS. The anatomic basis of femoral component design. Clin Orthop Relat Res. 1988; 235:148–165.

[43] Massin P, Geais L, Astoin E, Simondi M, Lavaste F. The anatomic basis for the concept of lateralized femoral stems: a frontal plane radiographic study of the proximal femur. J Arthroplasty. 2000; 15:93–101.

9

Vascular Injury in Total Hip Replacement: Management and Prevention

Nishant Kumar Singh, Sanjay Rai and Amit Rastogi

Abstract

This chapter analyzed the vascular complications in total hip replacement. Vascular injuries are the uncommon but well recognized and serious issue. During total hip replacement, laceration of major blood vessels has been reported which even cause morbidity and mortality. The injury to vascular structures occurs due to the placement of screws to fix acetabular components, structural grafts, and protrusio cages or rings. Massive hemorrhage resulting in immediate exsanguination may be caused due to the damage of any of these vessels by processes such as drilling, reaming, retraction, or dissection. The majority of these vascular injuries might be better prevented or even more proficiently treated by comprehensive preoperative assessment, better instrumentation, and careful postoperative monitoring.

Keywords: vessel injury, uncemented total hip replacement, reaming, bone screws, acetabulum, iliac artery, acetabular cup, obturator artery, reaming

1. Introduction

This chapter gives an etiology, management, and prevention of common injuries that occur at the time of total hip replacement surgeries or postoperative period. A total hip replacement has become one of the most successful procedures with minimal complications and long-term result [1]. According to the data published by various major national and international joint registries, an increasing number of total hip replacements are performed each year. The incidence of vascular injury occurs at the time of hip surgery or immediate postoperatively or in the late postoperative period, which is quite rare (0.2–0.3%), but the inevitable and serious issue may cause morbidity and even mortality [1, 2]. The most common pattern of vessel injuries include lacerations, pseudoaneurysms, thromboembolic and arteriovenous fistula [3–5].

Contiguous arteries to the acetabulum that are susceptible to be injured during total hip replacement are mostly branches of common iliac vessels; external iliac vessels, obturator vessels, superior and inferior gluteal artery, and internal pudendal arteries and veins as shown in **Figure 1** [6–12]. Indeed, many vascular structures surrounding the acetabulum may be injured by direct and indirect trauma have been reported [12, 13]. In particular, the primitive cause of injuries includes reaming during acetabular preparation, and retractor induced injury, drilling holes for fixation of screws in cementless acetabular cups, excessive traction in surgery, postoperative cup migration (**Figure 2a** and **b**). Also, cement erosion, excessive local heating by methyl methacrylate in cemented total hip replacement are further reasons of occurrence of arterial injuries during total hip replacement [4, 14–20]. However, there are many reported reasons in which symptoms of vessel injury were not evident. The possible reasons might be bone fragments or contamination caused due to soft tissue defect, result in infections [21].

Vessel injuries giving immediate symptoms of total hip replacement are the severe hemorrhage. The most common ischemic symptoms in the delayed postoperative period include pain, the decrease of hemoglobin, swelling, reduced blood pressure and hypovolemic shock [1, 2, 4, 6, 10, 11, 22, 23]. Other presenting signs and symptoms of vessel injury in revision surgeries include excessive bleeding, loss of pulse and instability during extraction of hip prosthesis [19].

In some reports, gender biasing has also been observed as one of the causes of vessel injury. In several retrospective studies, the female dominance of vessel injury as compared to male (3:2) has been confirmed [1, 4, 5, 16, 24].

At present, the participating physicians in total hip replacement are increasing, and indeed, vessel injury is a credit to those who are engaged in these types of surgeries. The relationship of pelvic vascular structures surrounding the acetabulum has been described in several studies [7, 9, 25]. Currently, substantial work by researchers has been carried out to visualize the

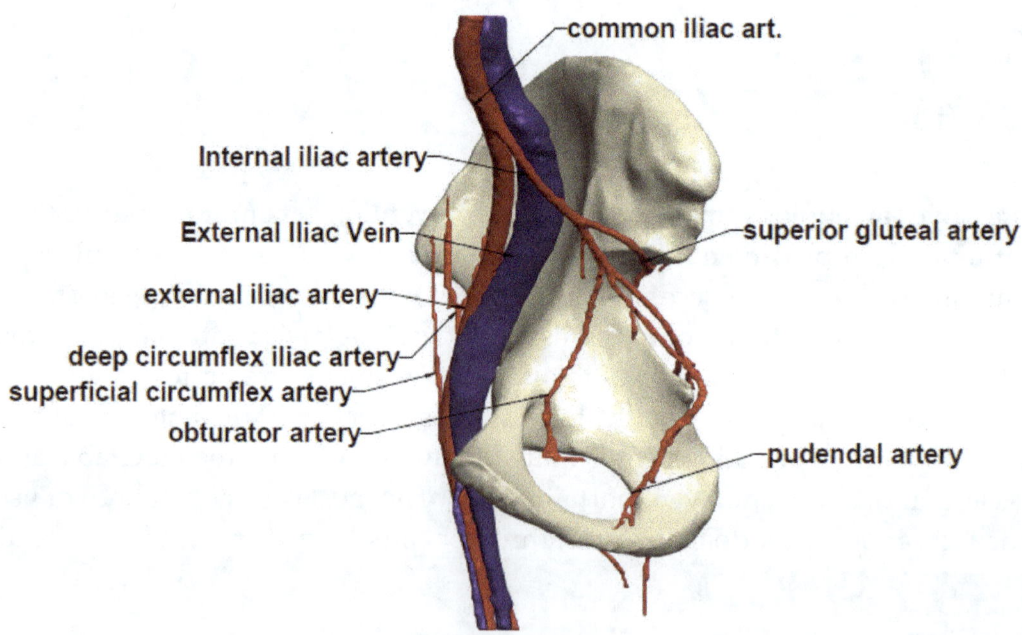

Figure 1. Three-dimensional construction of pelvis and vessel structures using computed tomographic images.

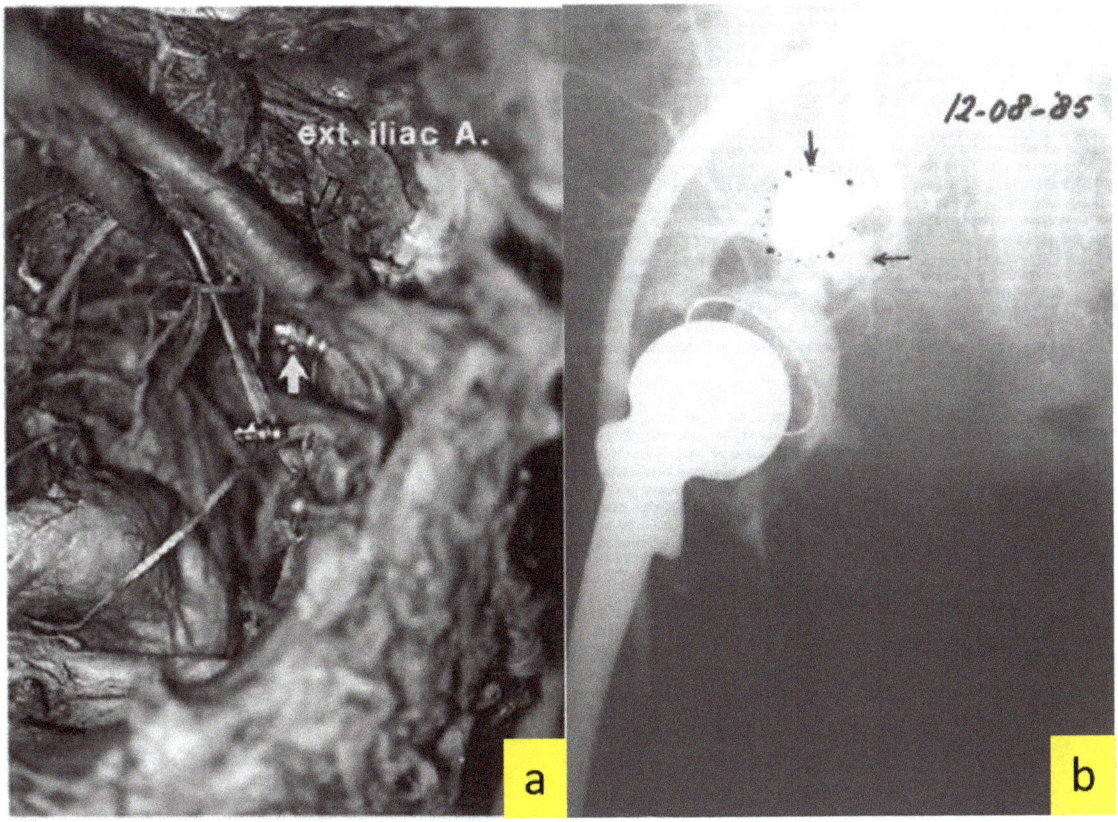

Figure 2. Vessel injury. (a) Photograph illustrating inserted acetabular screw close to external iliac artery and vein (arrow) (reprinted with permission from Hwang [25]). (b) Postoperative false aneurysm of superior gluteal artery (circled lines) by protruding cement to fix acetabular component (horizontal arrow) (reprinted with permission from Bakker and Gast [10]).

detailed vascular structures surrounding the acetabulum with the use of three-dimensional computed tomographic angiography (3DCT-A) [26–30]. These studies identified the actual distance of vessel structures to the osseous surface of the acetabulum to prevent the injuries caused by fixation of screws in cementless total hip replacement.

2. Prevention of vascular injuries

2.1. Obey quadrant system

Earlier, in continuation to prevent these injuries during fixation of acetabular screws, a simple method of acetabular quadrant system was described by Wasielewski et al. and accepted widely till date [9]. Various anatomical studies have shown the fixation of screws in cementless primary total hip replacement, particularly in revision surgeries being most prominent reason for vascular injuries.

Wasielewski et al. defined the acetabular-quadrant system for managing safe placement of screws during primary and revision total hip replacement surgeries. The quadrant system is proposed to explain the relationship between the osseous structure of acetabulum and surrounding vascular structures to prevent the vascular structures.

Acetabular quadrant system consists of four parts of acetabulum by dividing acetabulum with two mutually perpendicular lines. The first line A originates from the anterior superior iliac spine (ASIS) and passes straight to the center of the acetabulum, dividing the acetabulum into two halves and named collectively as anterior and posterior quadrants. The second line B originates from center of acetabulum and perpendicular to the first line, resulting in the two superior and inferior halves (**Figure 3**). To this end, these two perpendicular lines together form four quadrants by intersecting each other at the center of acetabulum, which is collectively named as an anterior superior quadrant, anterior inferior quadrant, posterior superior quadrant and posterior inferior quadrant. Most of the work published on vascular injury has been carried out on the cadaveric bone; the authors tried to give a clear picture of quadrant system by developing the three dimensional computational model of the pelvis and surrounding vascular structure with the help of angiographic computed tomography (A-CT). In the development of three-dimensional models of vascular structures, some of the arteries and veins are not visible because of imaging limitations of computed tomographic machine.

Quadrant system specifies the safe zones to fix the proper sized acetabular screws that are carefully considered at the time of total hip replacement surgery. The relationship between vascular structures and four quadrants with lines passing and center of acetabulum respectively mimic the safe and dangerous zones, which are as follows:

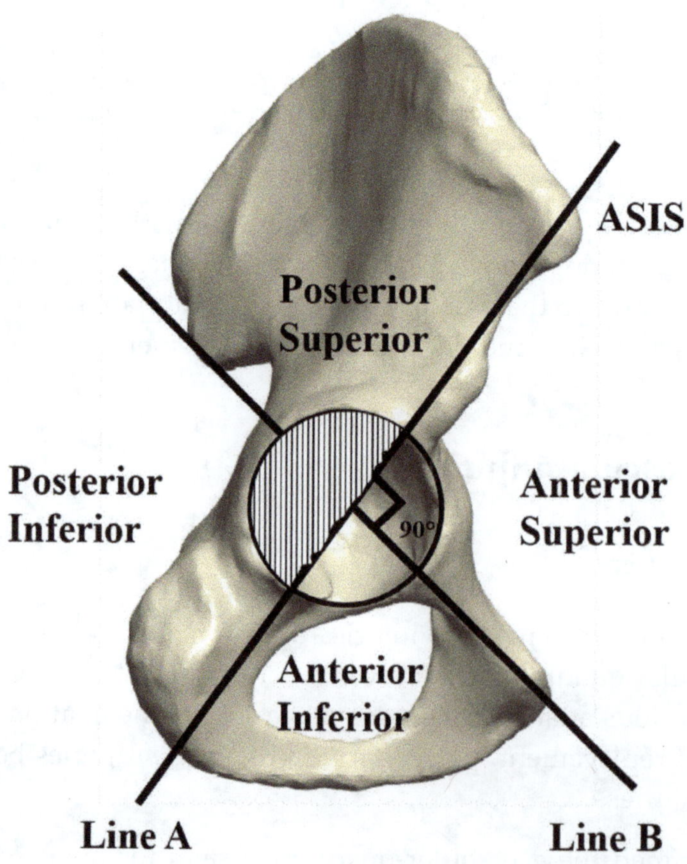

Figure 3. Demonstration of quadrant system used for placement of screws in total hip surgery.

2.1.1. Anterior-superior quadrant

This quadrant contains the external iliac artery and vein. The acetabular screws fixed in this quadrant will be directed towards these vessels. However, it was found that external iliac vein is lying down in more medial position than an artery and therefore is in more risky as compared to the artery.

2.1.2. Anterior-inferior quadrant

Obturator artery is present in this quadrant, and the bone stock is thin in respect of other quadrants. This order will increases the possibility of vessel injury during screw placement.

2.1.3. Posterior-superior quadrant

From the previous literature of dissection and a considerable amount of three-dimensional studies, it is evident that superior posterior quadrant has good bone stock. This quadrant contains the superior gluteal artery and vein, as they pass to the pelvis through the greater sciatic notch. The proper sized screw may be considered for safe placement as the bone stock in the central zone of this quadrant is more than 25 mm.

2.1.4. Posterior-inferior quadrant

Screws that are fixed in this quadrant are directed towards inferior gluteal and pudendal vessels. The quadrant is considered safe for screw placement as the central zone has a good bone purchase, and therefore a proper size of a screw may not touch the vessel structure thereby preventing the vessels from injury.

2.1.5. Center of the acetabulum

Line A and line B intersect each other at the center of the acetabulum. This position is very close to the obturator artery and is always avoided for placement of screws.

However, screws placed along line A in the superior portion of the acetabulum are directed towards the external iliac artery and may not be appreciated. Screws placed along line A in the inferior portion of acetabulum lie close to obturator vessel.

From the above discussion on quadrant system, it must be pointed out that external iliac vessels, obturator vessel and superior gluteal artery seem to have the most frequent injury. The anterior quadrant must be avoided for the placement of screw during total hip procedures, as these vessels mostly lie in this quadrant. In the exposure of posterior quadrants, the superior posterior quadrant is typically safer for proper sized screw placement as it has good bone purchase regardless of the presence of vessel structures.

In view of above, to give a clear picture of the quadrant system to prevent vascular structures from injury, the acetabular cups with 12 holes and additional central screw fixation is demonstrated along with vessel structures in **Figure 4**.

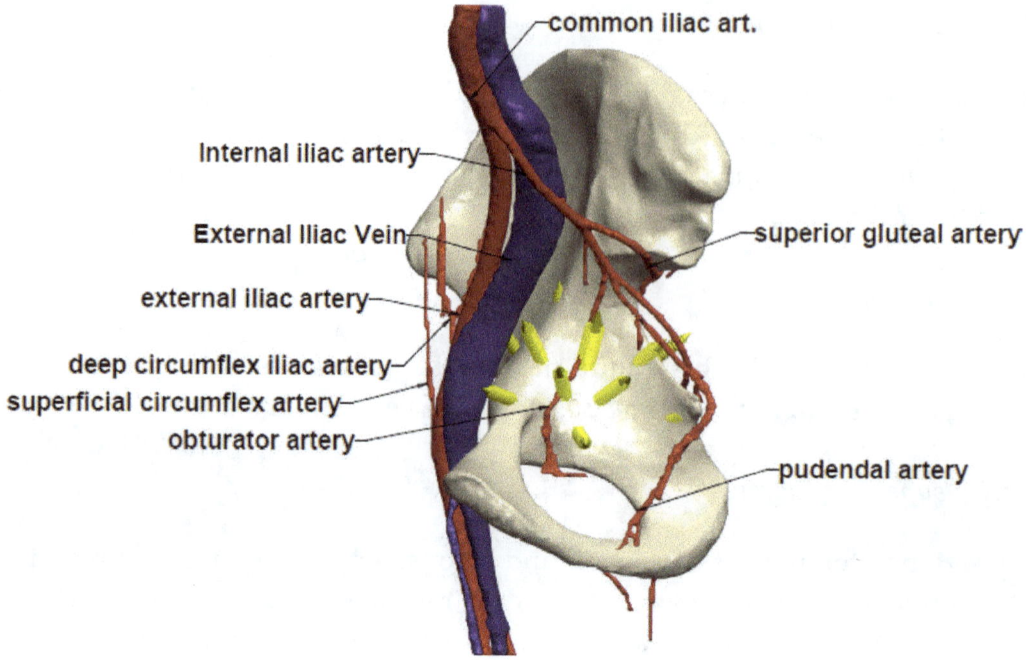

Figure 4. Visualization of vessels surrounding the pelvis which are prone to injury from screw placement.

2.2. High hip center

In cases of high hip center, the quadrant system serves as in normal hips but it is constructed in different ways. In the high hip, posterior superior and inferior posterior quadrants are found safe for screw placement with good bone stock at the periphery of the acetabulum as shown in **Figure 5** [31].

Besides, a rare case of the aberrant anatomy of vessels was found, in such cases, care must be taken during fixation of screws as they are more susceptible to injury [9, 32–34].

In the cases of revision surgeries where there is a bone loss in posterior quadrants, placement of screws is necessary in anterior quadrant. To place proper sized screws in the anterior columns, Lewallen proposed a technique in which screws and drill bits may be passed by visual perception and palpation of the careful dissection of soft tissues in anterior quadrant [7].

The quadrant system described by Wasielewski et al. is prevalent among total hip arthroplasty surgeons, until the normal hips are taken into account. In the technical demand for total hip replacement of Crowe type-IV developmental dysplasia, the posterior superior quadrant system is condemned. The reason behind this is that center of the acetabulum is shifted anteroinferiorly in the hip with a high, complete dislocation (**Figure 6**). Screws lying in the safe quadrant (proposed by Wasielewski et al. for normal hips) may frequently injure the obturator blood vessels. In such type of cases, modified quadrant system must be used on surgeon recommendations [26].

2.3. Acetabular retractors positioning

Retractors are placed around the acetabulum for proper exposure of acetabulum during total hip arthroplasty. It has been found that surgical approaches adopted by surgeons, are not only the appropriate causes of injury. Consequently, appropriate retractor positioning and

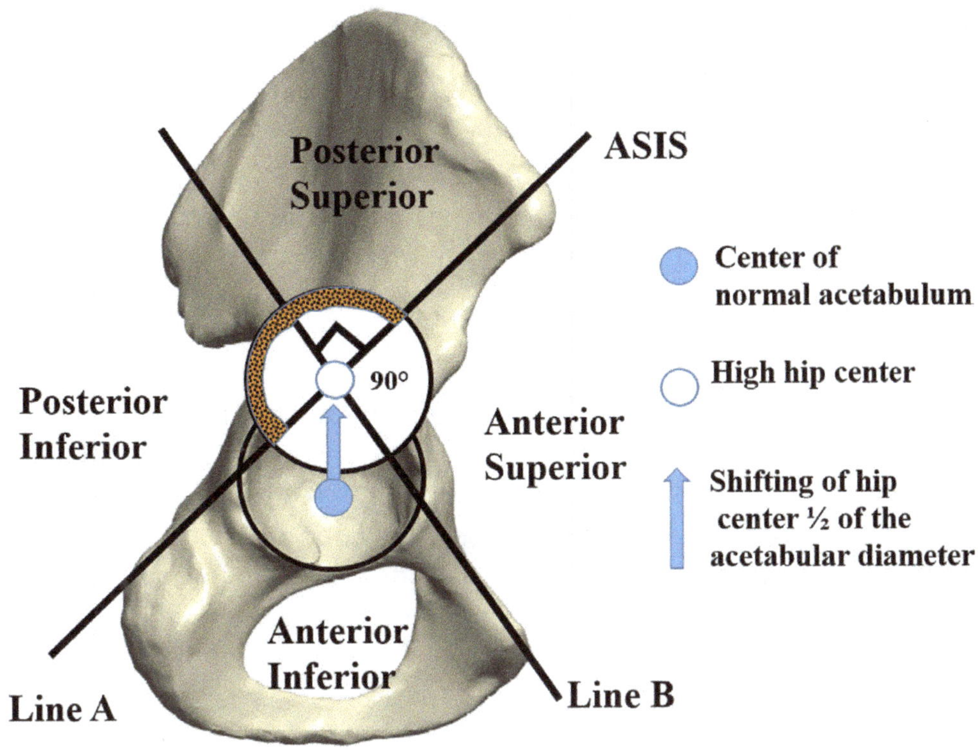

Figure 5. Illustration of screw placement zones in the high hip center.

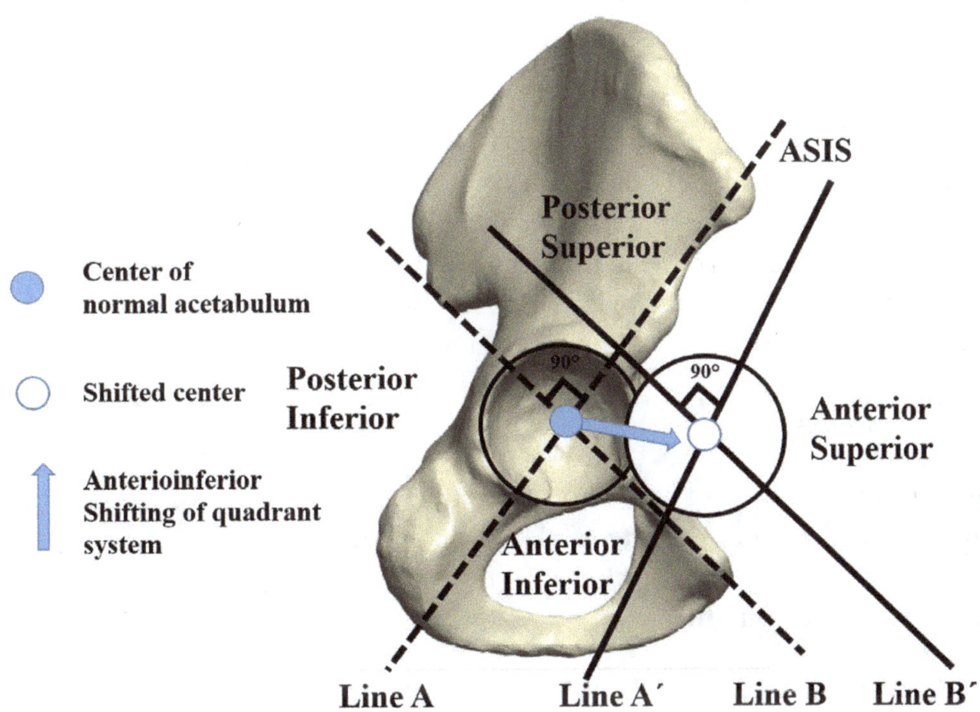

Figure 6. Illustration of shifted quadrant system anteroinferiorly in Crowe type-IV developmental dysplasia.

compression is critical to minimizing the vascular injury during total hip arthroplasty. Placing the anterior acetabular retractor at anterior inferior iliac spine and inferior acetabular retractor to the anterior wall is the safest position to avoid vascular injury during total hip arthroplasty.

2.4. Acetabular reinforcement ring and antiprotrusio cage

Acetabular reinforcement ring and antiprotrusio cages are generally used in traumatic hips and revision surgeries [35]. These prosthesis enable to fix the screws to actualize the pre-existing anatomical conditions of acetabulum. Avoiding the risk of vascular injuries, screw positioning in ventral and dorsal type of prosthesis is generally avoided. However, in such critical anatomical situations, radiological interventions must be required during surgery.

2.5. Cement

During cemented total hip replacement surgeries, cement must be allowed to reach lesser pelvis. Postoperative vascular complications occur due to cement extrusion in defect of acetabular wall can put external iliac vessels at risk. Excessive use of cement (methyl-methacrylate) can cause exothermic reaction, resulting in vessel thrombosis. Cement spiculae can erode through the artery and result in perforation and pseudoaneurysm formation in postoperative duration. The vessels are susceptible to avulsion if a revision surgery becomes necessary and intrapelvic cement is unwisely extracted.

3. Management

3.1. Preoperative management

3.1.1. Preoperative clinical investigation

The preoperative clinical examination of vessels must be carefully performed. Knowledge and local anatomy of vessel status surrounding the pelvis before surgery is essential and if necessary, surgeons must use the easier method like Doppler scan to measure the arterial occlusion pressure. Few arteries like femoral artery defects are easily identified in these examinations, while artery defects for the arteries like obturator and superior gluteal artery are often difficult to diagnose in early preoperative period.

3.1.2. Preventive measures

In case of revision total hip surgeries and traumatized hip, an appropriate vascular surgeon must be intimated prior to performing total hip replacement surgeries.

3.2. Intraoperative management

A high index of disbelief and careful intraoperative inspection are fundamental to immediate diagnosis and treatment of most intraoperative vessel injuries, both in primary and revision total hip surgeries. Sudden vascular injury at the time of surgery may be caused my many means for example instrumentation, broken bone edges, implants etc. Prompt recognition of vessel injury is important. In these injuries, the essential step is of course bleeding control.

Surgeon must not underestimate the urgency of vessel injury even in slight signs of bleeding. There are many steps that must be followed in such types of situation, which are listed below

- In open massive bleeding or slight signs of bleeding, immediate bleeding sights must be identified visually, and operated to stop the hemorrhage. Additionally, ultrasonography is the easiest and immediate way to recognize the site of bleeding in closed or open cases.
- In acute hemorrhage at first site, surgeons must put pressure for local control at either end of injured vessels.
- Additional supplies of blood and fresh frozen plasma must be done.
- Coagulation and legation technique for smaller vessels can be useful for temporary control of bleeding.
- Compression technique if unsuccessful at first attempt must be followed by surgical legation, endovascular stenting, and bypass as the next step for sites of vessel injury.
- Without time delay, vascular surgeons must be intervened to take the operative actions and stop the bleeding immediately.
- The operating orthopedic surgeon must be familiar with the advanced operative techniques like ilioinguinal and Stoppa approach for intrapelvic exposure, generally used in major injured vessel repair.

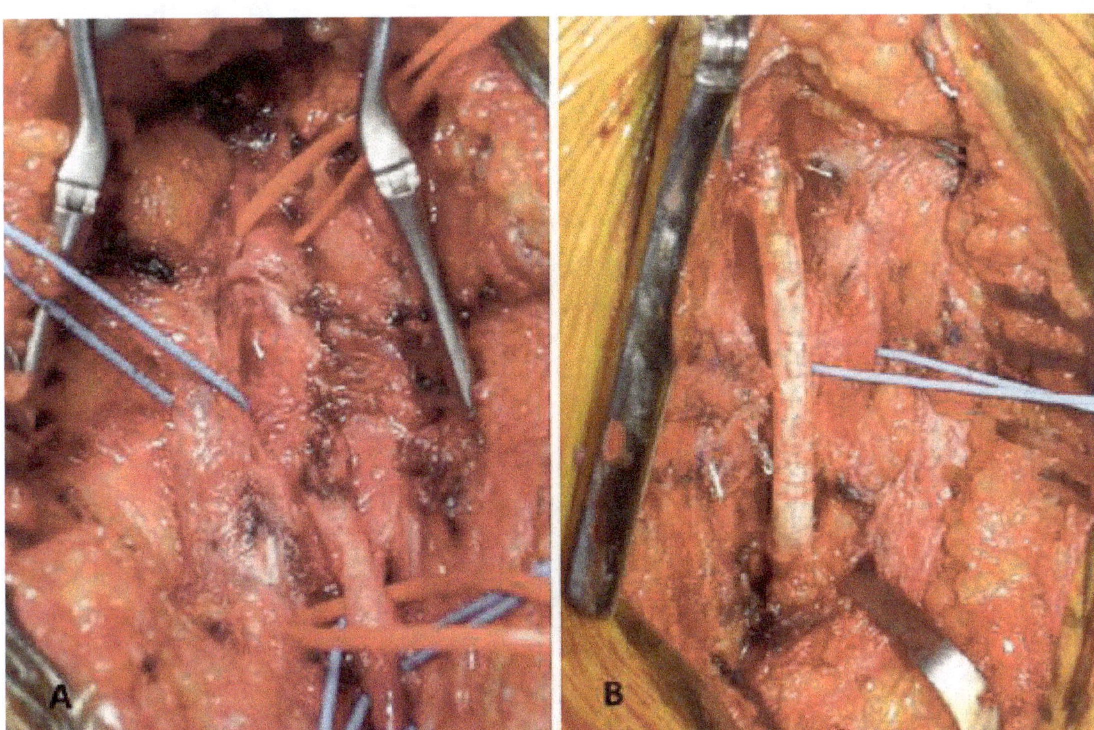

Figure 7. Photograph showing postoperative vessel injury. (A) Arterial injury between the distal external iliac artery and the femoral artery to the origin of deep femoral artery. (B) Arterial bypass (reprinted with permission from Barbier et al. [36]).

3.3. Postoperative management

Postoperative insult of vessel injury by surgeons, which is the slightly lesser common cause of unexplained pathological complications, might even result in death. Immediate after surgery to few days of recovery, careful monitoring of vessel status is essential to avoid postoperative vessel complications. After surgery and in the late postoperative period there are many sign and symptoms, the surgeons, and even individual must not circumvent, of course, it may be the sign of late vascular injury. Unexplained hypotension, tachycardia, nerve palsy, hypovolemic shock and decreased hemoglobin and blood pressure are the signs of vascular injury, postoperatively. In postoperative cases with the above signs and symptoms, immediate axial imaging or radiography, contrast-angiography, color ultrasonography are the more natural way to diagnose the bleeding source. Monitoring of these signs wisely is better and can be treated with open repair, stenting, bypass, coiling, or chemoembolization without any delay (**Figure** 7) [37–39]. The late symptoms from false aneurysm formation might be in the broad range of spectrum and very confusing and can be treated by surgical intervention, once the vascular injury is determined by diagnosis [13, 19].

Total hip replacement surgery is largely performed in aged patients and possibility of arterio-sclerosis vessel must be taken into account, as these vessels are more vulnerable to injury [29].

4. Conclusion

Conclusively, vascular injuries are rare in hip replacement surgeries. Careful preoperative planning, better instrumentation, knowledge of anatomical structures and meticulous surgical technique are necessary to avoid vascular injury. In advent screw penetration leading to vascular injuries can present early as hemorrhage during surgery, in the intermediate term as postoperative bleeding, hypotension, etc., and late as pseudoaneurysms. Further, management of these complications is beyond the scope of this chapter which focuses on prevention of these injuries rather than its management.

Acknowledgements

The authors would thank Professor P.P. Bansod, Head of Department, Department of Biomedical Engineering, SGSITS, Indore, India, for facilitating in preparation of this chapter.

Conflict of interest

The authors declare no conflict of interest.

Author details

Nishant Kumar Singh[1], Sanjay Rai[2]* and Amit Rastogi[3]

*Address all correspondence to: skrai.bme@iitbhu.ac.in

1 Department of Biomedical Engineering, National Institute of Technology, Raipur, India

2 Biomechanics Lab, School of Biomedical Engineering, Indian Institute of Technology, Banaras Hindu University, Varanasi, India

3 Department of Orthopedics, Institute of Medical Sciences, Banaras Hindu University, Varanasi, India

References

[1] Ethgen O, Bruyère O, Richy F, Dardennes C, Reginster JY. Health-related quality of life in total hip and total knee arthroplasty. Journal of Bone and Joint Surgery. 2004;**86**(5): 963-974. DOI: 10.2106/00004623-200405000-00012

[2] Nachbur B, Meyer RP, Verkkala K, Zürcher R. The mechanisms of severe arterial injury in surgery of the hip joint. Clinical Orthopaedics and Related Research. Jun 1979;**141**:122-133. DOI: 10.1097/00003086-197906000-00014

[3] Wilson JS, Miranda A, Johnson BL, Shames ML, Back MR, Bandyk DF. Vascular injuries associated with elective orthopedic procedures. Annals of Vascular Surgery. 2003;**17**(6): 641-644. DOI: 10.1007/s10016-003-0074-2

[4] Bergqvist D, Carlsson AS, Ericsson BF. Vascular complications after total hip arthroplasty. Acta Orthopaedica Scandinavica. 1983;**54**(2):157-163. DOI: 10.3109/17453678308996548

[5] Shoenfeld NA, Stuchin SA, Pearl R, Haveson S. The management of vascular injuries associated with total hip arthroplasty. Journal of Vascular Surgery. 1990;**11**(4):549-555. DOI: 10.1067/mva.1990.18087

[6] Bach CM, Steingruber I, Wimmer C, Ogon M, Frischhut B. False aneurysm 14 years after total hip arthroplasty. The Journal of Arthroplasty. 2000;**15**(4):535-538. DOI: 10.1054/arth.2000.4807

[7] Keating EM, Ritter MA, Faris PM. Structures at risk from medially placed acetabular screws. The Journal of Bone and Joint Surgery. American Volume. 1990;**72**(4):509-511. DOI: 10.2106/00004623-199072040-00006

[8] Singh N, Rai S, Rastogi A. Possible vascular injury due to screw eccentricity in minimally invasive total hip arthroplasty. Indian Journal of Orthopaedic Surgery. 2017;**51**(4):447. DOI: 10.4103/ortho.IJOrtho_224_16

[9] Wasielewski RC, Cooperstein LA, Kruger MP, Rubash HE. Acetabular anatomy and the transacetabular fixation of screws in total hip arthroplasty. Journal of Bone and Joint Surgery. 1990;**72**(4):501-508. DOI: 10.2106/00004623-199072040-00005

[10] Bakker KW, Gast LF. Retroperitoneal haemorrhage from the superior glutaeal artery: A late complication of total hip arthroplasty. Clinical Rheumatology. 1990;**9**(2):249-253. DOI: 10.1007/BF02031979

[11] Bach CM, Steingruber IE, Ogon M, Maurer H, Nogler M, Wimmer C. Intrapelvic complications after total hip arthroplasty failure. American Journal of Surgery. 2002;**183**(1):75-79. DOI: 10.1016/S0002-9610(01)00845-5

[12] Hopkins N, Vanhegan J, Jamieson C. Iliac aneurysm after total hip arthroplasty. Surgical management. Journal of Bone and Joint Surgery. British Volume (London). 1983;**65-B**(3): 359-361. DOI: 10.1302/0301-620X.65B3.6841412

[13] Akizuki S, Terayama K, Kobayashi S. False aneurysm of the external iliac artery during total hip replacement. Archives of Orthopaedic and Trauma Surgery. 1984;**102**(3):210-211. DOI: 10.1007/BF00575237

[14] Mallory TH. Rupture of the common iliac vein from reaming the acetabulum during total hip replacement: A case report. Journal of Bone and Joint Surgery. 1972;**54**(2):276-277

[15] Mcconaghie FA, Payne AP, Kinninmonth AWG. The role of retraction in direct nerve injury in total hip replacement: An anatomical study. Bone and Joint Research. 2014; **3**(6):212-216. DOI: 10.1302/2046-3758.36.2000255

[16] Shubert D, Madoff S, Milillo R, Nandi S. Neurovascular structure proximity to acetabular retractors in total hip arthroplasty. The Journal of Arthroplasty. 2015;**30**(1):145-148. DOI: 10.1016/j.arth.2014.08.024

[17] Kirkpatrick JS, Callaghan JJ, Vandemark RM, Goldner RD. The relationship of the intrapelvic vasculature to the acetabulum. Implications in screw-fixation acetabular components. Clinical Orthopaedics and Related Research. Sep 1990;**258**:183-190. DOI: 10.1097/00003086-199009000-00023

[18] Ohmori H, Ito S, Suda H, Yoshida Y. A case of late iliac arterial thrombosis due to component migration after revision total hip arthroplasty. Journal of Cardiology Cases. 2014; **10**(5):196-199. DOI: 10.1016/j.jccase.2014.07.009

[19] Nehme AH, Matta JF, Moufarrej NM, Jabbour FC, Moucharafieh RC, Feghaly MA. False aneurysm of the external iliac artery caused by aseptic loosening and migration of a cemented cup. Hip International. 2010;**20**(1):123-125. DOI: 10.1177/112070001002000119

[20] Fukuhara S, Kanki S, Daimon M, Shimada R, Ozawa H, Katsumata T. Pseudoaneurysm of the external iliac artery is a rare late complication after total hip arthroplasty. Journal of Vascular Surgery Cases and Innovative Techniques. 2017;**3**(3):149-151. DOI: 10.1016/j.jvscit.2017.04.006

[21] Clarius M, Heisel C, Breusch SJ. Pulmonary embolism in cemented total hip arthroplasty. In: Breusch S, Malchau H, editors. The Well-Cemented Total Hip Arthroplasty. Berlin/Heidelberg: Springer-Verlag; 2006. pp. 320-331. DOI: 10.1007/3-540-28924-0_43

[22] Kickuth R, Anderson S, Kocovic L, Ludwig K, Siebenrock K, Triller J. Endovascular treatment of arterial injury as an uncommon complication after orthopedic surgery. Journal of Vascular and Interventional Radiology. 2006;**17**(5):791-799. DOI: 10.1097/01.RVI.0000217929.35607.15

[23] Doi S, Motoyama Y, Itoh H. External iliac vein injury during total hip arthroplasty resulting in delayed shock. British Journal of Anaesthesia. 2005;**94**(6):866. DOI: 10.1093/bja/aei561

[24] Lewallen DG. Neurovascular injury associated with hip arthroplasty. Journal of Bone and Joint Surgery. 1997;**79**(12):1870-1180. DOI: 10.2106/00004623-199712000-00013

[25] Hwang SK. Vascular injury during total hip arthroplasty: The anatomy of the acetabulum. International Orthopaedics. 1994;**18**(1):3-5. DOI: 10.1007/BF00180175

[26] Liu Q, Zhou Y, Xu H, Tang J, Guo S, Tang Q. Safe zone for transacetabular screw fixation in prosthetic acetabular reconstruction of high developmental dysplasia of the hip. Journal of Bone and Joint Surgery. 2009;**91**(12):2880-2885. DOI: 10.2106/JBJS.H.01752

[27] Galat DD, Petrucci JA, Wasielewski RC. Radiographic evaluation of screw position in revision total hip arthroplasty. Clinical Orthopaedics and Related Research. 2004;**419**:124-129. DOI: 10.1097/00003086-200402000-00020

[28] Sakellariou V, Christodoulou M, Sasalos G, Babis G. Reconstruction of the acetabulum in developmental dysplasia of the hip in total hip replacement. Archives of Bone and Joint Surgery. 2014;**2**(3):130-136. DOI: 10.22038/abjs.2014.3353

[29] Tomé Bermejo F, Pajares Cabanillas S, Bonilla Madiedo L, Doblas Dominguez M, Flores Herrero Á, Criado E. Endovascular management of iliac vessel injury during revision of total hip replacement. European Journal of Orthopaedic Surgery and Traumatology. 2007;**17**(3):305-309. DOI: 10.1007/s00590-006-0161-5

[30] Kawasaki Y, Egawa H, Hamada D, Takao S, Nakano S, Yasui N. Location of intrapelvic vessels around the acetabulum assessed by three-dimensional computed tomographic angiography: Prevention of vascular-related complications in total hip arthroplasty. Journal of Orthopaedic Science. 2012;**17**(4):397-406. DOI: 10.1007/s00776-012-0227-7

[31] Wasielewski RC, Galat DD, Sheridan KC, Rubash HE, editors. Acetabular anatomy and transacetabular screw fixation at the high hip center. Clinical Orthopaedics and Related Research. Sep 2005;**438**:171-176. DOI: 10.1097/01.blo.0000165855.76244.53

[32] Pai MM, Krishnamurthy A, Prabhu LV, Pai MV, Kumar SA, Hadimani GA. Variability in the origin of the obturator artery. Clinics. 2009;**64**(9):897-901. DOI: 10.1590/S1807-59322009000900011

[33] Feugier P, Fessy MH, Béjui J, Bouchet A. Acetabular anatomy and the relationship with pelvic vascular structures implications in hip surgery. Surgical and Radiologic Anatomy. 1997;**19**(2):85-90. DOI: 10.1007/s00276-997-0085-8

[34] Marmor M, Lynch T, Matityahu A. Superior gluteal artery injury during iliosacral screw placement due to aberrant anatomy. Orthopedics. 2010;**33**(2):117-120. DOI: 10.3928/01477447-20100104-26

[35] D'Angelo F, Piffaretti G, Carrafiello G, et al. Endovascular repair of a pseudo-aneurysm of the common femoral artery after revision total hip arthroplasty. Emergency Radiology. 2007;**14**(4):233-236. DOI: 10.1007/s10140-007-0605-1

[36] Barbier O, Pierret C, Bazile F, De Kerangal X, Duverger V, Versier G. Vascular complications following total hip arthroplasty: A case study and a review of the literature. European Journal of Orthopaedic Surgery and Traumatology. 2012;**22**(S1):121-125. DOI: 10.1007/s00590-011-0880-0

[37] Sethuraman V, Hozack WJ, Sharkey PF, Rothman RH. Pseudoaneurysm of femoral artery after revision total hip arthroplasty with a constrained cup. The Journal of Arthroplasty. 2000;**15**(4):531-534. DOI: 10.1054/arth.2000.4332

[38] Zhou W, Bush RL, Terramani TT, Lin PH, Lumsden AB. Treatment options of iatrogenic pelvic vein injuries: Conventional operative versus endovascular approach. Vascular and Endovascular Surgery. 2004;**38**(6):569-573. DOI: 10.1177/153857440403800612

[39] Rossi G, Mavrogenis AF, Angelini A, Rimondi E, Battaglia M, Ruggieri P. Vascular complications in orthopaedic surgery. Journal of Long-Term Effects of Medical Implants. 2011;**21**(2):127-137. DOI: 10.1615/JLongTermEffMedImplants.v21.i2.30

10

Perioperative Management of Hip Fracture Patients Undergoing Total Hip Replacement

Bharati Rajdev and Subash Sivasubramaniam

Abstract

Patients with hip fractures have high morbidity and mortality, which has not changed significantly since last two decades. There are various national guidelines in UK, which give guidance to help improve outcomes in these patients such as National Institute for Health and Clinical Excellence's guidelines (NICE), Guidelines from Anaesthetists of Great Britain and Ireland (AAGBI) and Scottish intercollegiate guideline network (SIGN). NICE guidelines recommend total hip replacement (THR) rather than hemiarthroplasty in patients with a displaced intracapsular hip fracture in selected patients. AAGBI has produced guidelines for *Management of Proximal Femoral Fractures 2011*.

Keywords: total hip replacement, hip fracture, AAGBI, spinal anaesthesia, nerve block

1. Introduction

Patients with osteoporotic hip fracture have poor outcomes, which have not changed significantly in the last 20 years. Rates of morbidity and mortality are high in these patients and also there is decline in function and loss of independence. NICE, AAGBI, and SIGN have provided guidelines to help improve outcomes in these patients [1–3]. New approaches to treatment aim to improve outcomes. In older adults, hemiarthroplasty (or 'partial' hip replacement) has largely replaced internal fixation for displaced intracapsular hip fractures and this is associated with lower rates of revision surgery and better overall outcomes. Lately, in this population, there has been a thrust to enhance the use of total hip replacement (THR) because there are better chances of returning to functional mobility and, therefore, independence. THR is used more commonly for arthritis of the hip.

NICE guidelines [1] recommend total hip replacement (THR) rather than hemiarthroplasty to patients with a displaced intracapsular hip fracture if they were:

- able to walk independently out of doors with no more than the use of a stick;
- are not cognitively impaired; and
- are medically fit for anaesthesia and the procedure.

Outcomes after THR for displaced fractures of hip are similar to those after THR for elective surgery. Careful selection of patients is essential to achieve this success.

Perioperative care of patients with proximal femoral fractures can be challenging, as it involves care of large numbers of older patients with significant comorbidities. Risk of significant morbidity and mortality in these patients can be reduced by early surgical fixation of the fracture and early, effective rehabilitation.

The Department of Health has suggested the following targets for patients with hip fracture [4]:

i. All patients should be admitted within 4 h of arrival in the emergency department; and

ii. Patients should be operated on by an experienced clinical team within 24 h of a decision that the patient is fit for surgery.

Multidisciplinary care improves the quality and efficiency of hip fracture care. The multidisciplinary team includes trauma co-ordinators, general practitioners, nurses, emergency staff, bed managers, orthopaedic nursing staff and surgeons, anaesthetists, orthogeriatricians, physio- and occupational therapists, social workers and rehabilitation services.

2. Preoperative management

2.1. Initial management

'Fast-track' triage systems should be in place as most of these patients are admitted via the emergency department. These will enable early clinical recognition of hip fracture with early radiography and diagnosis, allowing rapid ward admission. The use of a care pathway pro forma ensures basic quality standards are met and helps in patient care.

Patients who have a clinical suspicion or confirmation of a hip fracture should have the 'Big Six' interventions/treatments before leaving the Emergency Department [5].

1. *Provision of pain relief.* All patients should be offered analgesia. The use of a nerve block helps to reduce pain, opioid requirement and delirium. Painkillers such as paracetamol should be prescribed on regular basis. Opioids should be prescribed with caution. Non-steroidal anti-inflammatory drugs and codeine to be avoided due to its side effects
2. *Screening for delirium.*
3. *Early warning score (EWS) system.*

4. *Full blood investigation and electrocardiogram*

5. *Intravenous fluids therapy*: Many hip fracture patients are fluid deplete at presentation. Assessment of hydration is difficult in elderly patients as they may not exhibit typical physiological responses such as tachycardia or hypotension. These patients tolerate hypovolemia poorly, risking cardiovascular instability and organ hypoperfusion. All patients should have a documented assessment of fluid status and resuscitation with IV fluids where appropriate. Preoperative administration of colloid solution intravenously before hip fracture surgery does not improve outcome, compared with a conventional IV fluid regime with a crystalloid solution.

   A literature review to identify relevant evidence supporting the use of blood resuscitation in adult patients aged 65 years and over who have presented within 24 h of sustaining a fracture of the proximal femur when compared with crystalloid or colloid resuscitation did not yield any articles [6].

6. *Pressure area care.*

2.2. Preoperative assessment

The assessment by anaesthetist allows pre-optimisation, planning of anaesthetic techniques and communication of perioperative risks to the patient and relatives.

Early involvement of orthogeriatrician has been shown to be useful in many ways such as medical pre-optimisation of patients, early rehabilitation and discharge planning.

One-fourth of these patients have moderate cognitive impairment and therefore tools such as abbreviated mental test score (AMTS) should be used to assess for cognitive impairment. Capacity assessment is vital for informed consent. Treatment may be provided according to the Mental Capacity Act 2005, if the patient lacks capacity and should be undertaken in the best interests of patients.

2.3. Nottingham hip fracture score

Nottingham hip fracture score (NHFS),a risk prediction tool [7], has been developed to predict postoperative mortality. It is summative score of seven variables—comorbidities and other factors (age, male sex, malignancy, preoperative cognitive function, place of residence and anaemia). NHFS is used to predict mortality at 30 days and it provides the information about outcome which may be discussed with the patient or their relatives (**Tables 1** and **2**).

2.4. Investigations

Full blood count, urea, electrolytes and ECG should be done in all patients. Anaemia is common in these patients due to various reasons and a lower threshold for blood transfusion should be considered in this group of patients.

Variable	Points
Age 66–85 years	3
Age 86 ≥ older	4
Male	1
Haemoglobin concentration ≤ 10 g.dl^{-1} on admission to hospital	1
Abbreviated mental test score ≤ 6/10 on admission to hospital	1
Living in an institution	1
More than one co-morbidity	1
Active malignancy within last 20 years	1

Table 1. Derivation of Nottingham hip fracture score (NHFS). Reproduced with kind permission of AAGBI [2].

Score	Predicted 30-day postoperative mortality
0	0
1	1%
2	2%
3	4%
4	6%
5	10%
6	15%
7	23%
8	22%
9	45%
10	57%

Table 2. Predicted 30-day mortality as per NHFS. Reproduced with kind permission of AAGB [2].

2.5. Special cases

2.5.1. Atrial fibrillation

All patients in AF should have ventricular rate less than 100 per min. Reversible causes such as electrolyte imbalance and hypovolemia should be corrected if rate is faster. Pharmacological treatment will be required if still remains high [8].

2.5.2. Anticoagulation

INR should be less than 2 for surgery and less than 1.5 for neuroaxial anaesthesia. Patients having warfarin should have vitamin K to reverse the effect.

If a patient is on clopidogrel, surgery should be done with expectation of higher blood loss.

Platelets should not be given prophylactically. The haematologist's opinion should be taken if required.

2.5.3. *Chest infection*

Patients with chest infection should have their surgery done under regional anaesthesia which will give the benefit of analgesia and help in early mobilisation and chest physiotherapy.

2.5.4. *Heart murmur*

The management of patients with hip fracture in whom a systolic murmur (indicating aortic stenosis) is heard remains debatable. If aortic stenosis is suspected and echo has not been done preoperatively, then the patient should be managed as having aortic stenosis.

2.5.5. *Implantable pacemakers*

Preoperative evaluation by cardiologist is necessary to know the type of device.

2.5.6. *DNA-CPR (do not attempt cardio pulmonary resuscitation)*

Resuscitation may not be in the best interests of the patient or not desired by the patients. DNA-CPR should be discussed with the patients where appropriate. Patients with pre-existing DNA-CPR orders must have perioperative modifications to that process prior to coming to theatre for having surgery [9] (As per recommendations from Resuscitation Council UK and Association of Anaesthetist of Great Britain & Ireland).

3. Intraoperative management

3.1. Surgical management

They can be broadly classified into extracapsular and intracapsular fractures.

Intracapsular fractures are further classified as subcapital, transcervical and basicervical fractures depending on the site of fracture. These may be displaced or undisplaced (**Table 3**).

Intracapsular	Extracapsular
Undisplaced fracture - internal fixation with multiple screws or a sliding hip screw.	Intertrochanteric fractures - a sliding hip screw
Displaced fractures - hemiarthroplasty or total hip replacement	Subtrochanteric fractures - proximal femoral intramedullary nail

Table 3. Surgical management of proximal hip fractures.

Cemented arthroplasty as compared to uncemented arthroplasty improves hip function and is associated with lower residual pain postoperatively.

3.2. Anaesthetic considerations

Both audit and meta-analysis of anaesthetic practice have not shown any great difference in outcome between general and regional (spinal) anaesthesia.

Parker and colleagues [10] in Cochrane review of 2004 analysed 22 trials (all of which were found to be methodologically flawed and many do not reflect current anaesthetic practice), involving 2567 patients, and concluded that regional anaesthesia may reduce the prevalence of acute postoperative confusion (9% *vs.* 19%); however, no difference in 30-day mortality after regional anaesthesia compared with general anaesthesia. Based on these findings, the Scottish Intercollegiate Guidelines Network (SIGN) has produced recommendation concerning choice of anaesthetic technique, namely that 'Spinal/epidural anaesthesia should be considered for all patients undergoing hip fracture repair, unless contraindicated'.

A meta-analysis [11] of 34 randomised controlled trials, 14 observational studies, and 8 meta-analyses, involving 18,715 patients, concluded that spinal anaesthesia is associated with significantly reduced early mortality, fewer incidents of deep vein thrombosis, less acute postoperative confusion, a tendency to fewer myocardial infarctions and fewer cases of pneumonia, fatal pulmonary embolism and postoperative hypoxia.

A further recent meta-analysis [12] of 47 clinical trials and 35 reviews/meta-analyses in geriatric patients undergoing non-cardiac surgery concluded that regional anaesthesia is associated with reduced early mortality and morbidity, for example, fewer incidents of deep vein thrombosis and less acute postoperative confusion, as well as a tendency towards fewer myocardial infarctions and fatal pulmonary embolisms.

Large observational studies in UK [13, 14] and US [15–17] show there is no difference in 30-day mortality between general and spinal anaesthesia.

NICE support the use of either spinal or general anaesthesia, + nerve block.

There are various problems attempting to perform the definitive outcome comparison study between general and regional anaesthesia, including, but not restricted to, definition of the primary endpoint.

For the time being, the AAGBI recommends that either method of anaesthesia (but not both together) may be used, but most importantly that they are administered with care to any patient, using reduced doses of anaesthetic agent combined with multimodal analgesia with an aim to minimise rapid fluctuations in arterial pressure and resultant changes in cerebral and coronary perfusion pressures. This is supported by a recent retrospective study of 1131 patients which showed that a reduced volume of intrathecal 0.5% hyperbaric bupivacaine was associated with a reduction in intraoperative hypotension, and therefore less reactive fluid administration avoiding consequent haemodilution [18].

3.2.1. *General anaesthesia*

Small doses of intravenous induction agents should be used. Alternatively, inhalational induction can be done. The advantages of inhalational induction are that it is well tolerated by the elderly patients and also allows for maintenance of spontaneous ventilation. The choice of using mechanical ventilation versus spontaneous ventilation remains controversial. The benefit of using mechanical ventilation is that there is reduced risk of aspiration and better control of carbon dioxide levels. On the other hand, there is greater physiological derangement with paralysis and tracheal intubation as compared to spontaneous ventilation.

3.2.2. *Regional anaesthesia*

Spinal anaesthesia: Lower doses of intrathecal bupivacaine (<10 mg) and unilateral subarachnoid anaesthesia may help to decrease hypotension. Use of intrathecal opioids helps for postoperative analgesia. As morphine or diamorphine is associated with greater respiratory and cognitive depression, it is preferable to use fentanyl.

Sedation should be used cautiously in elderly patients with spinal anaesthesia. If necessary for patient comfort, sedation should be restricted to propofol. Ketamine can cause postop confusion and delirium.

Epidural: It provides good postoperative analgesia, but may limit early mobilisation after surgery.

Nerve block: NICE recommends to consider intraoperative nerve blocks for all patients undergoing surgery.

The rational being, co-administration of a nerve block, reduces age-adjusted maintenance doses of general anaesthesia, helps in positioning of patient for spinal anaesthesia, enables the use of low-dose spinal anaesthesia as it provides analgesia during skin closure even if spinal starts wearing off and it helps in providing opioid sparing analgesia in early postoperative period.

Blockade of the three nerves—femoral, obturator and lateral cutaneous nerve of the thigh—can provide adequate analgesia. The most reliable method of blocking all three nerves is the psoas compartment block. The fascia iliaca block/femoral nerve blocks do not reliably block all three nerves but do provide some pain relief. Ultrasound guidance can be used for performing these nerve blocks.

3.3. Monitoring

As recommended by AAGBI, minimum standards for monitoring as for any other surgery include the continual presence of the anaesthetist, pulse oximetry, capnography, ECG and non-invasive blood pressure monitoring.

As elderly patients are prone to hypothermia, core temperature monitoring should be used routinely.

Further monitoring should be considered depending on the risk. This may include invasive blood pressure monitoring, central venous pressure (CVP) monitoring and cardiac output monitoring. Transoesophageal Doppler, Transthoracic Doppler or LIDCO can be used for cardiac output monitoring.

Bispectral index (BIS) monitors may be used to monitor the depth of anaesthesia as it will allow for dose reduction and hence avoid potential hypotension. Initial BIS levels may be abnormally low in alcoholic patients and patients with dementia.

Cerebral oxygen saturation: Postoperative cognitive dysfunction is associated with reduced cerebral oxygen saturation.

AAGBI emphasises the finding in the NCEPOD reports '*Extremes of Age* (1999)' and '*An Age Old Problem* (2010)' that, in spite of being among the sickest patients with the worst outcomes in hospitals, elderly hip fracture patients were not intensively monitored during surgery, and recommend a greater consideration be given to invasive arterial pressure monitoring and use of cardiac output (e.g. Doppler, LiDCO) and cerebral function (e.g., bispectral index, cerebral oxygen saturation) monitors.

3.4. Infection control

Antibiotic prophylaxis significantly reduces overall wound infections. Antibiotics should be administered within 1 h of skin incision according to AAGBI recommendations. Hospital antibiotic protocols should be followed.

3.5. Fluid management

Perioperative optimisation of fluid management helps to reduce morbidity. Cardiac output-guided fluid administration in this group of patients could reduce hospital stay and improve outcome [19].

3.6. Thromboprophylaxis

The following strategies will help reduce the risk of deep vein thrombosis-thromboprophylactic stockings or intraop usage of intermittent calf compressors, regional anaesthesia, early surgery and early mobilisation.

3.7. Prevention of hypothermia

Active warming techniques like body warmers and warm IV fluids should be used as elderly patients are prone to intraoperative hypothermia.

3.8. Tranexamic acid

Patients with hip fractures can have significant blood loss. The rate of blood transfusion in the perioperative period for hip fracture patients is reported between 20 and 60%.These patients have multiple comorbidities making them more susceptible to adverse events from blood loss.

Antifibrinolytics, such as tranexamic acid (TXA), have been used to limit bleeding in orthopaedic surgery and prevent the need for blood transfusion.

It acts as a competitive inhibitor in the activation of plasminogen to plasmin, therefore preventing the degradation of fibrin. Despite its proven efficacy in patients undergoing elective orthopaedic surgery, including total joint replacement and spine surgery, there is clinical uncertainty and a lack of high-quality evidence regarding the use of TXA in hip fracture patients.

Four of five studies [20–24] identified a significant decrease in rate of transfusion in patients who received TXA compared to those that did not. Some of these studies were underpowered for detecting significant differences in thromboembolic events. Also, patients were only followed perioperatively, and differences in 6-month and 1-year mortality rates and late-onset complications were not assessed.

A systematic review of tranexamic acid in hip fracture surgery showed moderate quality evidence that TXA reduces blood transfusion in hip fracture surgery and low-quality evidence suggesting no increased risk of thrombotic events. A randomised controlled trial on the efficacy of tranexamic acid in reducing blood loss in hip fracture patients is being done. The immediate goal of this trial is to provide high-quality evidence that can be used to develop clinical guidelines for use of TXA in patients with hip fractures [25].

3.9. Bone cement implantation syndrome (BCIS)

This is characterised by hypoxia, hypotension, or both, and/or unexpected loss of consciousness [26]. This occurs at the time of cementation, prosthesis insertion and reduction of the joint or, occasionally, limb tourniquet deflation in a patient undergoing cemented bone surgery. Several mechanisms may contribute to a multimodal aetiology, including fat/platelet/fibrin/marrow emboli and stimulated release of vasoactive mediators. The treatment of BCIS includes delivery of 100% oxygen, fluid resuscitation (guided by CVP measurement) and vasoactive/inotropic support. AAGBI [27] has made several recommendations to reduce the risk of developing BCIS from cemented arthroplasty. They advocate a three-step check process to ensure we are prepared for such events and we are able to manage them in a proactive manner.

4. Postoperative care

AAGBI recommends use of point-of-care Hb analysers (e.g., Hemocue or similar) routinely at the end of surgery to assess the degree of anaemia and guide blood transfusion. Haemoglobin and electrolytes need to be monitored postoperatively. An analysis of postoperative haemoglobin levels in patients with a fractured neck of femur demonstrated that a haemoglobin value taken on D2 postoperatively represents the largest drop in a patient's circulating haemoglobin with statistical and also clinical significance [28]. Certain groups will require close daily monitoring of haemoglobin levels such as patients with chronic renal, cardiac disease and patients taking any form of anticoagulation.

Good nursing care with regular input from orthogeriatricians, adequate analgesia, hydration and nutrition are all important for good postoperative outcomes.

Early rehabilitation helps return the patient to their pre-morbid level of activity.

4.1. Postoperative cognitive dysfunction

This is common in this group of patients. Management includes adequate analgesia, nutrition and hydration, electrolyte balance, appropriate medication, optimising bowel habit, mobilisation and also identifying and treating any infection or silent myocardial ischaemia. Drugs such as haloperidol or lorazepam should only be used for short-term control of symptoms.

5. Conclusions

1. Patients with a hip fracture have a relatively high risk of perioperative morbidity and mortality.
2. High-quality care of these patients requires multidisciplinary care and protocol-driven care pathways
3. Early surgery aids in providing analgesia and allows early mobilisation, and is associated with reduced morbidity and mortality.
4. The mode of anaesthesia provided is less important than the manner with which it is delivered with regard to the age and pathophysiological status of the individual patient.
5. Surgery and anaesthesia must be undertaken by appropriately experienced surgeons and anaesthetists.

Conflict of interest

None declared.

Author details

Bharati Rajdev* and Subash Sivasubramaniam

*Address all correspondence to: bharati.rajdev@nhs.net

Sandwell and West Birmingham Hospitals NHS Trust, Birmingham, United Kingdom

References

[1] National Institute for Health and Clinical Excellence. The Management of Hip Fracture in Adults. 2011. http://www.nice.org.uk/nicemedia/live/13489/54918/54918.pdf

[2] Association of Anaesthetists of Great Britain and Ireland. Management of proximal femoral fractures 2011. Anaesthesia. 2012;**67**:85-98

[3] Scottish Intercollegiate Guidelines Network. Management of Hip Fracture in Older People. National Clinical Guideline 111, 2009. http://www.sign.ac.uk/pdf/sign111.pdf

[4] NHS Institute for Innovation and Improvement. Delivering Quality and Value. November. 2005. http://www.dh.gov.uk/prod_consum_dh/groups/dh_digitalassets/@dh/@en/documents/digitalasset/dh_4122355.pdf [Accessed: 30 Aug 2011]

[5] Scottish Standards of Care for Hip Fracture Patients. 2016. www.shfa.scot.nhs.uk/_docs/20161109_SSC_for_Hip_Fracture_Patients.pdf

[6] Rocos B, Whitehouse MR, Kelly MB. Resuscitation in hip fractures: A systematic review. BMJ Open. 2017;**7**:e015906. DOI: 10.1136/ bmjopen-2017-015906

[7] Wiles MD, Moran CG, Sahota O, Moppett IK. Nottingham hip fracture score as a predictor of one year mortality in patients undergoing surgical repair of fractured neck of femur. British Journal of Anaesthesia. 2011;**106**:501-504

[8] The Task Force for the Management of Atrial Fibrillation of the European Society of Cardiology (ESC). Guidelines for the management of atrial fibrillation. European Heart Journal. 2010;**31**:2369-2429

[9] Association of Anaesthetists of Great Britain and Ireland. DNAR Decisions in the Perioperative Period. May, 2009. http://www.aagbi.org/publications/guidelines/docs/dnar_09.pdf

[10] Parker MJ, Handoll HHG, Griffiths R. Anaesthesia for hip fracture surgery in adults. Cochrane Database of Systematic Reviews. 2004;**18**:CD000521

[11] Luger TJ, Kammerlander C, Gosch M, et al. Neuroaxial versus general anaesthesia in geriatric patients for hip fracture surgery: Does it matter? Osteoporosis International. 2010;**21**(Suppl 4):S555-S572

[12] Luger TJ, Kammerlander C, Luger MF, Kammerlander-Knauer U, Gosch M. Mode of anesthesia, mortality and outcome in geriatric patients. Zeitschrift für Gerontologie und Geriatrie. 2014;**47**:110-124

[13] White SM, Moppett IK, Griffiths R. Outcome by mode of anaesthesia for hip fracture surgery. An observational audit of 65, 535 patients in a national dataset. Anaesthesia. 2014;**69**:224-230

[14] White SM, Moppett IK, Griffiths R, et al. Outcomes after anaesthesia for hip fracture surgery. Secondary analysis of prospective observational data from 11,085 patients included in the UK Anaesthesia Sprint Audit of Practice (ASAP 2). Anaesthesia. 2016;**71**:506-514

[15] Neuman MD, Silber JH, Elkassabany NM, Ludwig JM, Fleisher LA. Comparative effectiveness of regional versus general anesthesia for hip fracture surgery in adults. Anesthesiology. 2012;**117**:72-92

[16] Neuman MD, Rosenbaum PR, Ludwig JM, Zubizarreta JR, Silber JH. Anesthesia technique, mortality, and length of stay after hip fracture surgery. Journal of the American Medical Association. 2014;**311**:2508-2517

[17] Patorno E, Neuman MD, Schneeweiss S, Mogun H, Bateman BT. Comparative safety of anesthetic type for hip fracture surgery in adults: Retrospective cohort study. British Medical Journal. 2014;**348**:g4022

[18] Wood RJ, White SM. Anaesthesia for 1131 patients undergoing proximal femoral fracture repair: A retrospective, observational study of effects on blood pressure, fluid administration and perioperative anaemia. Anaesthesia. 2011;**66**:1017-1022

[19] Sinclair S, James S, Singer M. Intraoperative intravascular volume optimisation and length of hospital stay after repair of proximal femoral fracture: Randomised controlled trial. British Medical Journal. 1997;**315**:909-912

[20] Sadeghi M, Mehr-Aein A. Does a single bolus dose of tranexamic acid reduce blood loss and transfusion requirements during hip fracture surgery? A prospective randomized double blind study in 67 patients. Acta Medica Iranica. 2007;**45**:437-442

[21] Emara WM, Moez KK, Elkhouly AH. Topical versus intravenous tranexamic acid as a blood conservation intervention for reduction of post-operative bleeding in hemiarthroplasty. Anesthesia, Essays and Researches. 2014;**8**:48-53

[22] Zufferey PJ, Miquet M, Quenet S, et al. Tranexamic acid in hip fracture surgery: A randomized controlled trial. British Journal of Anaesthesia. 2010;**104**:23-30. DOI: 10.1093/bja/aep314

[23] Lee C, Freeman R, Edmondson M, et al. The efficacy of tranexamic acid in hip hemiarthroplasty surgery: An observational cohort study. Injury. 2015;**46**:1978-1982. DOI: 10.1016/j.injury.2015.06.039

[24] Vijay BS, Bedi V, Mitra S, et al. Role of tranexamic acid in reducing postoperative blood loss and transfusion requirement in patients undergoing hip and femoral surgeries. Saudi Journal of Anaesthesia. 2013;**7**:29-32. DOI: 10.4103/1658-354X.109803

[25] Gausden EB, Garner MR, Warner SJ, et al. Tranexamic acid in hip fracture patients: A protocol for a randomised, placebo controlled trial on the efficacy of tranexamic acid in reducing blood loss in hip fracture patients. BMJ Open. 2016;**6**:e010676. DOI: 10.1136/bmjopen-2015-010676

[26] Donaldson AJ, Thomson HE, Harper NJ, Kenny NW. Bone cement implantation syndrome. British Journal of Anaesthesia. 2009;**102**:12-22

[27] Association of Anaesthetists of Great Britain and Ireland. Safety guideline: Reducing the risk from cemented hemiarthroplasty for hip fracture 2015. Anaesthesia. 2015;**70**:623-626

[28] Nagra et al. An analysis of postoperative hemoglobin levels in patients with a fractured neck of femur. Acta Orthopaedica et Traumatologica Turcica. October 2016;**50**(5):507-513

11

Hip Fracture: Anatomy, Causes, and Consequences

Masoud Nasiri Sarvi

Abstract

Fall-induced hip fracture is a major worldwide health problem among the elderly population. Nowadays, hip replacement surgery represents a big part of the orthopedic surgeons' workload and has associated remarkable clinical and social cost implications. Hip fractures have several complications including medical and surgical treatment. A significant number of biomechanical models have been introduced to study hip fracture risk. The purpose of proposing the biomechanical models for predicting the hip fracture risk is to introduce prevention and protection activities that may reduce the number of hip fractures. For accurate prediction of hip fracture risk, the fracture procedure and the parameters that affect the risk of hip fracture should be well studied. The objective of this study is to investigate in-depth the hip fracture anatomy, causes, and consequences.

Keywords: hip fracture causes, hip anatomy, fall, hip impact force, hip fracture consequences

1. Introduction

Low-trauma hip fracture has become a common health problem among the elderly all over the world [1–21], mainly due to the population aging and the prevalence of osteoporosis. Of all osteoporotic fractures, hip fracture has the highest morbidity and mortality rate [22]. Approximately 50% of patients have permanent functional disability greater than that before fracture [23, 24]. The incidence of hip fracture appears to be increasing in many countries [10], and the total number of hip fractures is estimated to be more than five million by 2050 [25]. Socioeconomic impacts of hip fracture are twofold. On the one hand, hip fracture increases the morbidity and mortality in the elderly [26–28]; on the other hand, it is a substantial source of healthcare expenditure [29, 30]. Therefore, there is an urgent need to accurately assess hip fracture risk and then develop preventive and protective measures. In this chapter, hip anatomy is first reviewed, and hip fractures are classified by anatomic location. Then, prevalence of hip fracture is presented, followed by a description of the significance of accurately assessing hip fracture risk.

2. Hip fracture anatomy

Hip fracture is a medical condition in which there is a break in the continuity of the femoral bone. Hip fracture is generally affected by hip anatomy [31], the applied forces to the hip [32], and bone mechanical properties [33]. In this section, hip anatomy is explained to show why the hip is likely to experience fracture in a fall.

The hip joint is one of the most important joints in the human body. It is also one of the most flexible joints allowing a great range of motions. To better understand hip fracture, it helps to know the anatomy of the hip joint. The hip is a joint formed by the ball-shaped head of the femur and the socket of the pelvis. The femurs are the longest and the strongest bones in the human body, extending from the hip to the knee. Important geometric features of femur bones include the head, neck, and greater and lesser trochanters, as shown in **Figure 1(a)**. A femur is composed of two types of bones, cortical and cancellous. The cortical bone forms the outer layer of the femur and withstands most of the forces and moments. Cancellous bone is mostly enclosed by the cortical bone and mainly absorbs the shock energy produced in walking and running [34]. The hip joint is a stable ball-and-socket joint, much more stable than the shoulder joint. The stability in the hip mainly attributes to the deep socket, i.e., the acetabulum. Additional stability is provided by the strong joint capsule and its surrounding muscles and ligaments. The high level of stability of the hip joint is required to support the upper body [34].

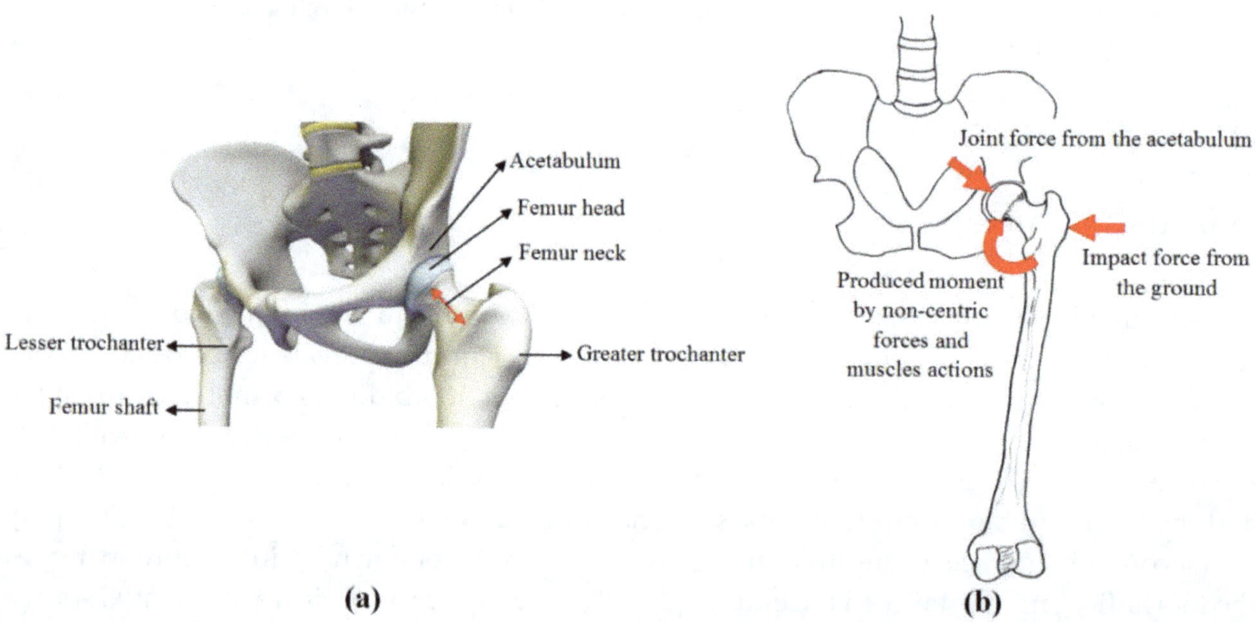

Figure 1. (a) Anatomic structure of the hip [35]. (b) Concentration of applied forces on the proximal femur in a lateral fall which increases the risk of fracture.

More than 90% of all hip fractures occur in falls [36] as the femur is subjected to a high-level impact force. As shown in **Figure 1(b)**, in a sideways fall, the greater trochanter and the femoral head are subjected to the impact and the joint force, respectively, from the ground and the acetabulum. The forces produce a moment at the intersection of the neck-shaft axes. Muscles that are attached to the femur also produce forces during the fall. As it is shown in **Figure 1(b)**, the applied forces in a fall are mainly on the proximal femur, and it may explain why the majority of fall-induced hip fractures occur at the proximal femur [37]. A hip fracture refers to any fracture of the proximal femur down to a level of approximately 5 cm below the lower border of the lesser trochanter [38]. The extent of the break depends on the forces that are involved.

3. Hip fracture causes

Hip fracture is usually caused by an applied force that exceeds the strength of the femur bone [39]. Therefore, any situation that either induces a high level of force on the femur bone or decreases the bone strength should be considered as a hip fracture cause.

The main cause of hip fracture is falling (90–92%) [36, 40–42], in particular falling in sideways direction (63–69% in fall-related fractures) [8, 43], as it induces a high level of force on the femur. Parameters that increase the risk of fall and apply a high level of force on the femur, especially in the elderly, are:

- Mental impairment and confusion
- Impaired vision
- Impaired muscle reactions
- Slow reflex response
- Inability to effectively use the arms to reduce the energy of the fall
- Impaired neuromuscular coordination and neurological diseases (e.g., hemiplegia, Parkinson's disease)
- Reduced soft tissue padding over the hip [44, 45]

In the elderly, most fractures occur after a low-trauma fall, which would not cause any severe injury to a healthy individual. Therefore, low bone strength is another main cause of hip fracture. Osteoporosis as a progressive bone disease, which is characterized by decreases in bone mass and density, has been identified as one of the main contributors of hip fracture [46, 47]. Osteoporosis advances when bone resorption exceeds bone formation, and therefore it is more common among the elderly [48]. Approximately three to four out of ten women over the age of 50, and one in eight men, suffer osteoporotic fracture in their lifetime [49].

Apart from osteoporosis, several other causes may reduce the strength of the bone such as bone cancer and medical side effects [38]. Other factors associated with reduction in bone strength include [38]:

- Genetic and family history
- Sedentary lifestyle
- Impaired nutrition
- Smoking
- Excess alcohol
- Medications (including tranquilizers, hypnotics, anticonvulsant drugs, and steroids)
- Osteomalacia from vitamin D deficiency, malabsorption, and liver or renal disease
- Cardiovascular disease and cardiac arrhythmias
- Underlying bone disease (e.g., Paget's disease, bone tumors, and secondary bone tumors)
- Endocrine abnormalities: hyperthyroidism, hyperparathyroidism, or hypercortisolism

In addition to the mentioned causes, high-trauma falls and accidents such as car and motorcycle accidents can lead to hip fracture [50]. But they are not studied in this dissertation. **Figure 2** shows how different factors contribute to the hip fracture [6, 38].

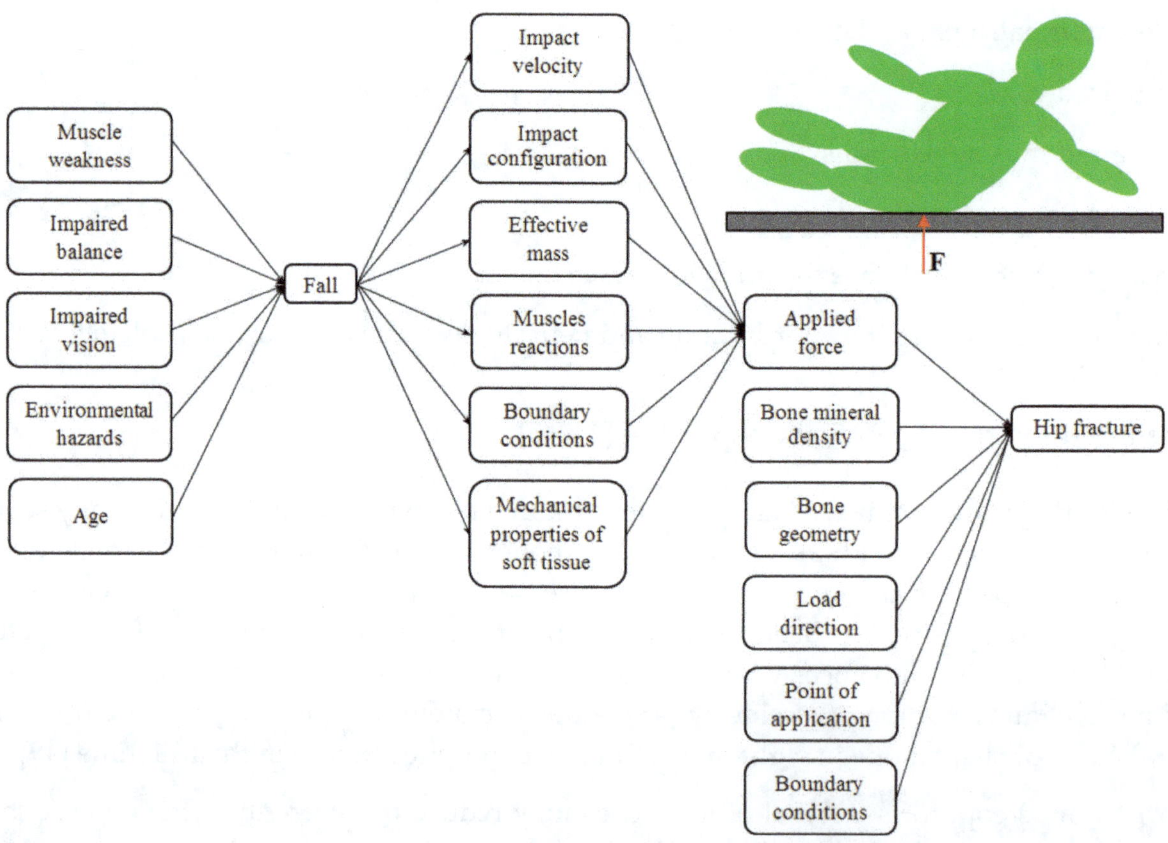

Figure 2. Conceptual model of the fall-induced hip fracture procedure and associated effective factors [15].

4. Hip fracture consequences

Hip fractures are associated with significant morbidity, mortality, loss of independence, and financial burden [3, 9, 25, 42, 51–53]. It has been reported that approximately 20% of hip fracture patients died within 1 year of the fracture [54]. Generally, the first year after hip fracture appears to be the most critical time. A recent meta-analysis revealed that women sustaining a hip fracture had a fivefold increase and men almost an eightfold increase in relative likelihood of death within the first 3 months compared with age- and sex-matched controls [29]. The relative death risk decreases substantially over the second year but still much higher than that of the controls [55]. Many lose their ability to walk mainly due to the pain caused by the hip fracture. In fact, only 40–79% of patients regain their previous ambulatory function a year after the fracture, and less than half return to their pre-fracture status of daily activities [56].

In addition to functional impairments, hip fracture can have a negative impact on self-esteem, body image, and mood [57], which may lead to psychological problems [58]. Individuals who suffer fractures may be immobilized by a fear of falling again and suffering more fractures. They may feel isolated and helpless. The National Osteoporosis Foundation conducted a survey [59] among 1000 women with osteoporotic fracture in the United States to investigate the psychological effects of the fracture on the patients. Eighty-nine percent of said they feared breaking another bone; 80% were afraid that they would be less able to perform their daily activities and lose their independence; 73% worried that they would have to reduce activities with family and friends; and 68% were concerned that another fracture would result in their having to enter a nursing home [59]. If not addressed, fear about the future and a sense of helplessness can produce significant anxiety and depression. These problems may be compounded by an inability to fulfill occupational, domestic, or social duties, thus leading to further social isolation.

The disability, reduced functional status, and poor mental health caused by hip fracture can have a profound impact on the quality of the individual's life. Survivors of hip fracture reported a 52% reduction in the quality of life in the first 12 months and a 21% reduction after 2 years [60].

Also, hip fracture is a major cause of the need for long-term nursing home care and a major contributor to healthcare costs [30, 61, 62]. There are approximately 23,000 cases of hip fracture every year in Canada with associated treatment costs of about $1 billion [63]. In the United States, 310,000 hip fractures occurred in 2003, and the total Medicare cost was estimated between $10.3 and $15.2 billion, including acute medical care and nursing home services [53, 64, 65]. As the population of the elderly is still continuously increasing, the number of hip fractures is expected to rise dramatically, and it will put more burdens on the community healthcare system [2, 66].

5. Classification of hip fractures

In general, there are three types of hip fractures, depending on what region of the proximal femur is involved [67]:

1. Femoral neck fractures occur in the narrow section of the proximal femur that lies between the femoral head and the intertrochanteric cross section. Most femoral neck fractures occur within the capsule surrounding the hip joint and are, therefore, termed intracapsular fracture. The blood supply to the femoral head is carried by a number of arteries that pass through the femoral neck region. Therefore, femoral neck fractures may disrupt the blood supply to the femoral head, causing death of the femoral head bone tissues, called osteonecrosis or avascular necrosis. Femoral neck fractures are further grouped into nondisplaced and displaced fractures by the alignment of the fractured segments in relation to the original anatomic position of the femur [68].

2. Intertrochanteric fractures occur at a lower location than femoral neck fractures, in the area between the greater and lesser trochanters. The trochanters are bony projections where major hip muscles are attached. Intertrochanteric hip fractures occur outside of the joint capsule and are therefore also called extracapsular fracture in the literature. Intertrochanteric fractures are complicated by the pull of the hip muscles on the bony muscle attachments, which can exert competing forces against fractured bone segments and pull them out of alignment. Thus, healing of the fracture in a misaligned position is considered as a complication for intertrochanteric fractures. Intertrochanteric fractures may be further grouped into stable and unstable fractures, depending on the location, number, and size of the fractured bony segments [68].

3. Subtrochanteric fractures occur in the zone about 5 *cm* below the lesser trochanter of the proximal femur. The blood supply to the bone of the subtrochanteric region is not as good as the blood supply to the bone of the intertrochanteric region, and thus subtrochanteric fracture heals more slowly [68]. Similar to the intertrochanteric fractures, subtrochanteric fractures are likely to cause femur misalignment [68].

In more complicated cases, the fracture of the bone can involve more than one of these zones. **Figure 3** shows different types of proximal femur fracture.

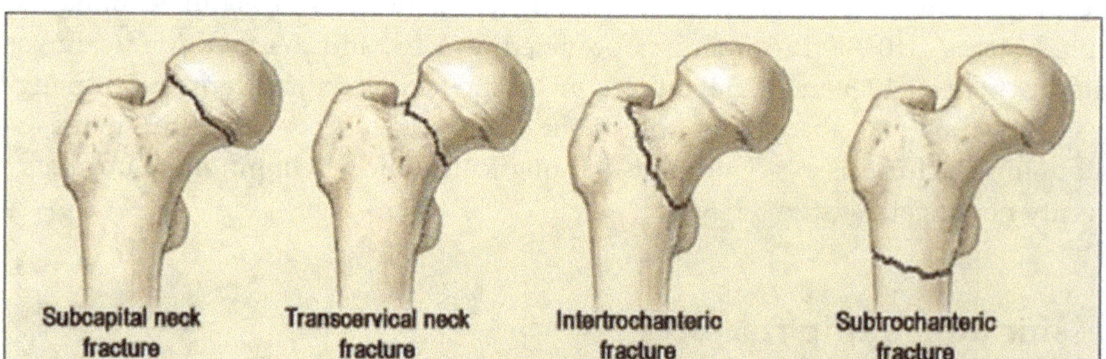

Figure 3. Three main types of hip fractures: femoral neck fracture (subcapital and transcervical fractures), intertrochanteric fracture, and subtrochanteric fracture [69].

6. Demographic feature of hip fractures

A variety of studies have examined hip fracture rates in different regions of the world [10, 51, 52, 70]. Greater than tenfold differences have been found on the basis of studies undertaken at a regional or national level for different calendar years. The studies show that the main demographic risk factors for hip fractures include increased age and female gender [10, 25]. The geographic distribution by fracture risk is shown for men and women combined in **Figure 4**. Heterogeneity in hip fracture risk in countries can be seen in this figure. Based on statistical results [10], for women, the lowest annual incidences are found in Nigeria (2/100,000), South Africa (20), Tunisia (58), and Ecuador (73). The highest rates were observed in Denmark (574/100,000), Norway (563), Sweden (539), and Austria (501). The incidence of hip fracture in men is approximately half of that noted in women. The highest annual incidence in men has been found in Denmark (290/100,000) and the lowest in Ecuador (35/100,000) [10].

As it is shown in **Figure 4**, the high-risk countries are Iceland, the United Kingdom, Ireland, Denmark, Sweden, and Norway in Northwestern Europe; Belgium, Germany, Austria, Switzerland, and Italy in Central Europe; Greece, Hungary, Czech Republic, Slovakia, and Slovenia in southwestern Europe; Lebanon, Oman, Iran, Hong Kong, Singapore, Malta, and Taiwan in Asia; and Argentina in South America. Regions of moderate risk include North America, Oceania, the Russian Federation, and southern countries of Latin America. Low-risk regions include the northern regions of Latin America, Africa, Jordan, Saudi Arabia,

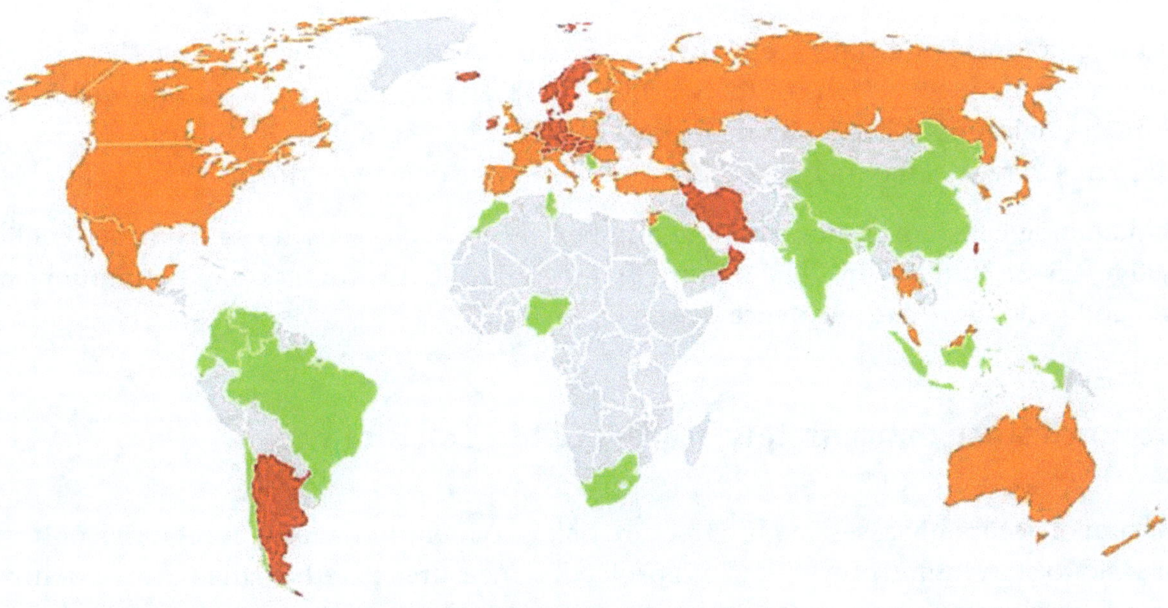

Figure 4. Hip fracture rates (men and women combined) in different countries of the world categorized by risk. Where estimates are available, countries are color-coded red (annual incidence >250/100,000), orange (150–250/100,000), or green (<150/100,000) [10] (reproduced with permission).

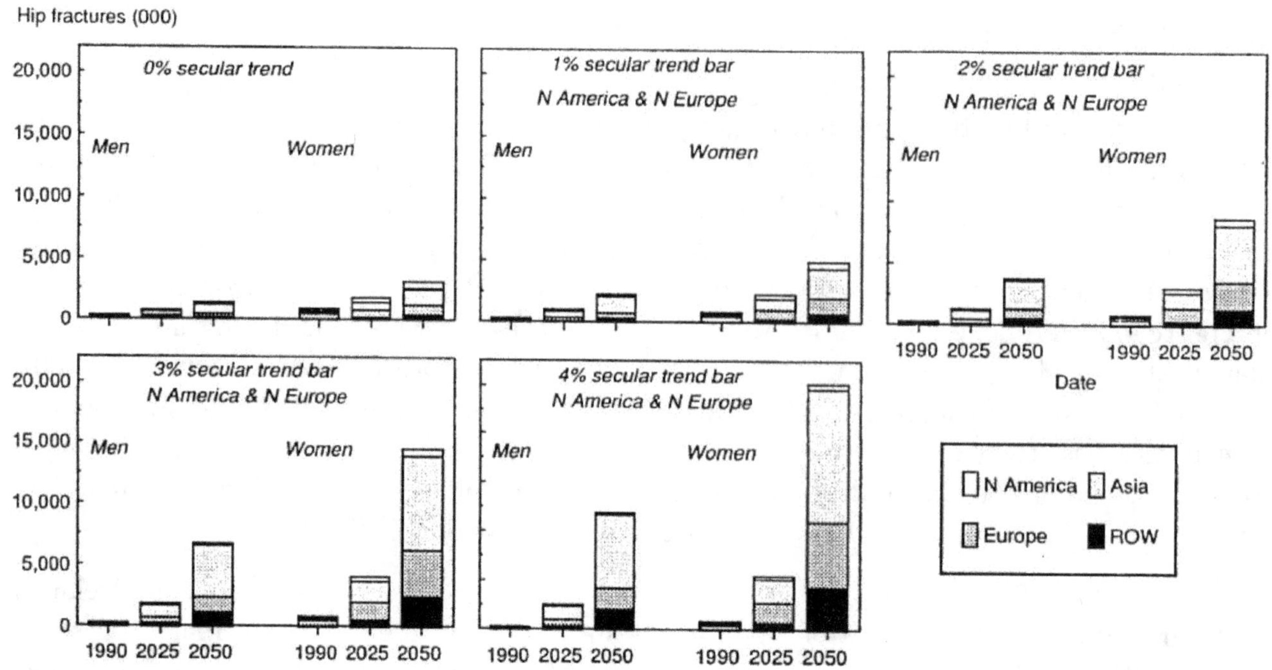

Figure 5. Estimated number of hip fractures by sex in the year 1990 and the number expected in 2025 and 2050 by region assuming no increase in age- and sex-specific rates, a 1% annual increase worldwide, or no increase in North America and northern Europe but an increase in age- and sex-specific incidence elsewhere of 2, 3, or 4%. (ROW is rest of world) [25] (reproduced with permission).

India, China, Indonesia, and the Philippines. It is notable that in Europe, the majority of countries are categorized as high or moderate risk. Low risk is identified only in Croatia and Romania [10].

Hip fracture incidence rates are known to increase exponentially with age in both men and women for the most regions of the world [71–74]. The increasing rate of hip fracture in the elderly is mainly associated with their slower reflex response and the inability to effectively use their arms to reduce the energy of the fall and low bone density of the proximal femur [44, 45].

Epidemiological studies show that the number of hip fractures will rise from 1.66 million in 1990 to 4.5–21.3 million by 2050 (**Figure 5**) depending on the underlying assumptions about age- and gender-specific incidence trends [9, 25, 51, 75].

7. Significance of accurately assessing hip fracture risk

The aim of accurately assessing hip fracture risk is to identify patients at high risk of hip fracture and to start intime prevention and protection measures to reduce the number of hip fractures. These measures are accepted by the patients only after they are accurately diagnosed with the high fracture risk. Also, accurate assessment of hip fracture risk is the prerequisite step before starting a therapy. For example, during the process of osteoporosis treatment, it is required to monitor the change of fracture risk and subsequently track the effectiveness of the therapy. By knowing the risk of fracture, people can improve their bone health and change their environment to reduce the likelihood of the fall.

Patients diagnosed with high fracture risk may consider the following prevention measurements:

- Individualized exercise programs:
  - Muscle-strengthening exercises [76]
  - Practicing balance exercises [77]
  - Increasing the lower extremity joint function [32]
- Management of visual impairment:
  - Obtaining maximum vision correction [6, 78]
- Examination of basic neurological function, including mental status, muscle strength, lower extremity peripheral nerves, and reflexes [79]
- Using mobility assisting devices (e.g., walking stick, frames)
- Implementing surveillance and observation strategies

Protection measurements must be provided to patients with high fracture risk, for example:

- Remembering that sideways falling is more likely to result in a hip fracture than falling in other directions [8]:
  - Trying to fall forward or backward not from sides
- Taking steps to reduce the potential energy and subsequently decrease the risk of fracture [80]
- Landing with the aid of hands or rea`chable objects around to break the fall [81]
- Using hip protectors [82–87]
- Environmental modification (e.g., flooring) [31]
- Medication and nutritional improvement:
  - Consuming a calcium-rich diet that provides about 1000 mg (milligrams) daily for men and women up to age 50 [88]. Women over age 50 and men over age 70 should increase their intake to 1200 mg daily from a combination of foods and supplements.
  - Obtaining 600 **IU** (international units = 0.025 μg) of vitamin D daily up to age 70 [88]. Men and women over age 70 should increase their uptake to 800 **IU** daily.
  - 5–15 min' exposure to sunlight 4–6 times per week [89].

8. Bone fracture criterion and hip fracture risk measurement

From biomechanics point of view, assessment of hip fracture under stance loading or lateral impact force has been performed using three criteria: factor of safety (FOS) [90], risk factor

(RF) [70], and fracture risk index (FRI) [91]. In this section, a review is performed on previously adopted bone fracture criteria in both 2D and 3D FE models.

Keyak et al. [90] assessed FOS under two loading conditions: one representing loading during the stance phase of gait and the other simulating the impact from a fall. Their study was based on a 3D FE model generated from CT data of the patient. They calculated FOS to compare the actual element strength with the applied von Mises stress.

Schileo et al. [92] applied maximum principle strain, von Mises stress, and maximum principle stress criteria to calculate risk factor and to predict fracture location of the femur. RF compares the applied stress/strain with the yield one to predict the bone fracture. Lotz et al. [93, 94] also used von Mises stress yield criterion for the cortical bone and crushing-cracking stress criterion for the trabecular bone. The performance of nine stress- and strain-based failure theories in assessment of hip fracture is investigated by Keyak and Rossi [95]. They evaluated the distortion energy (DE), maximum normal stress, maximum normal strain, maximum shear strain, maximum shear stress, Coulomb-Mohr, modified Mohr, Hoffman, and strain-based Hoffman failure theories, using CT-based FE models of the femur [95].

The abovementioned fracture risk measurements are all derived from CT images. The most recent DXA-based fracture risk criterion is proposed by Luo et al. [91]. They calculated the averaged FRI as a ratio between the effective stress (von Mises stress) by applied forces and the allowable stress (yield stress) of the bone over a region of interest (ROI). FRI is a local fracture risk measurement, while FOS and RF are global ones.

Acknowledgements

This chapter is concluded from a research that was supported by Dr. Yunhua Luo, and therefore, he is gratefully acknowledged.

Conflict of interest

Masoud Nasiri Sarvi declares that he has no conflict of interest.

Author details

Masoud Nasiri Sarvi[1,2]*

*Address all correspondence to: nasirism@myumanitoba.ca

1 Faculty of Engineering, Department of Mechanical Engineering, University of Manitoba, Canada

2 AI Incorporated, Toronto, Canada

References

[1] Shao CJ, Hsieh YH, Tsai CH, Lai KA. A nationwide seven-year trend of hip fractures in the elderly population of Taiwan. Bone. 2009;**44**:125-129

[2] Green C, Molony D, Fitzpatrick C, ORourke K. Age-specific incidence of hip fracture in the elderly: A healthy decline. The Surgeon. 2010;**8**:310-313

[3] Gronskag AB, Forsmo S, Romundstad P, Langhammer A, Schei B. Incidence and seasonal variation in hip fracture incidence among elderly women in Norway. The HUNT study. Bone. 2010;**46**:1294-1298

[4] Alvarez-Nebreda ML, Jimenez AB, Rodriguez P, Serra JA. Epidemiology of hip fracture in the elderly in Spain. Bone. 2008;**42**:278-285

[5] Wilson RT, Chase GA, Chrischilles EA, Wallace RB. Hip fracture risk among community-dwelling elderly people in the United States: A prospective study of physical, cognitive, and socioeconomic indicators. American Journal of Public Health. 2006;**96**:1210-1218

[6] Marks R, Allegrante JP, Ronald MacKenzie C, Lane JM. Hip fractures among the elderly: Causes, consequences and control. Ageing Research Reviews. 2003;**2**:57-93

[7] Testi D, Viceconti M, Baruffaldi F, Cappello A. Risk of fracture in elderly patients: A new predictive index based on bone mineral density and finite element analysis. Computer Methods and Programs in Biomedicine. 1999;**60**:23-33

[8] Greenspan SL, Myers ER, Kiel DP, Parker RA, Hayes WC, Resnick NM. Fall direction, bone mineral density, and function: Risk factors for hip fracture in frail nursing home elderly. The American Journal of Medicine. 1998;**104**:539-545

[9] Cooper C, Campion G, LJ MI. Hip fractures in the elderly: A world-wide projection. Osteoporosis International. 1992;**2**:285-259

[10] Kanis JA, Oden A, McCloskey EV, Johansson H, Wahl DA, Cooper C. A systematic review of hip fracture incidence and probability of fracture worldwide. Osteoporosis International. 2012;**23**:2239-2256

[11] Nasiri Sarvi M, Luo Y. Sideways fall-induced impact force and its effect on hip fracture risk: A review. Osteoporosis International. 2017;**28**:2759-2780

[12] Nasiri M, Luo Y. Study of sex differences in the association between hip fracture risk and body parameters by DXA-based biomechanical modeling. Bone. 2016;**90**:90, 98

[13] Nasiri Sarvi M, Luo Y. A two-level subject-specific biomechanical model for improving prediction of hip fracture risk. Clinical biomechanics. 2015;**30**:881-887

[14] Luo Y, Nasiri Sarvi M. A subject-specific inverse-dynamics approach for estimating joint stiffness in sideways fall. International Journal of Experimental and Computational Biomechanics. 2015;**3**:137-160

[15] Nasiri Sarvi M. Assessment of hip fracture risk by a two-level subject-specific biomechanical model. Ph.D. thesis. Canada: Mechanical Engineering, University of Manitoba; 2015. p. 164

[16] Nasiri SM, Luo Y. Development of an image-based biomechanical model for assessment of hip fracture risk. In: ASME 2015 International Design Engineering Technical Conferences and Computers and Information in Engineering Conference, IDETC/CIE; Boston; 2015

[17] Nasiri SM, Luo Y. A compound risk indicator for subject-specific prediction of hip fracture in sideways falls. In: ASME 2015 International Design Engineering Technical Conferences and Computers and Information in Engineering Conference, IDETC/CIE 2015; Boston, 2015

[18] Luo Y, Nasiri Sarvi M, Sun P, Ouyang J. A subject specific dynamics model for predicting impact force in elderly lateral fall. Applied Mechanics and Materials. 2014;**446-447**:339-343

[19] Luo Y, Nasiri Sarvi M, Sun P, Leslie WD, Ouyang J. Prediction of impact force in sideways fall by image-based subject-specific dynamics model. International Biomechanics. 2014:1-14

[20] Nasiri Sarvi M, Luo Y, Sun P, Ouyang J. Experimental validation of subject-specific dynamics model for predicting impact force in sideways fall. Journal of Biomedical Science and Engineering. 2014;**7**:405-418

[21] Nasiri Sarvi M, Luo Y. Estimation of body segment masses using whole-body DXA image. In: 24th CANCAM Conference, June 2-6, 2013; Saskatoon

[22] WHO. Assessment of fracture risk and its application to screening for osteoporosis. WHO technical report series 843 1994; Geneva

[23] Sernbo I, Johnell O. Consequences of a hip fracture: A prospective study over 1 year. Osteoporosis International. 1993;**3**:148-153

[24] Chrischilles E, Butler C, Davis C, Wallace R. A model of lifetime osteoporosis impact. Archives of Internal Medicine. 1991;**151**:2026-2032

[25] Gullberg B, Johnell O, Kanis JA. World-wide projections for hip fracture. Osteoporosis International. 1997;**7**:407-413

[26] Roche JJW, Wenn RT, Sahota O, Moran CG. Effect of comorbidities and postoperative complications on mortality after hip fracture in elderly people: Prospective observational cohort study. British Medical Journal. 2005;**331**:1-5

[27] Boonen S, Autier P, Barette M, Vanderschueren D, Lips P, Haentjens P. Functional outcome and quality of life following hip fracture in elderly women: A prospective controlled study. Osteoporosis International. 2004;**15**:87-94

[28] Lieberman D, Friger M, Fried V, Grinshpun Y, Mytlis N, Tylis R, Galinsky D. Characterization of elderly patients in rehabilitation: Stroke versus hip fracture. Disability and Rehabilitation. 1999;**21**:542-547

[29] Phy MP, Vanness DJ, Melton L, Long KH, et al. Effects of a hospitalist model on elderly patients with hip fracture. Archives of Internal Medicine. 2005;**165**:796-801

[30] Huddleston JM, Whitford KJ. Medical care of elderly patients with hip fractures. Mayo Clinic Proceedings. 2001;**76**:295-298

[31] Majumder S, Roychowdhury A, Pal S. Hip fracture and anthropometric variations: Dominance among trochanteric soft tissue thickness, body height and body weight during sideways fall. Clinical biomechanics. 2013;**28**:1034-1040

[32] Van den Kroonenberg AJ, Hayes WC, McMahon TA. Hip impact velocities and body configurations for voluntary falls from standing height. Journal of Biomechanics. 1996;**29**:807-811

[33] Roberts BJ, Thrall E, Muller JA, Bouxsein ML. Comparison of hip fracture risk prediction by femoral aBMD to experimentally measured factor of risk. Bone. 2010;**46**:742-746

[34] Marieb EN, Mallatt J. Human Anatomy and Physiology. Pearson plc; 2002

[35] Hirshorn K. http://stpetehipandknee.com/anatomy-hip-joint/. 2014

[36] Cumming R, Klineberg R. Fall frequency and characteristics and the risk of hip fractures. Journal of the American Geriatrics Society. 1994;**42**:774-778

[37] Ford CM, Keaveny TM, Hayes WC. The effect of impact direction on the structural capacity of the proximal femur during falls. Journal of Bone and Mineral Research. 1996;**11**:377-383

[38] Parker MJ. Fractures of the hip. Surgery (Oxford). 2003;**21**:221-224

[39] Zioupos P, Wang XT, Currey JD. Experimental and theoretical quantification of the development of damage in fatigue tests of bone and antler. Journal of Biomechanics. 1996;**29**:989-1002

[40] Youm T, Koval KJ, Kummer FJ, Zuckerman JD. Do all hip fractures result from a fall? American Journal of Orthopedics. 1999;**28**:190-194

[41] Teppo LNJ, Harri S, Karim MK, Ari H, Pekka K. Shifting the focus in fracture prevention from osteoporosis to falls. BMJ. 2008;**336**:124-126

[42] Cummings SR, Melton LJ. Epidemiology and outcomes of osteoporotic fractures. The Lancet. 2002;**359**:1761-1767

[43] Kannus P, Leiponen P, Parkkari J, Palvanen M, Jarvinen M. A sideways fall and hip fracture. Bone. 2006;**39**:383-384

[44] Greenspan SL, Myers ER, Maitland LA, Resnick NM, Hayes WC. FAll severity and bone mineral density as risk factors for hip fracture in ambulatory elderly. JAMA. 1994;**271**:128-133

[45] Sabick MB, Hay JG, Goel VK, Banks SA. Active responses decrease impact forces at the hip and shoulder in falls to the side. Journal of Biomechanics. 1999;**32**:993-998

[46] Kanis JA. Diagnosis of osteoporosis and assessment of fracture risk. The Lancet. 2002;**359**:1929-1936

[47] Carpintero P, Caeiro JR, Carpintero R, Morales A, Silva S, Mesa M. Complications of hip fractures: A review. World Journal of Orthopedics. 2014;**5**:402-411

[48] Rizzoli R, Bruyere O, Cannata-Andia JB, Devogelaer JP, Lyritis G, Ringe JD, Vellas B, Reginster JY. Management of osteoporosis in the elderly. Current Medical Research and Opinion. 2009;**25**:2373-2387

[49] Jee W. Integrated bone tissue physiology: Anatomy and physiology. In: Cowin Bone Mechanics Handbook. New York: Informa Healthcare; 2001

[50] Cummings SR, Nevitt MC, Browner WS, Stone K, Fox KM, Ensrud KE, Cauley J, Black D, Vogt TM. Risk factors for hip fracture in white women. New England Journal of Medicine. 1995;**332**:767-774

[51] Fisher AA, O'Brien ED, Davis MW. Trends in hip fracture epidemiology in Australia: Possible impact of bisphosphonates and hormone replacement therapy. Bone. 2009;**45**:246-253

[52] Johnell O, Kanis JA. An estimate of the worldwide prevalence and disability associated with osteoporotic fractures. Osteoporosis International. 2006;**17**:1726-1733

[53] Brauer CA, Coca-Perraillon M, Cutler DM, Rosen AB. Incidence and mortality of hip fractures in the United States. The Journal of the American Medical Association. 2009;**302**:1573-1579

[54] Leibson CL, Tosteson ANA, Gabriel SE, Ransom JE, Melton LJ. Mortality, disability, and nursing home use for persons with and without hip fracture: A population-based study. Journal of the American Geriatrics Society. 2002;**50**:1644-1650

[55] Haentjens P, Magaziner J, Colon-Emeric CS, Vanderschueren D, Milisen K, Velkeniers B, Boonen S. Meta-analysis: Excess mortality after hip fracture among older women and men. Annals of Internal Medicine. 2010;**152**:380-390

[56] Greendale G, Barrett-Connor E. Outcomes of Osteoporotic Fractures. 2nd ed. San Diego: Academic Press; 2001

[57] Ross PD. Clinical consequences of vertebral fractures. The American Journal of Medicine. 1997;**103**:S30-S43

[58] Gold D, Lyles K, Shipp K, Drezner M. Osteoporosis and its Nonskeletal Consequences: Their Impact on Treatment Decisions. 2nd ed. San Diego: Academic Press; 2001

[59] Gallup. Osteoporosis Prevalence Figures; State-By-State Report. Washington, D.C.: National Osteoporosis Foundation; 1997

[60] Tosteson ANA, Gabriel SE, Grove MR, Moncur MM, Kneeland TS, Melton Iii LJ. Impact of hip and vertebral fractures on quality-adjusted life years. Osteoporosis International. 2001;**12**:1042-1049

[61] Phillips S, Fox N, Jacobs J, Wright WE. The direct medical costs of osteoporosis for American women aged 45 and older. Bone. 1988;**9**:271-279

[62] Lonnroos E, Kautiainen H, Karppi P, Huusko T, Hartikainen S, Kiviranta I, Sulkava R. Increased incidence of hip fractures. A population based-study in Finland. Bone. 2006;**39**:623-627

[63] Wiktorowicz ME, Goeree R, Papaioannou A, Adachi JD, Papadimitropoulos E. Economic implications of hip fracture: Health service use, institutional care and cost in Canada. Osteoporosis International. 2001;**12**:271-278

[64] Dy CJ, McCollister KE, Lubarsky DA, Lane JM. An economic evaluation of a systems-based strategy to expedite surgical treatment of hip fractures. The Journal of Bone & Joint Surgery. 2011;**93**:1326-1334

[65] Hayes WC, Myers ER, Robinovitch SN, Van Den Kroonenberg A, Courtney AC, McMahon TA. Etiology and prevention of age-related hip fractures. Bone. 1996;**18**:S77-S86

[66] Kannus P, Parkkari J, Sievänen H, Heinonen A, Vuori I, Järvinen M. Epidemiology of hip fractures. Bone. 1996;**18**:S57-S63

[67] An YH, Draughn RA. Mechanical Testing of Bone and the Bone-Implant Interface. Florida: CRC Press; 2000. pp. 407-438

[68] Butler M, Forte M, Kane R. Treatment of common hip fractures. Evidence Report/Technology Assessment. 2009;**184**:1-85

[69] Peters M. http://advancedortho.net/info/hipfractureinfo.php. 2000

[70] Dhanwal D, Dennison E, Harvey N, Cooper C. Epidemiology of hip fracture: Worldwide geographic variation. Indian Journal of Orthopaedics. 2011;**45**:15-22

[71] Melton LJ. Hip fractures: A worldwide problem today and tomorrow. Bone. 1993;**14**:1-8

[72] Jacobsen SJ, Goldberg J, Miles TP. Hip fracture among the old and very old: A population-based study of 745 435 cases. The American Journal of Public Health. 1990;**80**:871-873

[73] Cummings SR, Black DM, Rubin SM. Lifetime risks of hip, colles, or vertebral fracture and coronary heart disease among white postmenopausal women. Archives of Internal Medicine. 1989;**149**:2445-2448

[74] Melton JL. Perspectives: How many women have osteoporosis now? Journal of Bone and Mineral Research. 1995;**10**:175-177

[75] Winner SJ, Morgan CA, Evans JG. Perimenopausal risk of falling and incidence of distal forearm fracture. BMJ. 1989;**298**:1486-1488

[76] Iwamoto J, Takeda T, Sato Y. Effect of muscle strengthening exercises on the muscle strength in patients with osteoarthritis of the knee. The Knee. 2007;**14**:224-230

[77] Wijlhuizen GJ, de Jong R, Hopman-Rock M. Older persons afraid of falling reduce physical activity to prevent outdoor falls. Preventive Medicine. 2007;**44**:260-264

[78] Chang WW, Friedman S. Hip fracture management. Hospital Medicine Clinics. 2013;**2**:e399-e421

[79] Kubota M, Uchida K, Kokubo Y, Shimada S, Matsuo H, Yayama T, Miyazaki T, Sugita D, Watanabe S, Baba H. Postoperative gait analysis and hip muscle strength in patients with pelvic ring fracture. Gait & Posture. 2013;**38**:385-390

[80] Groen BE, Weerdesteyn V, Duysens J. Martial arts fall techniques decrease the impact forces at the hip during sideways falling. Journal of Biomechanics. 2007;**40**:458-462

[81] Van der Zijden AM, Groen BE, Tanck E, Nienhuis B, Verdonschot N, Weerdesteyn V. Can martial arts techniques reduce fall severity? An in vivo study of femoral loading configurations in sideways falls. Journal of Biomechanics. 2012;**45**:1650-1655

[82] Derler S, Spierings AB, Schmitt KU. Anatomical hip model for the mechanical testing of hip protectors. Medical Engineering & Physics. 2005;**27**:475-485

[83] Holzer G, Holzer L. Hip protectors and prevention of hip fractures in older persons. Geriatrics. 2007;**62**:15-22

[84] Holzer LA, von Skrbensky G, Holzer G. Mechanical testing of different hip protectors according to a European standard. Injury. 2009;**40**:1172-1175

[85] Laing AC, Robinovitch SN. The force attenuation provided by hip protectors depends on impact velocity, pelvic size, and soft tissue stiffness. Journal of Biomechanical Engineering. 2008;**130**:1-9

[86] Li N, Tsushima E, Tsushima H. Comparison of impact force attenuation by various combinations of hip protector and flooring material using a simplified fall-impact simulation device. Journal of Biomechanics. 2013;**46**:1140-1146

[87] Robinovitch SN, Evans SL, Minns J, Laing AC, Kannus P, Cripton PA, Derler S, Birge SJ, Plant D, Cameron ID, Kiel DP, Howland J, Khan K, Lauritzen JB. Hip protectors: Recommendations for biomechanical testing-an international consensus statement (part I). Osteoporosis International. 2009;**20**:1977-1988

[88] Lilliu H, Pamphile R, Chapuy M-C, Schulten J, Arlot M, Meunier PJ. Calcium-vitamin D3 supplementation is cost-effective in hip fractures prevention. Maturitas. 2003;**44**:299-305

[89] Ascherio A, Munger KL, Simon KC. Vitamin D and multiple sclerosis. The Lancet Neurology. 2010;**9**:599-612

[90] Keyak JH, Rossi SA, Jones KA, Skinner HB. Prediction of femoral fracture load using automated finite element modeling. Journal of Biomechanics. 1998;**31**:125-133

[91] Luo Y, Ferdous Z, Leslie WD. Precision study of DXA-based patient-specific finite element modeling for assessing hip fracture risk. International Journal for Numerical Methods in Biomedical Engineering. 2013;**29**:615-629

[92] Schileo E, Taddei F, Cristofolini L, Viceconti M. Subject-specific finite element models implementing a maximum principal strain criterion are able to estimate failure risk and fracture location on human femurs tested in vitro. Journal of Biomechanics. 2008;**41**:356-367

[93] Lotz JC, Cheal EJ, Hayes WC. Fracture prediction for the proximal femur using finite element models: Part I-linear analysis. Journal of Biomechanical Engineering. 1991;**113**:353-360

[94] Lotz JC, Cheal EJ, Hayes WC. Fracture prediction for the proximal femur using finite element models: Part II-nonlinear analysis. Journal of Biomechanical Engineering. 1991;**113**:361-365

[95] Keyak JH, Rossi SA. Prediction of femoral fracture load using finite element models: An examination of stress- and strain-based failure theories. Journal of Biomechanics. 2000;**33**:209-214

12

Anterior Primary Total Hip Arthroplasty

Ulrich Bechler, Bernhard Springer and
Friedrich Boettner

Abstract

Total hip arthroplasty (THA) is the preferred treatment for end-stage osteoarthritis of the hip. The posterior, posterolateral, direct lateral, anterolateral, or the anterior approaches are the currently established surgical approaches for THA. Over the last decade, the anterior approach has gained increasing popularity. Its muscle-sparing nature and fluoroscopy-guided component positioning are the most important benefits. It has been suggested that postoperative recovery is facilitated by an anterior approach. Patients do not need to follow hip precautions, and can return to driving after 1 week. The anterior approach uses a muscle interval between the tensor fasciae latae and the rectus femoris to open the capsule without detachment of muscles. Especially, the external rotators and posterior capsule remain intact and reduce the risk of posterior dislocation. Accuracy of acetabular component positioning has an impact on postoperative dislocation rates, polyethylene wear, and impingement. When the operation is done in a supine position, fluoroscopy is available to check the acetabular component inclination and anteversion during THA as well as leg length and offset. The current chapter reports on the surgical approach, surgical technique, and results of anterior THA.

Keywords: primary total hip arthroplasty, minimally invasive surgery, anterior approach, osteoarthritis, intraoperative fluoroscopy, outcome

1. Introduction

THA is used to treat a variety of primary and secondary end-stage osteoarthritis, and has the primary goal to decrease pain, restore function, and increase joint mobility [1]. Depending on the specific patient there are various surgical techniques described to perform a THA. The general goal is to have an accurate and reproducible procedure and to avoid complications. Younger and more active patients have increased functional demands during early recovery. Utilizing an intramuscular approach allows for a faster return to activities of daily living, reduced pain, shortened recovery, and reduced costs [1].

The various available approaches are characterized by their own distinct advantages and risks. Extensions to these approaches have been described and allow for more extensive exposure and revision procedures.

In the USA, the most frequently used approach is the posterior approach. It provides easy access to the hip joint and minimizes the trauma to the hip abductor muscles. However, detachment of external rotator muscles and a complete capsulectomy results in an increased dislocation rate [2, 3]. Therefore, the repair of the external rotators and the capsule is of great importance in posterior THA [4]. In addition, the posterior approach is associated with an increased variance of acetabular component positioning [5–7]. Poor component positioning increases the risk of dislocation, facilitates increased polyethylene wear, and impingement [5, 8, 9]. Variations in the lateral patient position and the lack of intraoperative fluoroscopy might explain the less predictable cup positioning [10].

The lateral approach (anterolateral) with the patient lying in a supine position is a popular approach in Europe. The posterior part of the gluteus medius insertion can be preserved. However, injury or release of its anterior portion can result in limping [11]. Fractures of the greater trochanter are more likely using the lateral approach compared to the posterior approach [12, 13]. Postoperative patient-reported limping occurs twice as often using the lateral approach compared to the anterior approach [14]. Limping may be caused by trochanteric pain, leg length discrepancy, lack of offset restoration, nerve injury, or insufficiency of the gluteal muscles [15].

The anterior THA is unique because of its intramuscular and internervous exposure of the hip joint. A release of major muscular stabilizers is not necessary for most patients. First described by Smith-Peterson in 1949, the anterior approach became more popular in the USA over the last decade [16]. Rapid recovery, decreased dislocation rate, fluoroscopy controlled restoration of leg length, and offset as well as component position are its main benefits.

2. History

In 1881, Carl Hueter was the first surgeon to describe the anterior approach for resection of the femoral head. Smith-Peterson further developed the approach and described the extended exposure of the pelvis to perform a hip replacement. In 1978, Wagner preferred the approach for hip resurfacing procedures due to its preservation of the femoral blood supply and intermuscular dissection [17]. In 1947, the Judet table was developed and predominantly used in France. Ten years later, a special table was developed to optimize and ease the positioning of the operated leg in order to decrease injury to muscles and bone.

In the US, the anterior approach was originally combined with a lateral incision to facilitate the insertion of the femoral component and was marketed by Zimmer Biomet (Warsaw, IN, USA) in conjunction with Richard Berger as a "two incision" THA [1, 18]. Because of the higher complication rate, especially on the femoral side (fracture), the approach fell out of favor in the beginning of the twenty-first century [19]. At the same time, Joel Matta promoted an anterior approach without a second incision [20]. Matta soon realized that a special table similar to the Judet table was needed to improve exposure of the femur and provide elevation of the femur. Since the Judet table was not available in the USA, he pursued the development of the Hana® table (Mizuho OSI, Union City, CA, USA).

In 2004, large studies [20, 21] showed encouraging outcomes with low dislocation rate (<1%) and improved component positioning, but above all faster recovery pushed the interest in the anterior approach.

3. Anatomy and approach

The anterior approach classically described as Smith-Peterson approach uses an incision proximal and distal to the anterior superior iliac spine (ASIS) along the tensor fasciae latae [16]. While the proximal portion of the Smith-Peterson approach facilitates exposure of the pelvis, the distal portion is used during a direct anterior THA to expose the hip joint. The groin area usually has less subcutaneous fat than the lateral thigh, and therefore an anterior approach often has a more direct access to the fascial layer. The ASIS and greater trochanter are used as bony landmarks to guide placement of the incision. The incision usually starts

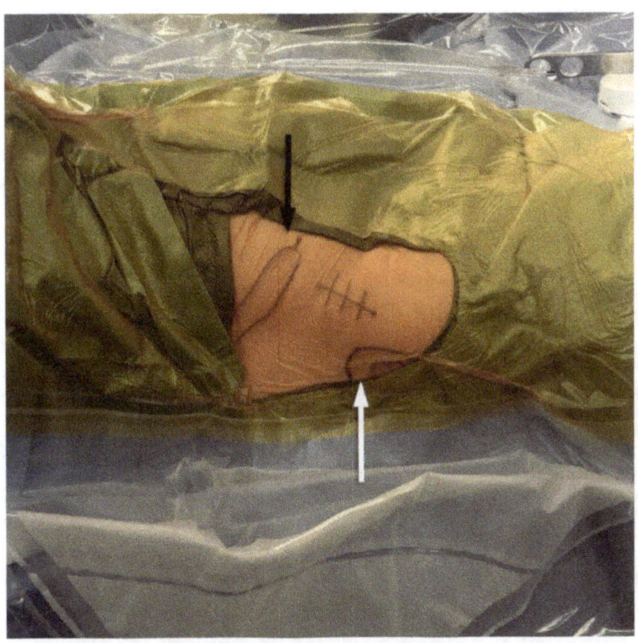

Figure 1. Patient in a supine position on a Hana® table. The skin incision, the anterior superior iliac spine (black arrow), and greater trochanter (white arrow) are marked.

two fingerbreadths lateral and distal of the ASIS and extends distally and posteriorly in line with the tensor fasciae latae muscle [20]. A slightly more lateral position can help to avoid the lateral femoral cutaneous nerve (LFCN) that enters the thigh medially to the ASIS (**Figure 1**).

The approach uses an intermuscular plane and does not require muscle releases. Medially, the interval borders to the Sartorius muscle (innervated by the femoral nerve) and laterally to the tensor fasciae latae muscle (innervated by the superior gluteal nerve) [22]. While the original Smith-Petersen approach entered between the sartorius muscle and the tensor fasciae latae, the modern anterior approach usually stays inside the fascia of the tensor fasciae latae to minimize the risk to injure the LFCN (**Figure 2**) [22]. Care should be taken not to confuse the medial located sartorius muscle and the more lateral tensor fasciae latae. Both can usually, easily be separated by the direction of the fibers. The tensor fasciae latae muscle fibers ran toward the lateral thigh in contrast to the sartorius muscle fibers, which run medially. After skin incision, the fascia of the tensor is split followed by deep finger dissection to separate the overlying fascia and the muscle belly of the tensor fasciae latae and progress toward its medial borders.

The deep intermuscular fat tissue between tensor and rectus femoris muscle contains the ascending branch of the lateral circumflex artery just proximal to the vastus lateralis muscle. At the level of the capsule, the interval is bordered by the gluteus medius (superior gluteal nerve) and medially by the rectus femoris muscle (femoral nerve). Ligations of the branches of the circumflex vessels are necessary to prevent perioperative bleeding and postoperative hematoma formation (**Figure 3**).

A Hohmann retractor is used to expose the anterior hip capsule. It is placed underneath the rectus muscle. A second blunt retractor is placed around the lateral femoral neck. The reflected head of the rectus femoris muscle is elevated and released to expose the capsule entirely. The released tendon can be marked to facilitate its identification and repair at the end of the procedure.

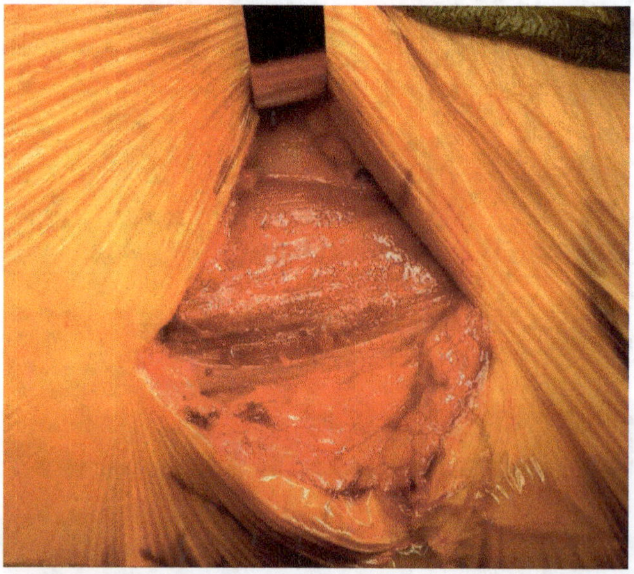

Figure 2. Incision of the fascia of the tensor fasciae latae muscle.

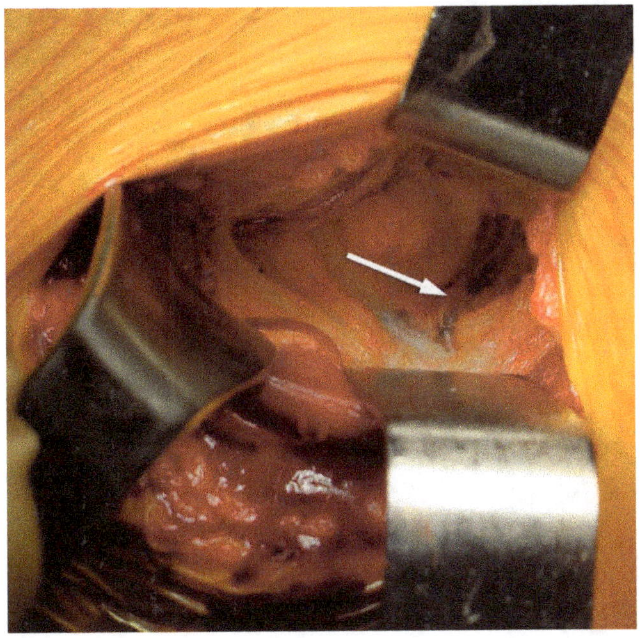

Figure 3. Image of the deep interval bordered laterally by the gluteus medius (superior gluteal nerve) and medially by the rectus femoris muscle (femoral nerve). The lateral femoral circumflex vessels (arrow) are visualized proximal to the vastus lateralis muscle.

4. Surgical technique

The procedure is performed under general or regional anesthesia. It can be performed with a standard operating table with an Omni-Tract® femur elevating system (Integra, Plainsboro, NJ, USA) or a specialized orthopedic table (Hana®, Mizuho OSI, Union City, CA, USA). The latter helps to control hip rotation, abduction, flexion, and traction of the affected extremity and facilitates exposure of the proximal femur for femoral component insertion. However, the costs, fracture risk, and limited ability to intraoperatively test the range of motion (ROM) are its main disadvantages. A number of alternative tables are currently available by other manufactures.

The authors recommend careful templating and implant selection. The primary goal of the templating is to guide acetabular reaming toward the most appropriate reamer size. On the femoral side, depending on the type of femur, shorter implants with less sizable distal dimensions might be preferred in a Dorr Type A Femur, while compression broaching for a longer implant with a collar might be preferred for a Dorr Type C femur [23]. In addition, careful planning of the femoral neck resection can help intraoperatively to restore the leg length.

The patient is lying supine on the table with a perineal post and both legs secured with the feet in boots. The pelvis and the nonsurgical hip are placed in a neutral position. After the standard anterior approach, as described above, a T-shaped capsulotomy is performed with medial and lateral extension at the level of the intertrochanteric ridge (**Figure 4**). The capsule can be tagged and preserved for later repair. Two Hohmann retractors are now placed within the capsule around the lateral and medial femoral neck. A napkin ring double osteotomy of the femoral neck is performed to ease removal of the head (**Figure 5**). The femoral head is removed with a corkscrew extractor. Additional traction and external rotation on the operated

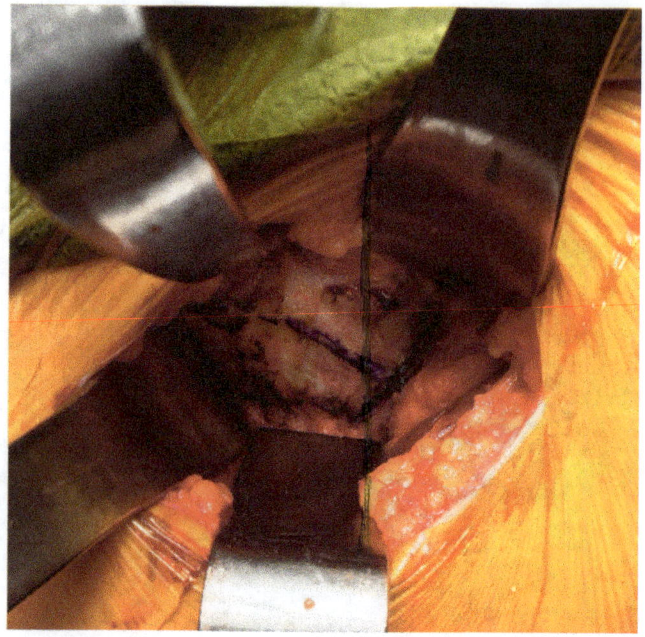

Figure 4. Markings for the T-shaped capsulotomy with medial and lateral extension.

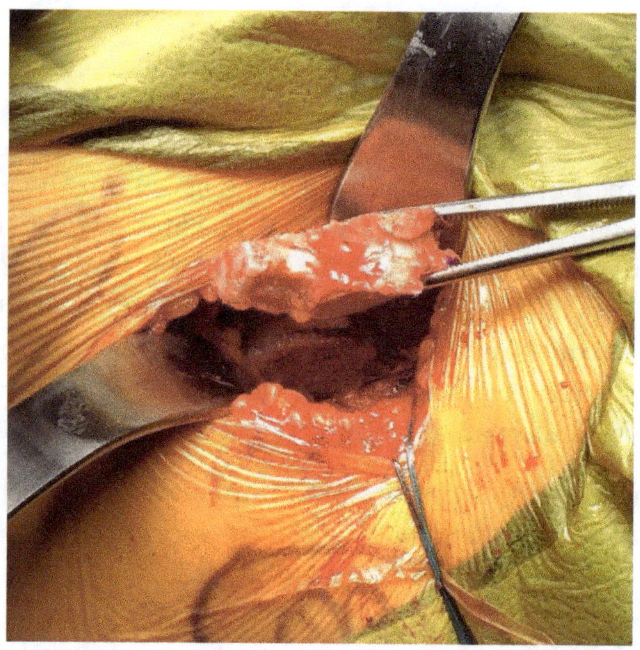

Figure 5. Photograph of a napkin ring double osteotomy of the femoral neck.

leg supports removal of the napkin ring and exposure of the acetabulum. Alternatively, to the *in situ* neck osteotomy, the hip can be dislocated using a corkscrew. The capsular releases are completed with the hip dislocated before the hip is reduced, the neck is cut, and the head removed (technique according to Matta et al. [20]).

Multiple retractors are used to facilitate acetabular exposure. First, an acetabular retractor is placed inferiorly to the fovea against the transverse acetabular ligament. This usually requires a short incision of the medial capsule. This is, followed by an anterior retractor, placed between the anterior labrum and capsule. A posterior retractor can be placed between the posterior labrum and capsule. The foveal tissue and labrum are removed. The acetabulum is either reamed under direct visualization or under fluoroscopy guidance. A press fit cup is placed and impacted (**Figure 6**). To facilitate cup alignment under the anterior acetabular bone, an implant less hemispherical then 180° is preferred. It also helps to medialize the center of rotation in comparison to a hemispherical cup.

The C-arm is used to guide intraoperative component positioning. An alternative to this technique is the use of intraoperative navigation. Because of the supine position and easy access to the iliac crest intraoperative navigation is usually fairly straightforward in anterior THA. Other techniques available for optimized cup position are based on C-arm images and include software programs like Radlink® (Radlink, El Segundo, CA, USA) and Jointpoint® (Jointpoint Inc., Belleair Bluffs, FL, USA).

The C-arm is positioned in 90° to the supine patient and centered over the pelvis to make sure the pelvis is in a neutral position (**Figure 7**). A neutral pelvis position is the requirement for any of the described C-arm based algorithms. If no software is available, the cup inclination can be checked with the C-arm centered in the middle of the pelvis. After reaching the target inclination of the acetabular component, the C-arm is moved over the operated hip. After estimating the cup anteversion based on the opening ellipse, the cup anteversion can be determined based on the C-arm tilt angle described by Boettner et al. and Zingg et al. [6, 24] (**Figure 8**). When aligned perfectly the elliptical shape of the cup presents as a line. The tilt angle can be measured on the C-arm and used to calculate the acetabular anteversion. Following correct acetabular implant positioning, the final liner is inserted and osteophytes are removed.

Exposure of the proximal femur can be facilitated by a standard release to minimize traction forces on the greater trochanter. This prevents intraoperative complications like fractures

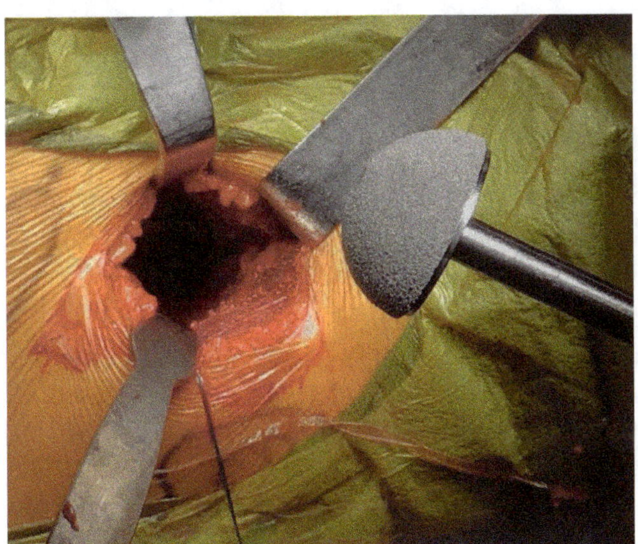

Figure 6. A press fit cup is placed and impacted into the reamed acetabulum.

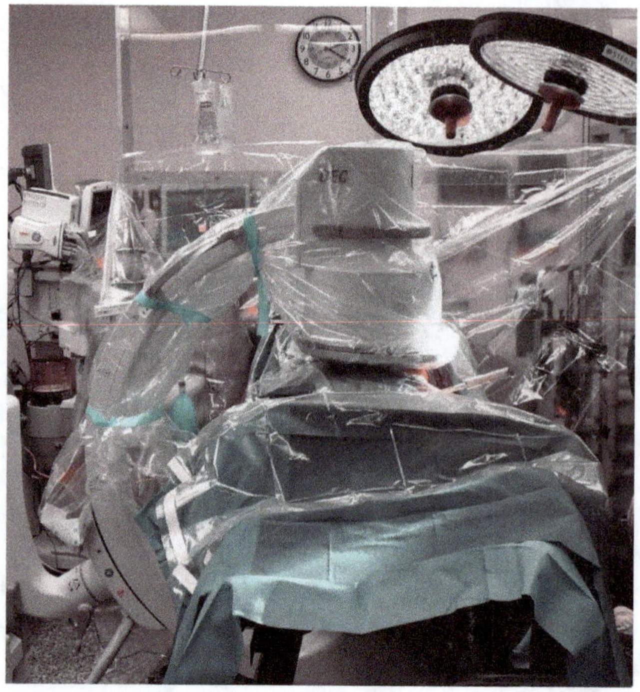

Figure 7. C-arm position in a 90° angle to the supine patient. The beam is centered over the neutral pelvis to assess inclination of the cup.

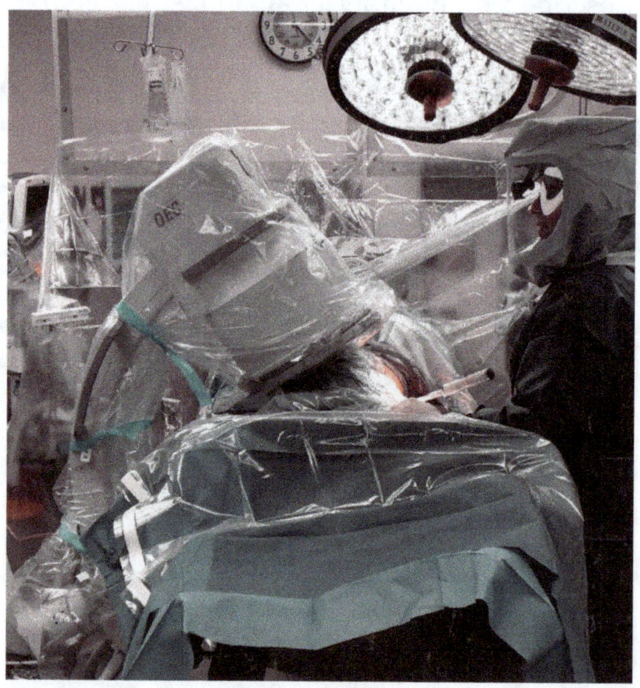

Figure 8. C-arm is tilted away from the operated hip until the ellipse of the positioned acetabular component is a straight line. The tilt angle is measured on the C-arm.

during anterior mobilization of the femur. The gluteus minimus muscle is elevated of the lateral capsule. The operated leg is positioned in extension, 90° external rotation and 20° adduction. In flexible patients adequate exposure might be possible without further releases;

however, the senior author favors the release of the conjoined tendon. The piriformis muscle insertion is preserved together with the posterior capsule, obturator externus muscle, and quadratus femoris muscle.

The Hana table® or Omni-tract® retractor provides a hook attached to a connector arm of the table. In combination with maximum extension of the leg, the hook elevates the femur anteriorly and provides better exposure for the preparation of the femoral component (**Figure 9**). Offset handles facilitate the broaching of the femur. Femoral preparation and broaching the femoral canal is done in a standardized fashion (**Figure 10**). The final trial stem is impacted into the femur with a trial head and neck.

Care should be taken not to injure the tensor fasciae latae. Good exposure to the femoral canal eases preparation and broaching. After adding the trial neck and head, the surgeon can reduce the dislocate hip with gentle traction and internal rotation. The surgeon guides the femoral head into the socket. Fluoroscopy can be used to assess leg length discrepancy, offset, and implant alignment.

For measurements of the leg length discrepancy, the inter-teardrop line is used as horizontal reference of the fluoroscopy image. The difference between the vertical distances from the reference line to the most prominent point on each lesser trochanter defines the leg length discrepancy with reference to the contralateral hip. Neutral pelvis position and equal leg abduction and rotation are required for accurate measurements. Alternatively, leg length and offset can be determined by overlaying two print-out images and comparing the contour of the operated hip to either the opposite normal or the preoperative image. Finally, the definite femoral component is implanted. The wound is irrigated and the anterior capsule closed using Vicryl #0 suture (**Figure 11**). The reflected head of the rectus can be repaired. Finally, the fascia of the tensor fasciae latae muscle is closed with #0 Vicryl sutures (**Figure 12**).

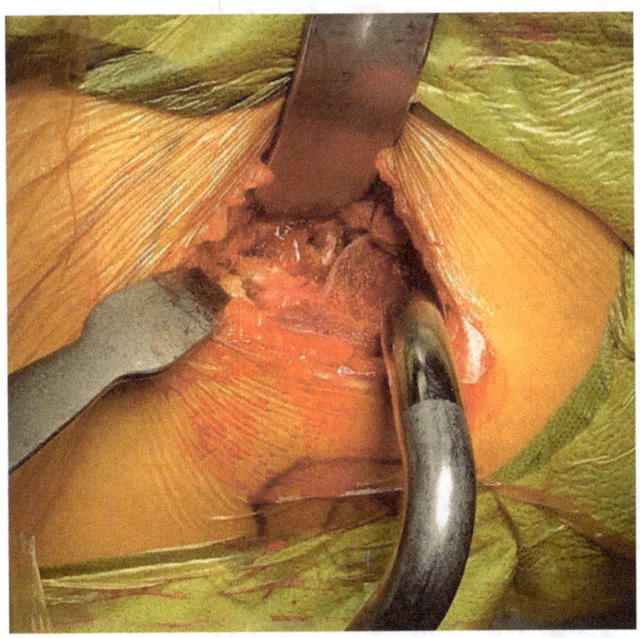

Figure 9. A hook attached to a connector arm of the table facilitates femoral exposure.

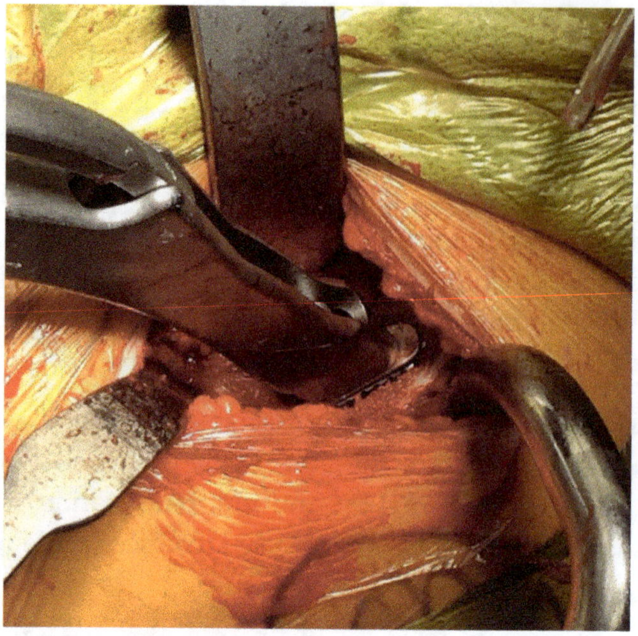

Figure 10. Photograph shows broaching of the femoral component.

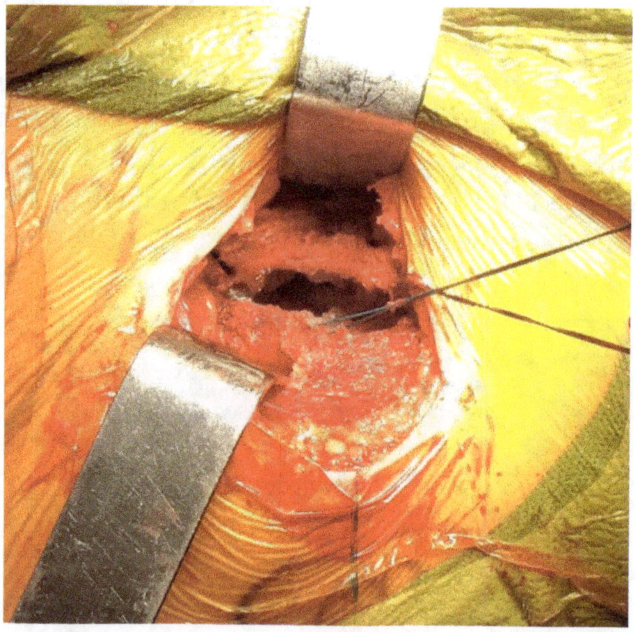

Figure 11. Tagging sutures in the medial and lateral capsular sleeve.

Many surgeons prefer a curved "Banana Type" stem for the anterior approach. Straight stem designs with a lateral shoulder require more aggressive releases including the piriformis tendon. There have been some concerns about increased femoral loosening rates and continued efforts are made to improve and develop femoral implant design. Due to the missing lateral shoulder, the curved stem provides no lateral support. As a result, lateralization and subsidence

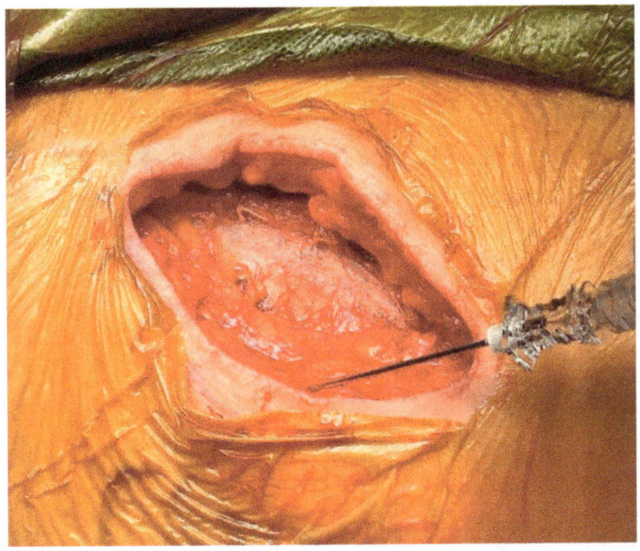

Figure 12. Photograph of the closed fascia of the tensor fasciae latae. A local anesthetic is injected into the subcutaneous layer.

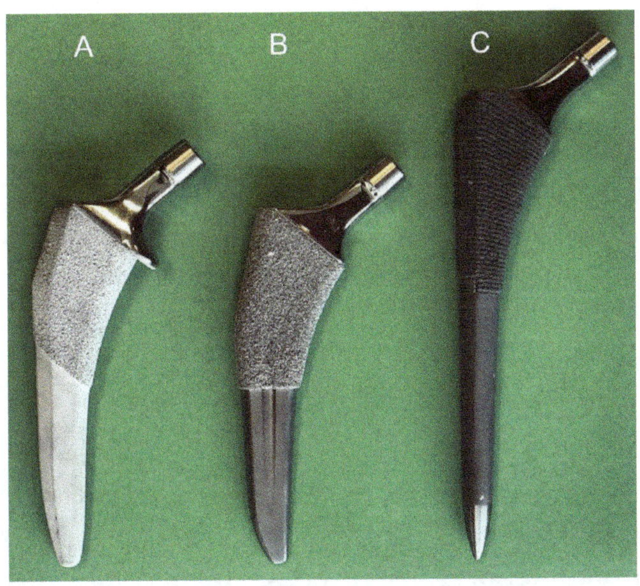

Figure 13. DePuy Synthes, Warsaw, IN, USA: (A) Medial collar and triple tapered ACTIS® Total Hip System. (B) Tapered-wedge TRI-LOCK® Bone Preservation Stem. (C) SUMMIT® Tapered Hip System.

with weight bearing can occur. The new stem designs often add a medial collar to augment primary stability for immediate weight bearing and reduced risk of subsidence (**Figure 13**).

To increase short and long-term stability, fully coated stems are preferred to achieve more reliable fixation. In addition, an overall more canal filling proximal stem design provides more proximal bone fixation compared to blade shaped medial-lateral implant fixation.

5. Standard table

Several advantages exist for the standard table in comparison to the Hana table. The ability to maneuver the legs allow for intraoperative assessment of leg length. The surgeon can directly manage the leg and no additional assistance is required to manage the table. In general, any operative table can be used that is radiolucent and allows for extension of the legs at the level of the hip joint. Regarding the surgical technique, there is no difference in the type of soft tissue releases between a standard or specialized table. The patient is positioned in a supine position with the hip joint at the level of the table break. It is necessary to hyperextend the operated hip during femoral preparation. Draping both lower extremities in a sterile fashion allows an intraoperative crossover of the operated leg for femoral exposure. The leg length discrepancy can be measured manually.

If an anterior retractor is used, the bone hook is inserted with the femur in neutral rotation. Afterward the leg is placed in a figure 4 position (external rotation) to release the medial capsule down to the lesser trochanter. There is no difference in the soft tissue release technique; however, the piriformis usually has to be released in heavy male patients. The distal part of the standard table is extended to 40° allowing hyperextension of the operated hip as well as adduction and external rotation while positioning the limb crossing under the contralateral side.

6. Outcome

Over the last couple of years, the anterior approach has become increasingly popular. Many advantages are described in comparison to the other approaches mentioned at the beginning of this chapter. Patients treated with the minimal invasive approach suffer less pain and consume fewer narcotics [25, 26]. This is usually explained by less soft-tissue damage while avoiding muscle splitting and detachment in comparison to the posterior or anterolateral approach.

An improved hip function and earlier return to normal gait are attributed to using an intermuscular and internervous interval [27, 28]. Rodriguez et al. have shown that patients reach certain milestones after an anterior THA earlier compared to a posterior THA. However, patients with a posterior approach had a similar result after 12 weeks [29].

The possibility of using intraoperative fluoroscopy when performing an anterior THA offers advantages over a posterior THA. The percentage of cup placed in the safe zone increases when using fluoroscopy routinely [6]. A higher precision and increased accuracy when implanting cup components can lead to a decreased dislocation rate [6, 21]. The anterior approach also improves relation of leg length and offset [7].

The majority of hip dislocations occur during the first 3 months after surgery. The healing of the posterior capsule and external rotator muscles release during a conventional posterior approach is considered the reason for early dislocation [30]. Hip precautions are recommended for 4–12 weeks to prevent any flexion and internal rotation after posterior THA [31].

The muscle sparing anterior approach avoids release of the piriformis and obturator externus tendon. No specific hip precautions are needed and the patient is able to return to his or her normal activities after surgery without limitations [32]. The dislocation rate for the anterior THA is described in literature ranges between 0.6 and 0.9% [20, 21]. It is lower in comparison to those reported for other approaches; however, comparative studies have failed to show a consistent benefit [33, 34]. The senior author has no reported dislocations at all after performing more than 500 THAs using an anterior approach.

7. Challenges with the anterior approach

Switching the surgical approach to an anterior THA is associated with a learning curve within the first 40–100 cases [35, 36]. Improvements in surgical and fluoroscopy times as well as differences in leg length have been reported during the learning curve [37, 38]. During the learning curve, it is recommended to carefully select patients. In general, preferred patients are thin and younger females with elongated femoral necks and a type B Dorr Femur.

The anterior approach has some specific complications. These include LFCN injury and greater trochanteric fracture. Injury of LFCN is most commonly encountered during exposure and retraction. The nerve is located in the intermuscular-internervous interval between the sartorius and tensor fasciae latae muscle and is at risk if the incision is extended distally. Its course varies in different branching patterns and is at risk in approximately one-third of the patients during an anterior approach [39]. The risk of an injury can be minimized when staying inside the tensor fascia rather than the interval between the tensor and sartorius muscle [40]. LCFN neurapraxia occurs in approximately 0–5% of patients [41, 42]. None of the patients experienced any hip-related functional limitations, while most symptoms resolving after 6–24 months [37, 43, 44].

Muscle damage has not been considered a major problem due to the intermuscular nature of the approach [45]. Nevertheless, incorrect placement or retraction may cause damage. During capsular exposure the rectus femoris muscle is elevated and at risk. Attention while placing the retractors or using specialized retractors developed for the anterior THA can reduce the risk of soft-tissue damage. During femoral exposure the tensor is at risk for injury as well.

Cup alignment is challenging when performing an anterior THA due to limited view of the anterior acetabular wall. When inserting the reamer into the acetabulum, the anterior aspect of the femur might block its entrance. This may lead to an anterior shift of the reamer and can violate the anterior wall. Careful retractor placement and use of intraoperative fluoroscopy can minimize the risk associated with reaming.

Fractures might occur during femoral preparation, while manipulating on a specialized table [20]. Aggressive extension and external rotation of the femur using the table can result in a fracture of the tip of the greater trochanter secondary to tension of the conjoined tendon. Calcar fractures are the results of medial force on the calcar during broaching and can be fixed with cerclages (**Figure 14**). A rare complication, which might only occur when using a specialized

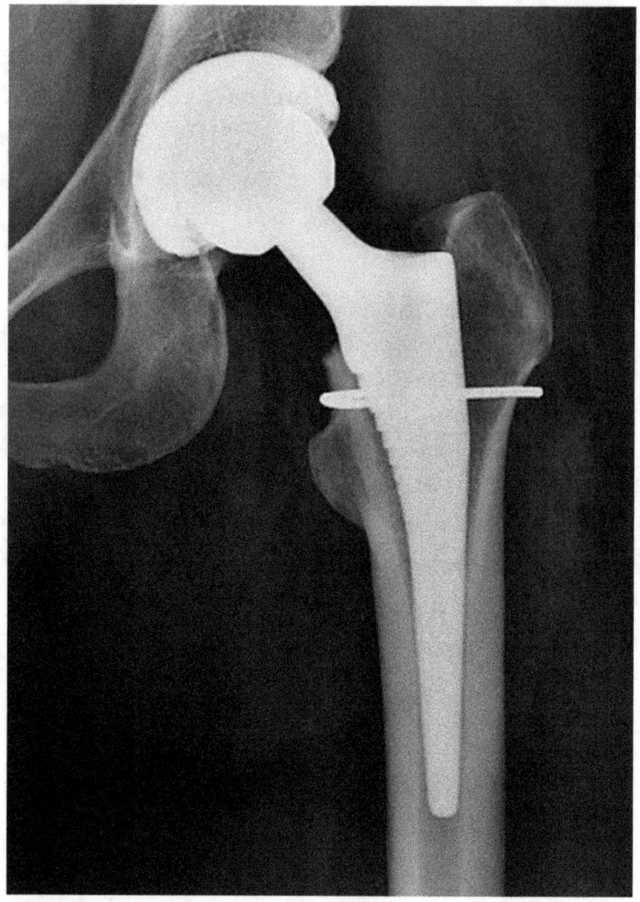

Figure 14. Intraoperative complication: calcar fracture fixed with two cerclages.

table, is a fracture of the ankle while performing external rotation in order to dislocate the operated hip. This is why close monitoring of the torque applied to the fixed leg is necessary.

In general, straight access to the femoral canal is limited in an anterior approach. The correct implant design and broaching instruments are essential and avoid malpositioning or fractures [46]. Perforation of the femur can occur when the direction of the femoral canal is not respected. The risk of postoperative complications in the hand of an experienced surgeon performing an anterior approach is comparable to other approaches.

The dislocation rate for the anterior THA is lower compared to the anterolateral and posterior approach [47]. Preserving the piriformis tendon, obturator externus tendon, and posterior capsule increases the stability when using the anterior approach. Therefore, the routine use of hip precautions for the anterior approach is not recommended [32].

The risk of postoperative hematoma can be minimized by routine exposure and proper ligation of the ascending branches of the lateral femoral circumflex vessels. The vessels are variable in number, location, and extend, but are usually found underneath the deep fascial layer of the tensor fasciae latae. At the end of the procedure, care should be taken for hemostasis. The risk of postoperative drainage can be reduced by meticulous capsular and tensor fasciae closure. Kasparek et al. describes the topical use of tranexamic acid (TXA) to reduce transfusion rates and increase postoperative Hb-levels [48]. For all patients undergoing anterior THA, intravenous TXA should be used as part of blood management. The location of the wound in the groin close to a natural skin fold can result in wound dehiscence and infections in patients with a larger soft tissue pannus overlaying the incision.

8. Conclusion

The popularity of the anterior approach has increased in the last decade. Its soft tissue sparing nature results in a faster recovery and a more stable hip joint. Postoperative precautions are not routinely applied. The use of intraoperative fluoroscopy has improved cup positioning and restoration of the leg length and offset.

Contribution statement

I attest to the fact that all authors have participated in the research, read the manuscript, attest to the validity and legitimacy of the data and its interpretation, and agree to its submission.

Conflict of interest

Dr. Boettner reports personal fees and royalties from Smith & Nephew, personal fees and royalties from Ortho Development Corporation and personal fees form DePuy, outside the submitted work.

We certify that we have not signed any agreement with commercial interest related to this book chapter, which would in any way limit publication for any reason.

Author details

Ulrich Bechler, Bernhard Springer and Friedrich Boettner*

*Address all correspondence to: boettnerf@hss.edu

Adult Reconstruction and Joint Replacement Division, Hospital for Special Surgery, New York, NY, USA

References

[1] Berry DJ, Berger RA, Callaghan JJ, Dorr LD, Duwelius PJ, Hartzband MA, et al. Minimally invasive total hip arthroplasty. Development, early results, and a critical analysis. Presented at the Annual Meeting of the American Orthopaedic Association,

Charleston, South Carolina, USA, June 14, 2003. The Journal of Bone and Joint Surgery. American Volume. 2003;**85-a**(11):2235-2246

[2] Woolson ST, Rahimtoola ZO. Risk factors for dislocation during the first 3 months after primary total hip replacement. The Journal of Arthroplasty. 1999;**14**(6):662-668

[3] L'Hommedieu CE, Gera JJ, Rupp G, Salin JW, Cox JS, Duwelius PJ. Impact of anterior vs posterior approach for total hip arthroplasty on post-acute care service utilization. The Journal of Arthroplasty. 2016;**31**(9 Suppl):73-77

[4] Kwon MS, Kuskowski M, Mulhall KJ, Macaulay W, Brown TE, Saleh KJ. Does surgical approach affect total hip arthroplasty dislocation rates? Clinical Orthopaedics and Related Research. 2006;**447**:34-38

[5] Lewinnek GE, Lewis JL, Tarr R, Compere CL, Zimmerman JR. Dislocations after total hip-replacement arthroplasties. The Journal of Bone and Joint Surgery. American Volume. 1978;**60**(2):217-220

[6] Boettner F, Zingg M, Emara AK, Waldstein W, Faschingbauer M, Kasparek MF. The accuracy of acetabular component position using a novel method to determine anteversion. The Journal of Arthroplasty. 2016;**32**(4):1180-1185

[7] Lin TJ, Bendich I, Ha AS, Keeney BJ, Moschetti WE, Tomek IM. A comparison of radiographic outcomes after total hip arthroplasty between the posterior approach and direct anterior approach with intraoperative fluoroscopy. The Journal of Arthroplasty. 2016

[8] Little NJ, Busch CA, Gallagher JA, Rorabeck CH, Bourne RB. Acetabular polyethylene wear and acetabular inclination and femoral offset. Clinical Orthopaedics and Related Research. 2009;**467**(11):2895-2900

[9] Malik A, Maheshwari A, Dorr LD. Impingement with total hip replacement. The Journal of Bone and Joint Surgery. American Volume. 2007;**89**(8):1832-1842

[10] Rathod PA, Bhalla S, Deshmukh AJ, Rodriguez JA. Does fluoroscopy with anterior hip arthroplasty decrease acetabular cup variability compared with a nonguided posterior approach? Clinical Orthopaedics and Related Research. 2014;**472**(6):1877-1885

[11] Hardinge K. The direct lateral approach to the hip. The Journal of Bone and Joint Surgery. British Volume. 1982;**64**(1):17-19

[12] Nakai T, Liu N, Fudo K, Mohri T, Kakiuchi M. Early complications of primary total hip arthroplasty in the supine position with a modified Watson-Jones anterolateral approach. Journal of Orthopaedics. 2014;**11**(4):166-169

[13] Hendel D, Yasin M, Garti A, Weisbort M, Beloosesky Y. Fracture of the greater trochanter during hip replacement: A retrospective analysis of 21/372 cases. Acta Orthopaedica Scandinavica. 2002;**73**(3):295-297

[14] Amlie E, Havelin LI, Furnes O, Baste V, Nordsletten L, Hovik O, et al. Worse patient-reported outcome after lateral approach than after anterior and posterolateral approach

in primary hip arthroplasty. A cross-sectional questionnaire study of 1,476 patients 1-3 years after surgery. Acta Orthopaedica. 2014;**85**(5):463-469

[15] Sueyoshi T, Meding JB, Davis KE, Lackey WG, Malinzak RA, Ritter MA. Clinical predictors for possible failure after total hip arthroplasty. Hip International: The Journal of Clinical and Experimental Research on Hip Pathology and Therapy. 2016;**26**(6):531-536

[16] Smith-Petersen MN. Approach to and exposure of the hip joint for mold arthroplasty. The Journal of Bone and Joint Surgery. American Volume. 1949;**31a**(1):40-46

[17] Wagner H. Surface replacement arthroplasty of the hip. Clinical Orthopaedics and Related Research. 1978;**134**:102-130

[18] Berger RA. Total hip arthroplasty using the minimally invasive two-incision approach. Clinical Orthopaedics and Related Research. 2003;**417**:232-241

[19] Desser DR, Mitrick MF, Ulrich SD, Delanois RE, Mont MA. Total hip arthroplasty: Comparison of two-incision and standard techniques at an AOA-accredited community hospital. The Journal of the American Osteopathic Association. 2010;**110**(1):12-15

[20] Matta JM, Shahrdar C, Ferguson T. Single-incision anterior approach for total hip arthroplasty on an orthopaedic table. Clinical Orthopaedics and Related Research. 2005;**441**:115-124

[21] Siguier T, Siguier M, Brumpt B. Mini-incision anterior approach does not increase dislocation rate: A study of 1037 total hip replacements. Clinical Orthopaedics and Related Research. 2004;**426**:164-173

[22] Unger AS, Stronach BM, Bergin PF, Nogler M. Direct anterior total hip arthroplasty. Instructional Course Lectures. 2014;**63**:227-238

[23] McLaughlin JR, Lee KR. Long-term results of uncemented total hip arthroplasty with the Taperloc femoral component in patients with Dorr type C proximal femoral morphology. The Bone & Joint Journal. 2016;**98-b**(5):595-600

[24] Zingg M, Boudabbous S, Hannouche D, Montet X, Boettner F. Standardized fluoroscopy-based technique to measure intraoperative cup anteversion. Journal of Orthopaedic Research: Official Publication of the Orthopaedic Research Society. 2017;**35**(10):2307-2312

[25] Alecci V, Valente M, Crucil M, Minerva M, Pellegrino CM, Sabbadini DD. Comparison of primary total hip replacements performed with a direct anterior approach versus the standard lateral approach: Perioperative findings. Journal of Orthopaedics and Traumatology: Official Journal of the Italian Society of Orthopaedics and Traumatology. 2011;**12**(3):123-129

[26] Miller LE, Gondusky JS, Bhattacharyya S, Kamath AF, Boettner F, Wright J. Does surgical approach affect outcomes in total hip arthroplasty through 90 days of follow-up? A systematic review with meta-analysis. The Journal of Arthroplasty. 2017;**33**(4):1296-1302

[27] Mayr E, Nogler M, Benedetti MG, Kessler O, Reinthaler A, Krismer M, et al. A prospective randomized assessment of earlier functional recovery in THA patients treated

by minimally invasive direct anterior approach: A gait analysis study. Clinical Biomechanics. 2009;**24**(10):812-818

[28] Nakata K, Nishikawa M, Yamamoto K, Hirota S, Yoshikawa H. A clinical comparative study of the direct anterior with mini-posterior approach: Two consecutive series. The Journal of Arthroplasty. 2009;**24**(5):698-704

[29] Rodriguez JA, Deshmukh AJ, Rathod PA, Greiz ML, Deshmane PP, Hepinstall MS, et al. Does the direct anterior approach in THA offer faster rehabilitation and comparable safety to the posterior approach? Clinical Orthopaedics and Related Research. 2014;**472**(2):455-463

[30] Prietzel T, Hammer N, Schleifenbaum S, Adler D, Pretzsch M, Kohler L, et al. The impact of capsular repair on the dislocation rate after primary total hip arthroplasty: A retrospective analysis of 1972 cases. Zeitschrift für Orthopädie und Unfallchirurgie. 2014;**152**(2):130-143

[31] Schmidt-Braekling T, Waldstein W, Akalin E, Benavente P, Frykberg B, Boettner F. Minimal invasive posterior total hip arthroplasty: Are 6 weeks of hip precautions really necessary? Archives of Orthopaedic and Trauma Surgery. 2015;**135**(2):271-274

[32] Restrepo C, Mortazavi SM, Brothers J, Parvizi J, Rothman RH. Hip dislocation: Are hip precautions necessary in anterior approaches? Clinical Orthopaedics and Related Research. 2011;**469**(2):417-422

[33] Maratt JD, Gagnier JJ, Butler PD, Hallstrom BR, Urquhart AG, Roberts KC. No difference in dislocation seen in anterior vs posterior approach total hip arthroplasty. The Journal of Arthroplasty. 2016;**31**(9 Suppl):127-130

[34] Tamaki T, Oinuma K, Miura Y, Higashi H, Kaneyama R, Shiratsuchi H. Epidemiology of dislocation following direct anterior total hip arthroplasty: A minimum 5-year follow-up study. The Journal of Arthroplasty. 2016;**31**(12):2886-2888

[35] de Steiger RN, Lorimer M, Solomon M. What is the learning curve for the anterior approach for total hip arthroplasty? Clinical Orthopaedics and Related Research. 2015;**473**(12):3860-3866

[36] Goytia RN, Jones LC, Hungerford MW. Learning curve for the anterior approach total hip arthroplasty. Journal of Surgical Orthopaedic Advances. 2012;**21**(2):78-83

[37] Seng BE, Berend KR, Ajluni AF, Lombardi AV Jr. Anterior-supine minimally invasive total hip arthroplasty: Defining the learning curve. The Orthopedic Clinics of North America. 2009;**40**(3):343-350

[38] Masonis J, Thompson C, Odum S. Safe and accurate: Learning the direct anterior total hip arthroplasty. Orthopedics. 2008;**31**(12 Suppl 2):129-143

[39] Rudin D, Manestar M, Ullrich O, Erhardt J, Grob K. The anatomical course of the lateral femoral cutaneous nerve with special attention to the anterior approach to the hip joint. The Journal of Bone and Joint Surgery. American Volume. 2016;**98**(7):561-567

[40] Homma Y, Baba T, Kobayashi H, Desroches A, Ozaki Y, Ochi H, et al. Safety in early experience with a direct anterior approach using fluoroscopic guidance with manual leg control for primary total hip arthroplasty: A consecutive one hundred and twenty case series. International Orthopaedics. 2016;**40**(12):2487-2494

[41] Lovell TP. Single-incision direct anterior approach for total hip arthroplasty using a standard operating table. The Journal of Arthroplasty. 2008;**23**(7 Suppl):64-68

[42] Restrepo C, Parvizi J, Pour AE, Hozack WJ. Prospective randomized study of two surgical approaches for total hip arthroplasty. The Journal of Arthroplasty. 2010;**25**(5):671.e1-679.e1

[43] Bhargava T, Goytia RN, Jones LC, Hungerford MW. Lateral femoral cutaneous nerve impairment after direct anterior approach for total hip arthroplasty. Orthopedics. 2010;**33**(7):472

[44] Goulding K, Beaule PE, Kim PR, Fazekas A. Incidence of lateral femoral cutaneous nerve neuropraxia after anterior approach hip arthroplasty. Clinical Orthopaedics and Related Research. 2010;**468**(9):2397-2404

[45] Agten CA, Sutter R, Dora C, Pfirrmann CW. MR imaging of soft tissue alterations after total hip arthroplasty: Comparison of classic surgical approaches. European Radiology. 2017;**27**(3):1312-1321

[46] Homma Y, Baba T, Ochi H, Ozaki Y, Kobayashi H, Matsumoto M, et al. Greater trochanter chip fractures in the direct anterior approach for total hip arthroplasty. European Journal of Orthopaedic Surgery & Traumatology: Orthopedie Traumatologie. 2016;**26**(6):605-611

[47] Higgins BT, Barlow DR, Heagerty NE, Lin TJ. Anterior vs. posterior approach for total hip arthroplasty, a systematic review and meta-analysis. The Journal of Arthroplasty. 2015;**30**(3):419-434

[48] Kasparek MF, Faschingbauer M, Waldstein W, Boettner CS, Boettner F. Topical tranexamic acid is equivalent to targeted preoperative autologous blood donation in total hip arthroplasty. The Journal of Arthroplasty. 2016;**32**(4):1176-1179

13

Ankara Oncology Training and Research Hospital

Guldeniz Argun

Abstract

Hip fracture is usually seen in advanced age. Due to the presence of metastases in elderly patients, the density of bones decreases, and the possibility of fracture increases. Cytokines, released from osteoclasts resulting in post-bony destruction, cause pain by activating pain receptors; hence, pain-related motion restriction may occur. Bone marrow suppression and medulla spinalis pressure may be seen in metastatic bone tumors. Three major complications can be observed in hip fracture operations: (1) perioperative bleeding, (2) bone cementum implantation syndrome and (3) thromboembolism. These indicate superiority of general anesthesia: 1 –controlled respiration. 2 –Invasive interventions to be performed during shock treatment can be made more easily and smoothly. 3 – The safest way to ensure that patients remain immobilized on the operating table. 4 – Hemodynamic parameters can be better controlled. Regional anesthesia has benefits such as allowing early mobilization and postoperative pain control and few complications such as hypoxia, deep vein thrombosis and consciousness blurring. Various regional anesthesia methods such as spinal, epidural, combined spinal-epidural and peripheral nerve blocks are applied. The knowledge and experience of the anesthetist, the general condition and the mental state of the patient, the skill of the surgeon and the type of surgery determine the type of the anesthesia.

Keywords: hip fracture, regional anesthesia, general anesthesia

1. Introduction

Hip fracture is an important medical problem, which is seen in elderly patients, and has a higher incidence related to increased life expectancy, causing increased economic burden. Substantial increase of hip fractures is seen due to increased incidence of age-related osteoporosis and decreased balance resulted in falling. Fractures are more common in women, since osteoporosis is seen frequently in women. About 15–30% of patients with hip fracture die in a year. In addition to osteoporosis, hip fractures due to bone metastases are too high to be neglected. Current treatment is to provide patient weight bearing as soon as possible. Hemiarthroplasties and locked hip nails are the first surgical treatment methods [1].

The most common problems faced in clinical practice are as follows:

- Periosteum stretching
- Intramedullary hypoxia
- Infiltration and compression in the nerve roots
- Reflex muscle spasm
- Pathological fracture formation
- Direct bone invasion and destruction
- Pain due to activation of pain receptors by cytokines (prostaglandin, etc.), released by osteoclasts due to bone destruction
- Limitation of movement due to pain
- Bone marrow suppression due to medulla spinalis pressure and bone marrow infiltration

Non-surgical treatment is only available to patients with poor general conditions that are too low to tolerate any of the anesthetic methods. Hip fracture treatment requires a treatment choice, which needs to be individualized at the highest level. The choice of treatment should be based on surgeon, type of fracture, patient's age and health status. In an elderly patient population, hip fractures due to falling are among the first causes of death. An important factor determining the mortality in these surgeries is an advanced age; 30% of these cases are above 85 years of age.

Complications due to hip fracture operations:

- Bone cement implantation syndrome
- Perioperative bleeding
- Thromboembolism

2. Bone cement

Bone cement is a chemical substance consisting of methyl methacrylate polymers, which tightly adheres prosthetic material to the patient's bone by filling in the slots of the spongiosa. The exothermic reaction followed by the placement of the cement causes the cement to harden and expand. As a result, a pressure greater than 500 mmHg is seen in the bone medullary. This pressure causes fat, bone marrow and air embolism in femoral deep veins. In addition, residual methyl methacrylate monomers cause vasodilatation and reduce systemic vascular resistance. Release of tissue thromboplastin triggers platelet aggregation that leads to micro thrombus formation in the lungs and cardiovascular instability due to vasoactive substances in circulation [2].

Clinical signs of complication related to bone cement are as follows:

- Hypoxia (increased pulmonary shunt).
- Hypotension.
- Arrhythmia (including heart block and sinus arrest).
- Pulmonary hypertension (increased pulmonary vascular resistance).
- Reduced cardiac output.
- Embolism most commonly occurs when a femoral prosthesis is placed.

Methods to reduce cement-related complications:

- Increasing oxygen concentration in inspiration before cement procedures
- Close monitoring of the patient's fluid balance
- Opening a hole in the distal region of the femur (vent hole)
- Cleaning the femoral shaft with high-pressure lavage to remove debris
- Using prosthesis without cement

3. Bleeding

Hip surgery is an operation causing significantly blood loss. Average loss of blood is about 1000–1500 ml. Bleeding cause depends on several factors. These factors are as follows:

- Experience of the surgeon.
- The surgical technique and the type of prosthesis.
- Controlled hypotension may reduce intraoperative bleeding.
- Some studies have shown that loss of blood in regional techniques (spinal and epidural) providing equal average blood pressure was 30–50% less than general anesthesia [3, 4].
- For bleeding control, preoperative embolization, autologous and allogeneic transfusions and hemodilution methods may be applied. Aprotinin, epsilon aminocaproic acid and tranexamic acid prevent blood loss without increasing thrombus formation risk [5].

4. Venous thromboembolism

Factors that increase the risk of thromboembolism are as follows:

- Previous thromboembolism history
- Previous venous surgery and/or varicose surgery history
- Previous orthopedic operations
- Advanced age
- Malignancy
- Congestive heart failure
- Chronic lower limb laceration
- Immobilization
- Obesity
- Oral contraceptive and estrogen
- Unnecessary blood transfusions

Regional anesthesia reduces the incidence of thrombus formation and pulmonary embolism [6]. Davis et al. found that the deep vein thrombosis was 13% in spinal anesthesia, while 27% in general anesthesia [7]. Other approaches that reduce the risk of thromboembolism are the use of devices providing intermittent compression to legs and low-dose anticoagulant prophylaxis.

Pulmonary artery and its branches are obstructed by venous thrombus from systemic veins. There is a close relationship between pulmonary embolism (PE) and deep vein thrombosis (DVT).

DTV is responsible for 90% PE. In 1856, Wirchow described clinical triad about the reasons of venous thromboembolism:

- Venous stasis
- Hypercoagulopathy
- Local injury at vessel walls (intraluminal damage)

Clinical impact of PE depends on several factors:

- Width of obstructed vessels bed
- Humoral factors released by serotonin and thromboxane A2
- Whether the patient has cardiopulmonary disorders or not
- Patient's age and general health status

4.1. Diagnosis

- Chest X-ray
- ECG
- Arterial blood gas analyses:
- Major findings include hypoxemia, hypocapnia, respiratory alkalosis, and alveolar-arterial gradient increase (PO_2 A-a).
- Biochemical investigations: While CPK-MB, D-dimer, FDP, SGOT are normal, LDH and bilirubin are high.
- Respiratory function tests:
- The physiological dead space (VD) and the tidal volumetric ratio (VD/VT) are increased.

4.2. Treatment

- Ventilation with 100% O_2.
- Heparinization.
- Inotropic agents.
- Surgical embolectomy is performed in the large embolus. The small embolus is anticoagulated. The best treatment is prophylaxis.
- Venous stasis should be avoided. For this purpose, the legs should be lifted up and early mobilization should be provided postoperatively. Advanced venous stasis causes deep vein thrombosis and pulmonary embolism.

5. Venous air embolism

Low venous pressure and open ventilation are required for the air to enter the venous system as compared with the atmospheric pressure.

This most often occurs during the neurosurgery operations in a sitting position.

In addition, poor surgical technique may increase the formation of air embolism.

Factors affecting air embolization are as follows:

- Intravascular air volume
- Air inlet velocity
- The use of nitrogen protoxide
- Foramen ovale presence
- General health status

Slowly entering a small air bubble has usually minimal physiological importance. In this case, venous air bubbles are taken out from lungs based on increased compensator pulmonary artery pressure (PAP). If this situation exceeds the capacity of lung removal, PAP increases, cardiac output (CO) decreases and hearth failure occurs. If balanced, namely, if venous air input is equal to pulmonary removal, PAP reaches a plateau.

300-ml air is fatal in adults. In animal trials, 1 ml/kg/min causes embolism signs; 3–8 ml/kg causes death. The earliest sign is cardiovascular collapse. Blood pressure decreases dramatically; sudden hypotension, tachycardia, arrhythmia and cardiac arrest occur in succession. CVP increases; a metallic sound is heard with the precordial or esophageal stethoscope. In case of this, characteristic "sound of the mill wheel" is heard. This sound can be heard in all precordium. Respiratory changes such as increased respiratory rate, irregularity and apnea can be seen.

5.1. Diagnosis

- Doppler ultrasonic flow meter
- PAP
- End-tidal CO_2
- Other methods: Monitoring should be done for patient in a sitting position. In these patients, continuous measurement of arterial blood pressure, CVP, end-tidal CO_2, Doppler ultrasound and esophageal stethoscope should be applied.

6. Fat embolism

6.1. Etiology

- Bone fractures
- Liver and kidney ruptures
- Rarely, after bone surgery

6.2. Diagnosis

With the presence of free fat in sputum and urine and in histological examination, petechiae and hyperlipidemia are diagnosed, with maximum level of free fat being reached in 3–4 days [8].

6.3. Treatment

Hypovolemia and shock should be treated. Clofibrate (atromid-S) and alcohol should be used for hyperlipidemia.

6.4. Preanesthesia assessment in arthroplasties

- Personal background.
- Physical examination:
- The patient's age, weight, body mass index and vital signs (blood pressure, heart rate, pulse rate, body temperature, number of breaths, (depth breathing)) of the patient are evaluated.
- In these patients, the underlying etiology is mostly osteoarthritis or rheumatoid arthritis. Therefore, examination of the cervical and lumbar vertebrae is especially important for anesthesia.
- The cervical spine mobility should be checked to evaluate any restriction and assessed for intubation difficulty. Also, under the anesthesia and during intubation, attempts should be avoided from excessive extension of the neck joint.
- Osteoarthritis may lead to nerve root compression in the spine. Cervical spine and temporomandibular joint may be involved in patients with rheumatoid arthritis. In the presence of atlantoaxial joint subluxation, diagnosis can be made radiologically. During intubation, subluxation of the atlantoaxial joint may cause foramen magnum protrusion to odontoid process, reducing vertebral blood flow and compressing the spinal cord or brain. Intubation must be done by stabilizing the neck. A vigilant intubation technique may be preferred in some patients. It may be easier to prefer regional anesthesia in this group of patients [9].
- Because of multiple joint involvements in rheumatoid arthritis, it should be taken into account when placing intravenous catheters to the hand, wrist, foot, etc.
- Since most of patients undergoing arthroplasty are older, having cardiac, respiratory, cerebral, renal and endocrine diseases, perioperative and postoperative morbidity and mortality increase. Therefore, evaluation of systems is very important.

6.4.1. The evaluation of cardiovascular system

MET's (classification of metabolic equivalent) meaning is that 40 years old, 70-kg man expresses oxygen consumption at rest. It is considered to be over 4 in the MET evaluation, can go uphill, go up 2 stories of stairs, walk straight on the road at 6 km/h, run short distance, do heavy work at home and participate in moderate activities. Patients with MET ≥4 are considered to be good in terms of functional capacity.

- 1 MET resting, eating, toilet needs
- 3 MET mild housework, walking at 2–3 mph
- 4 MET 2-story climbing stairs

- 7 MET heavy housework
- ≥10 MET heavy sports ability

6.4.2. Cardiovascular risk assessment: the Lee risk index is the most appropriate for orthopedic patients

Number of current risks and incidence of cardiac complications

- 0 0.4%
- 1 0.9%
- 2 7%
- >3 11%

6.4.3. Cardiovascular drug management

- Antihypertensive agents should not be discontinued until morning of the operation.
- Beta blockers should not be discontinued until an operation; the drug dose should be adjusted so that the heart rate is below 65/min.
- Aspirin reduces the risk of deep vein thrombosis and pulmonary embolism. The use of aspirin alone provides suboptimal protection for thromboembolic events associated with hip fractures. It is imperative that aspirin should be continued for stapled, drug-free stents.
- Thienopyridine (clopidogrel and ticlopidine) combined with dual use of aspirin is associated with the use of coronary stent. Dual use increases the possibility of bleeding by 0.4–1.0% compared with aspirin treatment alone. Three ways may be followed based on the type of stent and intervention time:
- Dual treatment is continued without interruption.
- Bridging therapy with antithrombotic agents (low molecular weight heparin, glycoprotein II b/III a inhibitors) can be applied.
- Thienopyridine treatment is discontinued 10 days before surgery and resumed in a safe period.

Antithrombotic agents; fondaparinux, unfractionated heparin (UFH) and low molecular weight heparin (LMWH).

7. Airway assessment

There is a risk of difficult mask ventilation and difficult intubation due to hardness in the neck, dental deterioration and cervical joint degeneration.

Hypoxia may be associated with pulmonary collapse and/or infection. Preoperative physiotherapy and spirometer may be beneficial to postoperative hypoxia.

Death, pneumonia, prolonged extubation and persistent bronchospasm can be seen in patients with COPD and smokers. The length of stay in intensive care unit is longer. The incidence of postoperative pulmonary complications is about 25–90% (If FEV1 < 65%, risk of complications >50%). Arterial blood gas analysis may be done. If the value of $PaCO_2$ is above 45 mmHg, it is a strong risk factor for preoperative pulmonary complication. In case of preoperative inhaler use, respiratory exacerbations and the presence of lung infection, antibiotic and supportive treatment should be provided with optimal conditions.

8. Neurological assessment

In the group of patients planned for arthroplasty, weakening of the memory, decrease in cognitive and intellectual functions, diminished movements, deterioration of sleep order, decrease in visual, acoustical, taste and smell sensation, autonomic nervous system imbalances, Parkinson, depression and dementia are common. If there is a suspicion of a mental condition of the patient, the mental status test (Mini Mental Status Test) can be planned.

9. Renal assessment

There is a risk of renal insufficiency and preoperative azotaemia related to age. Prerenal azotaemia should be corrected by hydration, by taking patients into dialysis program if necessary and by optimizing biochemical values.

10. Glycaemia control

Autonomic dysfunction, which is usually caused by diabetes mellitus in a long term, is an important actor for regional anesthesia and for control of perioperative hemodynamic. There is a possibility of silent myocardial ischemia. Oral antidiabetics should be stopped at least 24 hours before the operation.

11. Nutrition control

Because patients undergoing arthroplasty are geriatrics, preoperative nutritional status should be evaluated. Their nutritional status is assessed by Mini Nutritional Assessment Test. If albumin is <3.5 gr/dl, the patient should be supported. Reduced glomerular filtration rates due to age should be considered. Urea, serum creatinine and electrolytes should be examined.

12. Pain education

Preoperative training including surgical procedure and rehabilitation protocol, informing the prospective benefits of the procedure, postoperative pain level and pain management techniques (intravenous, epidural patient-controlled analgesia), is beneficial to reduce patient anxieties, increase patient satisfaction, and reduce rehabilitation and hospital stay. Pre-emptive administration of opioid analgesics, NSAII and COX-2 inhibitors can provide effective postoperative analgesia. However, it should be considered that opioid use is associated with increased postoperative nausea and vomiting risk. Pre-emptive epidural analgesia with an epidural catheter prior to arthroplasty can provide postoperative pain control at a significant level [10].

13. Approaches to oncological patients

Systematic evaluation of oncologic patients is important. Patients are questioned about whether they have received chemotherapy (RT) or radiotherapy (RT). In these patients, impaired health status and blood vessel changes due to bone marrow suppression may be seen.

Alkylating agents such as cyclophosphamide may cause prolongation of the neuromuscular block.

It should be kept in mind that oxygen therapy at high concentration increases interstitial pneumonia and interstitial fibrosis due to bleomycin.

Skin reactions related to RT and KT should be noted. Vascular access may be problematic. Most cancer patients are malnourished due to their illnesses and side effects of treatment. Loss of appetite, cachexia, hyperproteinemia and hypoalbuminemia are common. Preoperative nutritional support should be given. Immunonutrition is thought to be useful to reduce immunosuppression. Lung metastases may be found to impair respiratory functions. The cardiotoxic effects of KT and RT may extend to cardiomyopathy, pericardial effusion, pericarditis and congestive heart failure.

In the hepatobiliary system, hepatomegaly, deterioration in liver function tests and even cirrhosis can be seen. Decrease in coagulation factors and coagulopathy can be seen.

In the urinary system, radiation nephropathy can be seen.

In the hematopoietic system, immune system impairment may be seen.

Multidisciplinary examination of cancer patients should be done. After their clinical and laboratory values are improved, the patients should be given to surgery.

14. Anesthesia techniques in hip fracture operations

14.1. General anesthesia

- It may be possible for hip fracture operations to obtain safer results with general anesthesia.

- With controlled breathing, it may be possible to obtain the patient's alveolar oxygen pressure to the levels that meet the oxygen needs of the tissues.
- Invasive interventions to be done for the treatment of shock and monitoring of unconscious patient can be completed more easily and free of problems.
- It is the safest way for patients with restless and agitation due to shock and pain due to trauma to remain immobilized on the operating table.
- General anesthesia has some advantages (better control of hemodynamic parameters, given oxygen with higher concentration compared to regional anesthesia) [11].

Important points in general anesthesia:

- Firstly, enough volume should be replaced.
- Induction under appropriate monitoring conditions following a good pre-oxygenation to reduce hypoxemia risk.
- Hypnotics, narcotic agents and inhalation agents with balanced anesthesia usually minimize the potential problems in a perioperative period.
- It should be given attention for the position of the patient during anesthesia.

14.1.1. The general anesthesia management in elderly patients

Given that the vast majority of hip fracture surgeries are performed on elderly individuals, general anesthesia guidelines should be followed in geriatric patients. At first, the premedication to which the respiratory tract may be depressed should be avoided or the dose should be reduced.

When performing volume replacement, the cardiac load should be avoided and the mean arterial pressure should be preserved. Respiratory depression can be avoided by minimizing the opioid dose. The inotropic medicines can be necessary to treat hypotension. The preserve of renal function should also be supplied.

We must make sure that the neuromuscular block is completely turned. For postoperative analgesia, regional anesthesia techniques should be used and the dose should be adjusted.

14.2. Regional anesthesia

There is a long history for epidural and spinal block interventions and the use of these interventions for pain relief. Both techniques are widely used around the world. They have some advantages such as regional anesthesia interventions, early mobilization, postoperative pain relief and reduced risk of DVT, hypoxia and conscious problems [12]. There are a number of studies in geriatric patients that indicate the superiority of regional anesthesia in hip fracture operations.

Advantages of spinal anesthesia:

- Short acting time
- Provide better muscular relaxant effect
- More effective analgesia
- Rarely serious respiratory depression
- Cost-effective
- Easy to perform

Disadvantages:

- Provide low dose and toxicity.
- Rarely shaking.
- Hypotension is more frequent and sudden onset.
- The incidence of post-spinal headache is high.
- Upper level of blockage may be changed and cannot be adjusted.
- Postoperative analgesia cannot be obtained.
- Duration of the effect cannot be extended.

Advantages of epidural anesthesia:

- The desired block level can be titrated with the catheter.
- The duration of anesthesia can be extended with added doses.
- It is possible to obtain postoperative analgesia [13].
- No headache.
- The effect time is long.
- The depth of the block may vary depending on the agent.
- Lower boundary may vary; sacral distribution is limited.
- High dose is required.
- Shaking is often present.

Combined spinal-epidural anesthesia:

- It provides both spinal and epidural advantages as mentioned above in abdominal, lower extremity surgery and birth analgesia.
- It is possible to complete an inadequate spinal anesthesia.

- It provides longer analgesia with opioids and/or local anesthetics even in postoperative period.
- The incidence of headache due to postdural puncture is low, and it also provides autogenous blood injection to treat/protect headache due to incidental postdural puncture.

14.3. Peripheral nerve blockage

If neuro-axial blockage is contraindicated, fascia iliaca block, femoral nerve block and sciatic nerve block can be applied. Peripheral nerve blockage is particularly useful in tumor patients developing opioid intolerance and using anticoagulants.

Lumbosacral blocks and femoral and sciatic nerve blocks may be used in hip arthroplasty operations in geriatric patients. These blocks also provide postoperative pain treatment. Since peripheral nerve blocks do not have sympathetic blockade, sudden hypotension cannot occur.

Advantages:

- Protection of the patient's consciousness and unaffected respiration.
- Higher possibility of providing unilateral blockage.
- The respiratory system is not affected.
- The effect of them on central nervous system is minimal.
- Less sympathetic blockade than regional techniques.

The use of ultrasonography in peripheral blockage:

- The use of Stimuplex may not be needed, the number of punches is reduced, the dose is reduced, and the blockage application time is reduced. Vasculature may not be prevented, the duration of the blockage is not prolonged in adults, and the shortened neuropraxia does not decrease [14].

14.4. Evaluation after operation in hip fracture surgery

Decent postoperative evaluation and care after the surgery are important factors for the healing of the patient. Post-anesthetic care includes periodic follow-up, if necessary; the treatment of respiratory, cardiovascular and neuromuscular functions of the patient; and monitoring of blood level, body temperature, pain intensity, nausea, vomiting, drainage, bleeding and urinary output.

The respiratory system is followed by the pulse oximeter monitoring. It is useful for early detection of hypoxia. ASA recommends oxygen supplementation therapy at risk of hypoxemia, during transport and at collection facilities. Oxygen therapy for up to 24 hours is especially recommended in the elderly group at risk of myocardial ischemia undergoing the hip fracture surgery.

Cardiovascular system: ECG and blood pressure monitor should be continued during waking and compilation. It should not be forgotten that arthroplasty patients are elderly and cardiovascular comorbid diseases can be found and the risk of postoperative cardiac complications is high. The most important factor affecting mortality in geriatric patients is the current co-morbidities. Increase in troponin I is important in postoperative follow-up due to myocardial ischemia.

Assessment of neuromuscular functions (NMF) is done by physical examination and neuromuscular block monitors.

Body heat: Preservation of normothermia and periodic body temperature measurements should be made to prevent hypothermia, and heaters should be used if necessary. Both anesthesia recovery and postoperative patient comfort are important. In the treatment of thyroid disease, agents such as low-dose meperidine and tramadol can also be used.

Thromboemboli: Prophylactic anticoagulants, early mobilization, intermittent pneumatic compression devices, compression socks and neuro-axial anesthesia can reduce thromboembolic complications. Continuation of acetyl salicylic acid therapy is recommended in elderly patients. The use of regional anesthesia and anticoagulation is still controversial.

Nausea and vomiting: Periodic control of nausea and vomiting is important to detect complications. In the treatment of nausea and vomiting, 5-HT3 antagonists, tranquilizers/neuroleptics, scopolamine, dexamethasone, antihistamines or metoclopramide may be used.

Renal functions: Urinary retention is a common complication. It is especially more common after epidural anesthesia. This complication does not occur in peripheral nerve blocks.

Cognitive changes: Cognitive changes after hip fracture operations are common in elderly patients. There are studies showing that short-term cognitive changes are less frequent after spinal anesthesia. However, there was no difference in the long term.

15. Postoperative analgesia methods in hip fracture surgery

Pain management in hip fracture operations is multimodal. The combined use of different effect mechanistic analgesics provides less pain relief resulting in less opioid use and less complications [15].

Inadequate postoperative pain treatment causes prolonged hospitalization and additional malignancy. Inadequate pain management leads to the chronicity of the pain and the decrease in the quality of life of the patient.

Intraoperative analgesic treatment from the preoperative epidural catheter ensures that the patient does not have pain at the end of the operation. The patient can return to daily activities more quickly. Patient-controlled analgesia (PCA) technique is frequently used in postoperative pain management. It can be administered via peripheral intravenous or epidural catheter. Peripheral nerve blocks can also be provided with PCA using catheter.

Bupivacaine and opioid protocols. are mostly used in regionalized PCA. It should be noted that opioids administered by the epidural route may also cause sedation.

Periarticular injection and multimodality in patients with hip arthroplasty should be part of the treatment [16]. Periarticular injection solution includes; bupivacaine 0.5% 200–400 mg, morphine sulfate 4–10 mg, epinephrine 300 mcg, methylprednisolone 40 mg, cefuroxime 750 mg and 0.9% NaCl. The total volume is 60 ml.

Periarticular injection is applied in anterior capsule, iliopsoas tendon and inseriosion before reduction. After reduction,it is applied in abductor, fascia lata, snovia, gluteus maximus and insercius, posterior capsules, short external rotators.

Duration of hospital stay and ambulance: The average length of hospital stay is 3 days in hip arthroplasty. After a hip fracture repair, the average time for elderly patients is 20 days. Although there are many studies advocating that neuro-axial anesthesia is an advantage in ambulance [17], there are studies advocating that the anesthesia route is not effective.

Author details

Guldeniz Argun

Address all correspondence to: guldargun@yahoo.com

Departmant of Anesthesiology and Reanimation, Ankara, Turkey

References

[1] Patterson BM, Healy JV, Cornell CN, et al. Cardiac arrest during hip arthroplasty with a cemented long-stem component. The Journal of Bone and Joint Surgery. American Volume. 1991;**73A**:271

[2] Ranawat CS, Beaver WB, Sharrock NE, et al: Effect of hypotensive epidural anesthesia on acetabular cement-bone fixation in total hip arthroplasty. The Journal of Bone and Joint Surgery. British Volume 1991;**73B**:779

[3] Thompson GE, Miller RD, Stewans WC, Murray WR. Hypotensive anesthesia for total hip arthroplasty: A study of blood loss and organ function (brain, heart, liver and kidney). Anesthesiology. 1978;**48**:91

[4] Vazeery AK, Lunde O. Controlled hypotension in hip joint surgery: An assessment of surgical haemorrhage during sodium nitroprusside infusion. Acta Orthopaedica Scandinavica. 1979;**50**:433

[5] Weber RS et al. Anemia and transfusions in patients undergoing surgery for cancer. Annals of Surgical Oncology. 2008;**15**:34-35

[6] Modig J. The role of lumbar epidural anaesthesia as antithrombotic prophylaxis in total hip replacement. Acta Chirurgica Scandinavica. 1991;**151**:1721

[7] Davis FM, Laurenson VG, Gillespie WJ, et al. Leg blood flow during total hip replacement under spinal or general anaesthesia. Anaesthesia and Intensive Care. 1989;**17**:136

[8] Djelonah I, Lefevre G, Ozier Y, et al. Fat embolism in orthopedic surgery: Role of bone marrow fatty acid. Anesthesia and Analgesia. 1997;**85**:441

[9] Frestein GS: Etiology and pathogenesis of rheumatoid arthritis. In: Kelly WN, Harris ED Jr, Ruddy S, et al. Textbook of Rheumatology. 5th ed. Philadelphia: WB Saunders; 1997. p. 851

[10] Carli F, Halliday D. Continuous epidural blockade arrests the postoperative decrease in muscle protein fractional synthetic rate in surgical patients. Anaesthesiology. 1997;**86**:1033

[11] Dyson A, Henderson AM, Chamlley D, et al. An assessment of postoperative oxygen therapy in patients with fractured neck of femur. Anaesthesia and Intensive Care Medicine. 1988;**16**:405

[12] Williams-Russo P, Sharrock NE, Mattis S, et al. Cognitive effects after epidural vs general anaesthesia in older adults: A randomized trial. Journal of the American Medical Association. 1995;**274**:44

[13] Moiniche S et al. A qualitative and quantitative systematic review of pre-emptive analgesia for postoperative pain relief: The role of timing of analgesia. Anesthesiology. 2002;**96**(3):526-527

[14] Busoni P. Central or peripheral blocks? Techniques in Regional Anesthesia and Pain Management. 2002;**6**:95-98

[15] American Society of Anesthesiologist Task Force on Acute Pain Management. Practice guidelines for acute pain management in the perioperative setting: An updated report by the American Society of Anesthesiologist Task Force on acute pain management. Anesthesiology. 2012;**116**(2):248-273

[16] Lunn TH, Husted H, Solgaard S, Kristensen BB, Otte KS, Kjersgaard AG, Gaarn-Lansen L, Kehlet H. Intraoperative local infiltration analgesia for early analgesia after total hip arthroplasty: A randomized, double-blind, placebo controlled trial. Regional Anesthesia and Pain Medicine. 2011;**36**:424-429

[17] Lunn TH, Kristensen BB, Gaarn-Lansen L, Husted H, Kehlet H. Post-anaesthesia care unit stay after total hip and knee arthroplasty under spinal anaesthesia. Acta Anaesthesiologica Scandinavica. 2012;**56**:1139-1145

14

Complications of Total Hip Replacement

Chang Park and Irfan Merchant

Abstract

Total hip replacement is a highly effective surgical procedure for patients suffering from end stage osteoarthritis and its success in improving symptoms of osteoarthritis has meant that its use has increased across many healthcare systems. Although in experienced hands the procedure provides very effective outcomes one must be aware of the potential complications of the procedure. These can be divided into general and procedure specific. General complications include infections, postoperative pulmonary issues and thromboembolic complications. Procedural specific complications include a surgical site infection, haemorrhage, nerve injury, dislocation, leg length discrepancy, periprosthetic fractures and heterotrophic ossification. This chapter explores and describes the complications a surgeon may face when performing a total hip replacement and how one may avoid and address these.

Keywords: complication, hip, arthroplasty

1. Introduction

Total hip replacement is a highly effective surgical procedure for patients suffering from end stage osteoarthritis [1]. Its success in improving pain, mobility and quality of life for patients has meant its use has increased since its introduction [2, 3].

As like any surgical procedure however, total hip replacements have associated surgical complications. Thanks to advances in technology, surgical awareness and anaesthetic techniques the overall rates of complications have been declining despite an increasing burden of co-morbidities in the population [4]. The complications encountered can be divided into general and procedure specific. This chapter will explore both aspects of complications that the surgeon may encounter when performing total hip replacements.

2. General complications

2.1. Urinary tract infection

Urinary tract infections represent an approximately 13% of all healthcare-associated infection [5] and in the context of post total hip replacement is seen to be the most common minor postoperative compilation [6]. The estimated rates of postoperative urinary tract infections are at 3.26 [7]. Risk factors for the development of a urinary tract infection include female sex, increased age, ASA 3 or higher and the use of a general anaesthetic [6]. Of these in a recent multicentre study by Alvarez et al., increased age followed by female sex was the strongest variable in developing a postoperative urinary tract infection. As with respiratory tract infections to be discussed in the next section, urinary tract infection in the postoperative setting following total hip replacements have been linked to more significant adverse effects such as peri-prosthetic infections, implant failure and revision procedures along with the immediate prolonged hospital stay [8].

2.2. Postoperative pulmonary complications

Postoperative pulmonary complications are common after major surgeries and are defined as a collective of respiratory failure, pneumonia, pleural effusion, atelectasis, pneumothorax and aspiration pneumonia [9]. Postoperative pulmonary complications are a common complication after total hip replacement with 45.9% patients having some form of postoperative pulmonary complications on postoperative CT screening [10]. The symptoms of any postoperative pulmonary complication can vary greatly with many atelectasis following general anaesthesia being asymptomatic but as like urinary tract infections can cause more serious complications along with increased length of stay. The rate of in-patient pneumonia following total hip replacement is estimated to be between 0.74 and 0.86% [7].

2.3. Thromboembolic complications

2.3.1. Deep vein thrombosis

Deep vein thrombosis is a common complication following total hip replacements due to the venous stasis and hypercoagulability experienced both during and subsequent to the procedure, adversely influencing Virchow's triad towards a state of thrombus formation [11]. The subsequent results of deep vein thrombosis can vary from asymptomatic, chronic venous insufficiency and proximal propagation. Without the use of any prophylaxis the overall radiological diagnosed rates of deep vein thrombosis has been as high as 70% in total hip replacement cases [12].

With the introduction of modern thromboprophylaxis the overall rates of deep vein thrombosis has reduced to approximately 44% and in those that are symptomatic as low as 1.3% [13, 14]. Thankfully with prophylactic treatment the rate of symptomatic proximal propagation to form a pulmonary embolus is lower still at less than 0.6% [15].

Although half of patient who develop a deep vein thrombosis post total hip replacement have no identifiable risk factor there are numerous well recorded risk factors that alter Virchow's triad towards a state of thrombus formation [16]. These include associated fracture, malignancy, previous history of thromboembolism, immobility, obesity, pro-thrombotic conditions such as anti-phospholipid syndrome and the use of oral contraceptive pills. Furthermore an ASA grade of greater than 3 is an independent risk factor [16].

The prophylaxis for deep vein thrombosis is aimed at returning the pro-thrombotic state into equilibrium by adjusting the parameters of Virchow's triad. This is done by treating the stasis of flow in the lower limbs both by mechanical thromboprophylaxis but also by the choice of anaesthetic used. A regional anaesthetic has been shown to reduce the risks of deep vein thrombosis over that of general anaesthetic by 50% alone due to the relative improvement in the flow of venous blood in the lower limbs [17]. Furthermore chemical thromboprophylaxis can be used to reverse the hypercoagulability. Various agents are used for chemical thromboprophylaxis but include low molecular weight heparin and more recently oral factor Xa inhibitors. Mechanical and chemical prophylaxis are utilised both intra and postoperatively to reduce the overall risk of deep vein thrombosis.

2.3.2. *Pulmonary embolism*

Deep vein thrombosis has a risk of propagating proximally through the right sided cardiac circulation into the pulmonary system. If the thrombus passes into the lungs they result in pulmonary embolisms. The results of these pulmonary embolisms can vary from being asymptomatic to caused catastrophic respiratory failure and can be fatal and pulmonary embolus being one of the leading causes of mortality post total hip replacements. The overall rates of postoperative total hip replacements are 3% in the absence of chemical prophylaxis [15], and 0.21% when chemical prophylaxis is used from a recent large review [18]. The prevention of pulmonary embolism lies primarily in the prevention of deep vein thrombosis discussed in the previous section. The treatment of established pulmonary embolisms are by the use of therapeutic agents to inhibit the pro-thrombotic cascade and profibrinolytic agents to dissolve away the embolus.

2.3.3. *Fat embolism*

In the same way that a deep vein thrombus can pass into the pulmonary circulation, at the time of implant insertion the rise of intramedullary pressure from the prosthesis and cement can cause the embolization of medullary fat and marrow contents into the venous system [19, 20]. If the fat or marrow then passes into the pulmonary circulation in can pass in the pulmonary arteries in the same way as a venous thrombus causing much the same issues. These bodies of fat can also pass into the left sided circulation and cause cerebral embolisms and infarction causing neurological deficits [21]. By the same pattern the fat bodies can cause infarcts in the systemic circulation in tissues causing a classic upper body petechiae. As such the classic symptomatic triad of fat embolism is respiratory distress, neurological symptoms and upper body petechiae. To avoid such complications the intra-medullary canal is lavage cleaned prior to implant insertion to reduce the fat content. The treatment of fat embolism is supportive principally for the symptoms of respiratory compromise [22].

3. Procedure-specific complications

3.1. Surgical site infection

Surgical site infections can be classified as that of superficial and deep. Whereas superficial infections can be a nuisance and cause prolonged hospital stays and increased morbidity for patients and potential for wound dehiscence the sequelae of deep infection post total hip replacement can be catastrophic and challenging for the clinician to manage.

At the advent of its introduction the deep infection rates for total hip replacements were recorded to be as high as 9.4% [23]. However in modern practice with the widespread adoption of laminar flow operating theatres and prophylaxis antibiotics the current rates of deep infection are at between 0.3 and 1.5% [24, 25].

The prevention of deep infection is principally reducing the contamination of the surgical site from contaminants. These contaminants can arise from the patient's skin, the surgical personnel or the surgical instruments [26]. The use of laminar flow air circulation in theatres and the adaptation of rigorous sterile techniques and practices in the operating room is now standard practice to reduce the contamination of the surgical site. However despite these best practice the reality is that all surgical wounds are contaminated and even the most thorough of skin preparation will not decontaminate the micro-organisms in the deeper layers of the skin and the efficacy of laminar air flow can be easily influence by a variety of factors in the operating room [27–29].

As the contamination of the surgical site cannot be fully eliminated the use of prophylaxis antibiotics is standard practice with recognised benefits to reduce the risk of deep infection [30, 31]. The use of prophylaxis antibiotics in total hip replacements have been shown to reduce the absolute risk of infection by 81% [32]. Such use of prophylaxis antibiotics is not without its risks however and include both the direct side effects of its use but also the increasing concern of resistance. As such the choice of antibiotics is best directed by local protocols and guidelines and currently there is no clear consensus on the best regime [32].

Despite the effort to reduce the rates of deep infections however they do still occur and the diagnosis of a deep infection can be clinically challenging. The principal symptom is hip pain, but this along with more systemic symptoms such as fever, malaise and rigours are very variable. Further the clinical examination may show signs of local inflammatory changes along with reduced range of motion within the hip joint.

Biochemical marks such as CRP and ESR are widely used. However in the both markers are non-specific and can be elevated in the presence of any concurrent inflammatory process. In the absence of any concurrent conditions that may increase their levels the a CRP of greater than 10 mg/l has a sensitivity and specificity of 96 and 92% and an ESR of over 30 mm/h that of 82 and 85% [33].

Radiological investigations can aid the diagnosis with signs of osteopaenia and osteolysis however there is no clear way to distinguish these from aseptic loosening on plain radiographs alone. Radionucelotide scanning can identify areas of increased bone turnover and inflammatory foci and are more sensitive and specific to deep infection. More specialist radiological investigations such as labelled white cell scans and immunoglobin scans and modern PET scanning techniques are more sensitive and specific still, at 85.5 and 92.6% respectively for PET scans, but the availability remains challenging [34, 35].

Cytological and microbiological analysed sample can give both diagnostic information on the presence of infection but also the causative organism. Done radiologically under sterile conditions, a guided aspirate has been shown to have a sensitivity and specificity of 82 and 91% [36]. A surgically performed procedure allows the concurrent washout of the surgical site to furthermore reduce the organism load. Any such sample however should be taken with 2 weeks of antibiotic cleared time to avoid any false negative findings.

The treatment of deep infection in total hip replacement is based on the principles of eradication of infection and restoration of function [37]. If deep infection occurs in the acute period, in the first 2 weeks, then component retention may be possible with thorough debridement and antibiotic treatment. However such this only results in clearance of infection in 50–74% of patients [38]. More often the presence of deep infection requires a full revision of the total hip replacement. This can be performed as either a single or two stage procedure. A single stage procedure is the removal of the prosthesis with thorough clearance of the infection with the implantation of a new prosthesis and subsequent antibiotics therapy. This differs to that of a two stage procedure whereby the first stage is the removal of the infected prosthesis, soft tissue debridement and the insertion of an antibiotic loaded spacer. After an interval of approximately 6 weeks of antibiotic therapy and the patient undergoes a second stage procedure with the insertion of a new prosthesis [39, 40]. The benefits of a single stage procedure are that of reduced operative morbidity however the results of successful treatment of the infection is consistently better with a two stage procedure at 87–94% [41] (**Figure 1**).

3.2. Haemorrhage

Haemorrhage can be classified into intraoperative haemorrhage and postoperative. Arthroplasty surgery is associated with significant levels of haemorrhage and a relatively high demand of blood transfusion [42, 43]. Haemorrhage that is deemed to be clinically significant is difficult to determine and varies between clinician, centres and trails. One large multi-centered study defines important haemorrhage to be as *"bleeding that is recorded by the surgeon as being outside the range of 'typical expected levels' of bleeding following THA/TKA, or bleeding that is cited as the cause of prolonged hospital stay"* [44]. Rates of intraoperative haemorrhage vary from 2 to 3.6 unit [44–47]. Risk factors for increased intraoperative haemorrhage rates include increased operative time, with one study demonstrating a 1 min increase in operative time resulting in a 1.552 ml increase in intraoperative bleeding in total hip replacements [48]. Low and high BMI has been both associated with increased risk of haemorrhage [49, 50].

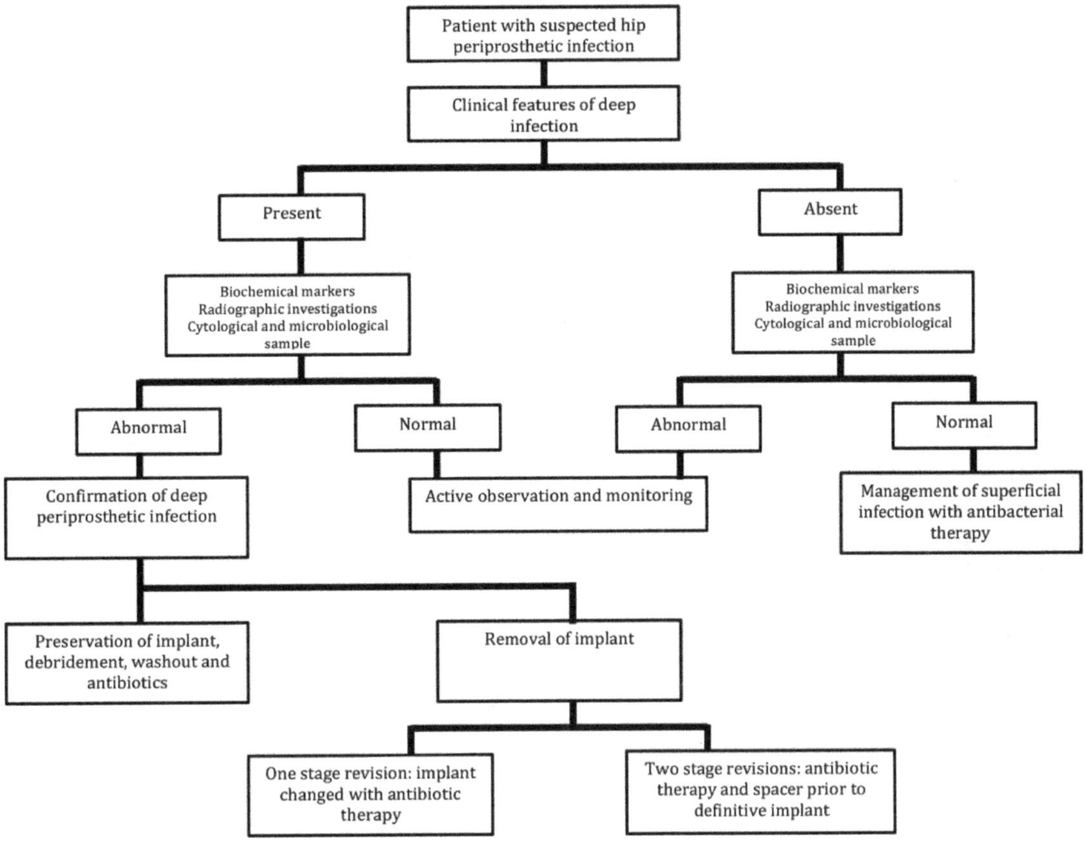

Figure 1. Management algorithm of peri-prosthetic infection.

Due to the high rates of intraoperative haemorrhage total hip replacement has a high rate of transfusion requirements. Median volume of allogenic transfusions in total hip replacements is 2 units [46, 47]. Autologous transfusion is also extensively used in total hip replacements with estimates at 20–80% of all total hip replacement patients requiring an allogenic transfusion [51–57]. When autologous transfusion is used the rates of requiring only autologous transfusions vary from 49 to 79% [47, 58–61]. Risk factors for intraoperative blood transfusion are low preoperative Hb, high age, female gender, large estimated volume of intraoperative blood loss and American Society of Anesthesiologists score of more than 2 [49, 62].

The risks of allogenic transfusions have been widely reported to include disease transmission, haemolytic reactions, fluid and haemodynamic overload, acute lung injury, coagulopathy, febrile non-haemolytic reactions as well as the a potential increased length of hospital stay and the financial cost [54, 63–65]. Various methods of blood management interventions are utilised to reduce the rates of autologous blood transfusions to include correcting any preoperative anaemia, ceasing antiplatelet and anticoagulant medications, intraoperative cell salvage and autologous transfusions and the use tranexamic acid [66–68].

Tranexamic acid in particular has been widely adopted as an agent to reduce intraoperative haemorrhage. As a synthetic lysine analogue tranexamic acid acts as an antifibrolytic agent by inhibiting plasminogen to plasmin and therefore delays the breakdown of fibrin containing blood clots. Studies have shown that the administration of tranexamic acid has reduced the proportion of patients requiring allogenic blood transfusions but not increasing the rates of complications including thromboembolic events and renal failure [68, 69].

3.3. Nerve injury

The incidence of nerve injury following a total hip replacement is approximately between 0.05 and 1.9% [70]. Damage to the sciatic and femoral nerve is most common, accounting for 79 and 13% respectively, with combined nerve palsy occurring in 5.8% cases. Obturator nerve palsies are more rare, occurring in 1.6% of cases [71].

Risk factors for nerve injury include revision surgery, female sex and developmental dysplasia of hip or acetabulum [72, 73]. The most common cause of nerve injury in total hip replacement is of unknown aetiology at 47%. Other recognised causes are iatrogenic with damage during the operative approach, though direct laceration is rare at 1%, or due to the mechanical effects of limb lengthening and offset mismatch [74]. If cement is used then the direct pressure effect or thermal injury can cause damage to the nerve. Haematoma formation can cause damage to the nerve and therefore meticulous haemostasis is important [72, 75].

There is no difference in the incidence of nerve palsy between the direct lateral or posterior approach [76]. When the sciatic nerve is affected it is usually the peroneal component, as it is more susceptible to traction and trauma [72]. Femoral nerve palsy is less common and is usually the result of direct compression intraoperatively by the retraction of soft tissues by surgical instruments.

Management of nerve injury can be challenging. The surgeon must ensure that the appropriate radiological imaging, usually an ultrasound to exclude a haematoma and possibly an MRI, is performed to exclude a reversible cause of injury and also other causes not related to the surgical intervention. Nerve conduction studies may be of benefit to assess the level and degree of injury. If the limb has been lengthened and there are no other causes of the injury identified, the leg length can be addressed to reduce the stretch of the sciatic nerve. If a haematoma is confirmed this may be an indication for surgery if symptoms do not resolve [72, 77–79]. However as most causes of nerve injuries are of unknown aetiology, generally in the absence of a clear cause, conservative management is advocated for a postoperative neuritis in a multi-disciplinary approach to ensure that all other causes of nerve injuries are excluded [80–82]. In this manner, one would ensure close observation and follow-up to ensure gradual improvement in function.

3.4. Dislocation

The rate of hip dislocations can range from 0.2 to 10% with 2% of patients dislocation within 1 year of their operation [83]. Of those who dislocate their total hip replacement, approximately one third will go on to have recurrent dislocations [84]. Risk factors are multifactorial and divided into patient, surgery and implant related.

3.4.1. Patient related factors

Cognitive disorders such as cerebral palsy, muscular dystrophy, dementia, advanced age and impaired compliance have showed increased chances of hip dislocations. Patients should avoid movements such as bending forward from a standing position or internal rotation of a flexed hip [76, 83]. Previous hip surgery have also shown to double the risk of dislocations [85].

3.4.2. *Surgical risk factors*

Surgical risk factors for dislocation of total hip replacements include the surgical approach, soft tissue tension, component design and orientation and surgeon experience. The majority dislocations occur posteriorly and therefore the posterior approach has the highest risk of dislocation. It has been documented in the literature a rate of 5.8% for the posterior approach in comparison to 2.3% for the anterolateral approach [85]. However recent research showing patients that have had a posterior capsular and external rotator repair have comparable rates to other approaches [76].

Implant alignment during hip replacement surgery is very important for stability of the joint. 'Safe zones' for acetabular cup position are defined as an abduction angle of 40 ± 10 degrees and anteversion of 15 ± 10 degrees, first defined by 6 in 1978 [86]. Recent studies have shown that although this range can be a useful guide to acetabular position, stability of a total hip replacement is multifactorial and should be assessed on an individual basis and therefore the 'Safe Zone' for a particular patient may lie outside this range [87].

3.4.3. *Implant related factors*

Component position and design can both influence the risk of dislocation. Head to neck ratio is very important for stability of the prosthesis and to allow a free range of movement without impingement. Larger femoral heads also allow a wide a mechanical range of motion when compare it to smaller head diameters [88]. In addition to this a larger femoral head has to move a greater distance away from the centre of the acetabular component before it can dislocate (jumping distance) therefore protecting against dislocation.

3.4.4. *Management*

Dislocations are initially managed by closed reduction in the majority of cases. In practice it is commonly seen that these patients are placed in an abduction brace though there is little evidence to support their use [76]. Patients who have recurrent or irreducible dislocations with correctly positioned components, can be managed with restrained liners. This has become a relatively more recent method of treatment that can be complicated with the increase risk of restricted range of movement due to impingement, osteolysis due to wear debris or early acetabular loosening. These should be used if a cause for instability has not been identified and can be used as a salvage procedure [89].

Recurrent dislocations can also be treated with a bipolar hemiarthroplasty due to the larger head size providing additional stability. This should be reserved for elderly low demand patients [89].

The use of dual mobility cups in unstable hips is becoming increasingly popular. Dual mobility cups have two points of articulation allowing increased stability with less restriction on range of movement [90].

Poor component position, soft tissue laxity and dislocations due to impingement may require surgical intervention to revise their total hip replacement.

3.5. Leg length discrepancy

Leg length discrepancy following a total hip arthroplasty is one of the most common reasons for patient dissatisfaction as it can cause nerve palsies, abnormal gait, lower back pain and reduced functional outcome. Inevitably this often leads to litigation against orthopaedic surgeons [91].

The incidence has been reported between 1 and 27% [92]. The measured leg length discrepancy have been reported to vary from 3 to 70 mm [93]. As previous covered, nerve palsies are one of the most serious complications of leg length discrepancy. Sciatic and peroneal nerve palsies have both been associated with limb lengthening [74].

Minor leg length discrepancy of less than 1 cm may be tolerated well by the patient but more than 2 cm may cause gait abnormalities as well as increase in physiological demand [91, 94]. It is important to assess the patient preoperatively and measuring true and apparent leg lengths can do this. True leg length is measured from the ipsilateral anterior superior iliac spine to medial malleolus whereas apparent leg length is measured from the umbilicus to medial malleolus. Apparent leg length discrepancies can be affected by pelvic abnormalities secondary to lumbar spine pathology or contractures around the hip. Leg length discrepancy that occurs secondary to chronic lumbar spine pathology can be very difficult to correct and may lead shortening or lengthening of the overall leg length.

Radiographs can be used for preoperative evaluation of leg length discrepancy and the use of a preoperative template to determine the level of the neck cut and position of acetabular component [95, 96]. However the reliance of preoperative templating alone has shown that its efficacy in avoiding any leg length discrepancy to be only 60% [96]. There are many intraoperative techniques using landmarks to ensure that the correct leg length is maintained. One review of the literature by Desai et al. has identified over 20 methods discussed in the literature [91]. These methods have in common the two constant reference points, one of the pelvis and the other on the femur intraoperatively to ensure the leg length is maintained and traditionally the greater trochanter is the reference point of the femur [97].

The achievement of absolute leg length equality is challenging to achieve [98]. There must be adequate time allowed for any contractures to resolve and any residual minor leg length discrepancies can be corrected with simple shoes raises. Although a simple intervention these are not always well received by patients [99]. In more significant discrepancies surgical intervention may be required to address the symptoms of pain and functional impairment then surgical correction may be required [100].

3.6. Peri-prosthetic fracture

With increasing life expectancy and an ageing population, resulting in more patients with poor bone quality and increase risk of falls, the number of total hip replacement is increasing. Thus the likelihood of patients who have had a total hip arthroplasty sustaining a peri-prosthetic fracture is on the rise. Furthermore with a broader indication for surgery, younger patients who are more active and therefore high energy trauma prone are increasingly undergoing such procedures, again increasing the risks of subsequent peri-prosthetic fractures [101].

Peri-prosthetic fractures can either occur in the intraoperative or postoperative period. Intraoperative and postoperative peri-prosthetic have been reported at 1 and 1.1% respectively. Cementless fixation are at higher risk for intraoperative peri-prosthetic fracture at 5.4% for primary total hip replacement and 21% for revision surgery [102]. For those sustaining a postoperative peri-prosthetic fracture the most significant risk factor is osteolysis with implant loosening [103]. The most common mechanism for peri-prosthetic fractures is a low energy movement accounting for over 75% of all peri-prosthetic fractures [104].

Peri-prosthetic fractures of the femur can be classified using the Vancouver classification (**Table 1**).

The management of peri-prosthetic fractures following total hip replacement is based not only on the fracture characteristics as defined by the Vancouver system but also patient factors including co-morbidities and bone quality. However the Vancouver classification does provide a well proven approach in considering the management of such injuries and we will briefly describe some of the approaches used in addressing such injuries.

Type A fractures are usually treated non-operatively unless a large part of the calcar is involved leading to instability of the prosthesis which would then require revision surgery. Type B fractures occur around or just distal to the stem and are most common representing 80% of all cases [101]. B1 fractures may be treated with open reduction internal fixation with a combination of plate and cerclage wire system. B2 type fractures have good bone stock and are commonly treated with revision total hip arthroplasty with a long stem, bypassing the fracture site in combination with plates and cerclage wires. B3 can be the most challenging to treat due to the poor bone stock. These may be treated with either revision hip arthroplasty with structural allografts, distally fixed long stem implants or custom proximal femoral replacements. Type C can be fixed using an open reduction internal fixation technique and there are numerous methods in use to include locking plates, screw and cable plates and intramedullary systems [101].

Various implants are available but treatment is very much dependent on the type of fracture, amount of bone stock along with taking into account patient factors. Dynamic compression plates (DCP) or locking compression plates (LCP) can be used in combination with cerclage wires and screws. Fixation of the plate can be done with either cerclage wires or unicortical screws. Proximal fixation with unicortical screws increases strength and therefore preferred

Type	Subtype	Description
A	A L	Lesser trochanter
	A G	Greater trochanter
B	B1	Well–fixed prosthesis
	B2	Loose prosthesis
	B3	Loose prosthesis with poor bone stock
C		Fracture well below the tip of prosthesis

Table 1. The Vancouver classification for periprosthetic fractures of total hip replacements [105].

over cerclage wires. Plates can also be biplanar to provide further stability. Various proximal femoral replacements are available and the choice depends on level of fracture, quality of bone and amount of bonestock remaining [106].

Acetabular peri-prosthetic fractures are uncommon but usually occur intraoperatively when inserting the acetabular component. The aim of treatment is to stabilise the fracture and prevent further propagation of the implant by plating the anterior or posterior columns, using bone grafts and, or using jumbo revision cups if there is significant bone loss [107].

3.7. Heterotopic ossification

Heterotopic ossification is the abnormal formation of lamellar bone in extra-skeletal soft tissue [108]. The reported rates of heterotopic ossification post total hip replacement varies greatly between 0.6 and 90% [108–112]. Risk factors include male gender, previous history of heterotopic ossification, pre-existing hip fusion, ankylosing spondylitis, Paget's disease, post traumatic osteoarthritis, osteonecrosis and rheumatoid arthritis [113]. Surgical factors may also play a role and include, extensive soft tissue dissection, haematoma formation, and excess bone debris [113].

Early changes of heterotopic ossification can be detected as early as 3 weeks on bone scan, 6 weeks on plain radiographs but can take up to 1 year for bone to fully mature [76]. Heterotopic ossification is usually asymptomatic and diagnosed on follow up radiographs. When symptomatic, patients most commonly present with pain and stiffness [108].

The abductor compartment is most commonly affected and is classified using the Brooker classification which is based on extent of heterotopic ossification seen on anteroposterior radiographs of the pelvis [114].

The management of heterotrophic ossification is divided into prevention and treatment once established. The prophylactic management was pioneered by Dhal with the administration of non-steroidal anti-inflammatory drugs [115]. Radiotherapy treatment in the form of 60Co gamma radiation or high energy X photons is also used to prevent the formation of heterotrophic ossification. The treatment of established heterotrophic ossification include physiotherapy during the maturation phase to prevent further propagation and no surgical intervention such as radiotherapy and extracorporeal shockwave therapy [116, 117]. Interventional procedures in the form of embolization of the nutrient arteries have been used to prevent the formation of further heterotopic ossification [118]. Surgical excision of the lesions may be considered to treat the symptoms of both pain and stiffness [119, 120].

3.8. Other complications

Osteolysis and subsequent aseptic loosening are complications that can occur as a late complication in total hip arthroplasty. Osteolysis is induced by several mechanisms to include; adaptive bone remodelling, fluid pressure and particulate debris [121]. The principle mechanism for osteolysis following total hip arthroplasty is particular debris, particularly polyethylene [122]. These particulates are dissolved in the surrounding joint fluid that can lead to chronic inflammation at the implant bone interface. This leads to a build-up of cells such as macrophages, fibroblasts, giant cells, neutrophils, lymphocytes and osteoclasts. The cellular response created by these cells lead to resorption of bone leading to aseptic loosening and failure of the arthroplasty [123]. This type of complication would be treated with a revision total hip replacement.

Trochanteric bursitis can be seen in 3–17% of patients following total hip arthroplasty. This can be a result of irritation due to over use, change in posture, leg length discrepancy or inappropriate offset. This is usually treated non operatively with simple analgesia, non-steroidal anti-inflammatory drugs or steroid injections [124].

Finally although more of an irritation rather than a complication with significant morbidity, some total hip arthroplasty can have issues with squeaking. Squeaking is an issue found on hard on hard bearings and rates have been reported between 0.3 and 24.6% in ceramic on ceramic arthroplasty [125]. The sound is thought to be produced from the friction created from hard on hard surfaces with insufficient fluid film lubrication. Although a nuisance, there is currently no clear consensus on the association of squeaking with ceramic failure, but patients should be counselled on the issue if hard on hard bearing surfaces are to be considered [126].

4. Conclusion

Complications following total hip replacement can be broadly divided into systemic and procedure specific complications. Overall, incidence of complications have improved over time as surgical and anaesthetic techniques have improved along with the diagnosis and management of such complications.

The most common systemic complication is a deep vein thrombosis. Infection is the most feared complication but the incidence have reduced with prophylactic antibiotics and improved theatre environment. Leg length is one of the most common causes of patient dissatisfaction and all complications can be challenging to manage for the hip surgeon. However despite these complications total hip replacements is one of the most successful orthopaedic procedures performed and continue to be widely performed across different healthcare systems with very positive patient satisfaction outcomes.

Conflict of interest

The authors have no conflicts of interest to declare.

Author details

Chang Park* and Irfan Merchant

*Address all correspondence to: changpark3@gmail.com

Royal Berkshire NHS Foundation Trust, Reading, UK

References

[1] Jones CA, Voaklander DC, Johnston DW, Suarez-Almazor ME. Health related quality of life outcomes after total hip and knee arthroplasties in a community based population. The Journal of Rheumatology. 2000 Jul;**27**(7):1745-1752

[2] Mancuso CA, Salvati EA, Johanson NA, Peterson MG, Charlson ME. Patients' expectations and satisfaction with total hip arthroplasty. The Journal of Arthroplasty. 1997 Jun;**12**(4):387-396

[3] National Joint Registry. Summary of Annual Statistics (England and Wales). National Joint Registry. UK: Northgate Public Service; 2017

[4] Liu SS, Gonzalez Della Valle A, Besculides MC, Gaber LK, Memtsoudis SG. Trends in mortality, complications, and demographics for primary hip arthroplasty in the United States. International Orthopaedics. 2009 Jun;**33**(3):643-651

[5] Magill SS, Edwards JR, Bamberg W, Beldavs ZG, Dumyati G, Kainer MA, Lynfield R, Maloney M, McAllister-Hollod L, Nadle J, Ray SM. Multistate point-prevalence survey of health care–associated infections. New England Journal of Medicine. 2014 Mar 27;**370**(13):1198-1208

[6] Alvarez AP, Demzik AL, Alvi HM, Hardt KD, Manning DW. Risk factors for postoperative urinary tract infections in patients undergoing total joint arthroplasty. Advances in Orthopedics. 2016;**2016**:7268985

[7] Rasouli MR, Maltenfort MG, Purtill JJ, Hozack WJ, Parvizi J. Has the rate of in-hospital infections after total joint arthroplasty decreased? Clinical Orthopaedics and Related Research®. 2013 Oct 1;**471**(10):3102-3111

[8] Poss RO, Thornhill TS, Ewald FC, Thomas WH, Batte NJ, Sledge CB. Factors influencing the incidence and outcome of infection following total joint arthroplasty. Clinical Orthopaedics and Related Research. 1984 Jan 1;(182):117-126

[9] Sabaté S, Mazo V, Canet J. Predicting postoperative pulmonary complications: Implications for outcomes and costs. Current Opinion in Anesthesiology. 2014 Apr 1;**27**(2): 201-209

[10] Song K, Rong Z, Yang X, Yao Y, Shen Y, Shi D, Xu Z, et al. Early pulmonary complications following total knee arthroplasty under general anesthesia: A prospective cohort study using CT scan. BioMed Research International. 2016;**2016**:4062043

[11] Jain V, Dhaon B, Jaiswal A, Nigam V, Singla J. Deep vein thrombosis after total hip and knee arthroplasty in Indian patients. Postgraduate Medical Journal. 2004;**80**(950):729-731. DOI: 10.1136/pgmj.2003.018127

[12] Kim YH, Oh SH, Kim JS. Incidence and natural history of deep-vein thrombosis after total hip arthroplasty. A prospective and randomised clinical study. Journal of Bone and Joint Surgery. British Volume (London). 2003 Jul;**85**(5):661-665

[13] Samama CM, Ravaud P, Parent F, Barre J, Mertl P, Mismetti P. Epidemiology of venous thromboembolism after lower limb arthroplasty: The FOTO study. Journal of Thrombosis and Haemostasis. 2007 Dec;**5**(12):2360-2367

[14] Mantilla CB, Horlocker TT, Schroeder DR, Berry DJ, Brown DL. Frequency of myocardial infarction, pulmonary embolism, deep venous thrombosis, and death following primary hip or knee arthroplasty. Anesthesiology. 2002 May;**96**(5):1140-1146

[15] NICE. Venous Thromboembolism: Reducing the Risk of Venous Thromboembolism (Deep Vein Thrombosis and Pulmonary Embolism) in Inpatients Undergoing Surgery. National Collaborating Centre for Acute Care; 2007

[16] Beksac B, Gonzalez Della Valle A, Salvati EA. Thromboembolic disease after total hip arthroplasty: Who is at risk? Clinical Orthopaedics and Related Research. 2006 Dec; **453**:211-224

[17] Davis FM, Laurenson VG, Gillespie WJ, Wells JE, Foate J, Newman E. Deep vein thrombosis after total hip replacement. A comparison between spinal and general anaesthesia. Journal of Bone and Joint Surgery. British Volume (London). 1989 Mar;**71**(2):181-185

[18] Lieberman JR, Cheng V, Cote MP. Pulmonary embolism rates following total hip arthroplasty with prophylactic anticoagulation: Some pulmonary emboli cannot be avoided. The Journal of Arthroplasty. 2017;**32**(3):980-986

[19] Kallos T, Enis JE, Gollan F, Davis JH. Intramedullary pressure and pulmonary embolism of femoral medullary contents in dogs during insertion of bone cement and a prosthesis. The Journal of Bone and Joint Surgery. American Volume. 1974 Oct;**56**(7):1363-1367

[20] Tronzo RG, Kallos T, Wyche MQ. Elevation of intramedullary pressure when methylmethacrylate is inserted in total hip arthroplasty. The Journal of Bone and Joint Surgery. American Volume. 1974 Jun;**56**(4):714-718

[21] Colonna DM, Kilgus D, Brown W, Challa V, Stump DA, Moody DM. Acute brain fat embolization occurring after total hip arthroplasty in the absence of a patent foramen ovale. Anesthesiology. 2002 Apr;**96**(4):1027-1029

[22] Wenda K, Degreif J, Runkel M, Ritter G. Pathogenesis and prophylaxis of circulatory reactions during total hip replacement. Archives of Orthopaedic and Trauma Surgery. 1993;**112**(6):260-265

[23] Charnley J. A clean-air operating enclosure. The British Journal of Surgery. 1964 Mar;**51**:202-205

[24] Blom AW, Taylor AH, Pattison G, Whitehouse S, Bannister GC. Infection after total hip arthroplasty. The Avon experience. Journal of Bone and Joint Surgery. British Volume (London). 2003 Sep;**85**(7):956-959

[25] Bannister G. Prevention of infection in joint replacement. Current Orthopaedics. 2002; **16**(6):426-433

[26] Hughes SP, Anderson FM. Infection in the operating room. Journal of Bone and Joint Surgery. British Volume (London). 1999;**81**(5):754-755

[27] Charnley J. Postoperative infection after total hip replacement with special reference to air contamination in the operating room. Clinical Orthopaedics and Related Research. 1972;**87**:167-187

[28] Hooper GJ et al. Does the use of laminar flow and space suits reduce early deep infection after total hip and knee replacement?: The ten-year results of the New Zealand joint registry. Journal of Bone and Joint Surgery. British Volume (London). 2011;**93**(1):85-90

[29] Zheng H et al. Control strategies to prevent total hip replacement-related infections: A systematic review and mixed treatment comparison. BMJ Open. 2014;**4**(3):e003978

[30] Classen DC et al. The timing of prophylactic administration of antibiotics and the risk of surgical-wound infection. The New England Journal of Medicine. 1992;**326**(5):281-286

[31] Prokuski L et al. Prophylactic antibiotics in orthopaedic surgery. Instructional Course Lectures. 2011;**60**:545-555

[32] AlBuhairan B, Hind D, Hutchinson A. Antibiotic prophylaxis for wound infections in total joint arthroplasty: A systematic review. Journal of Bone and Joint Surgery. British Volume (London). 2008;**90**:915-919

[33] Spangehl MJ, Masri BA, O'Connell JX, Duncan CP. Prospective analysis of preoperative and intraoperative investigations for the diagnosis of infection at the sites of two hundred and two revision total hip arthroplasties. The Journal of Bone and Joint Surgery. American Volume. 1999 May;**81**(5):672-683

[34] Zhuang H, Yang H, Alavi A. Critical role of 18F-labeled fluorodeoxyglucose PET in the management of patients with arthroplasty. Radiologic Clinics of North America. 2007 Jul;**45**(4):711-718, vii

[35] Love C, Marwin SE, Palestro CJ. Nuclear medicine and the infected joint replacement. Seminars in Nuclear Medicine. 2009 Jan;**39**(1):66-78

[36] Ali F, Wilkinson JM, Cooper JR, Kerry RM, Hamer AJ, Norman P, et al. Accuracy of joint aspiration for the preoperative diagnosis of infection in total hip arthroplasty. The Journal of Arthroplasty. 2006;**21**:221-226

[37] Tsukayama DT, Estrada R, Gustilo RB. Infection after total hip arthroplasty. A study of the treatment of one hundred and six infections. The Journal of Bone and Joint Surgery. American Volume. 1996 Apr;**78**(4):512-523

[38] Crockarell JR, Hanssen AD, Osmon DR, Morrey BF. Treatment of infection with debridement and retention of the components following hip arthroplasty. The Journal of Bone and Joint Surgery. American Volume. 1998 Sep;**80**(9):1306-1313

[39] Buchholz HW, Elson RA, Engelbrecht E, Lodenkamper H, Rottger J, Siegel A. Management of deep infection of total hip replacement. Journal of Bone and Joint Surgery. British Volume (London). 1981;**63-B**(3):342-353

[40] Younger AS, Duncan CP, Masri BA, McGraw RW. The outcome of two-stage arthroplasty using a custom-made interval spacer to treat the infected hip. The Journal of Arthroplasty. 1997 Sep;**12**(6):615-623

[41] Stockley I, Mockford BJ, Hoad-Reddick A, Norman P. The use of two-stage exchange arthroplasty with depot antibiotics in the absence of long-term antibiotic therapy in infected total hip replacement. Journal of Bone and Joint Surgery. British Volume (London). 2008 Feb;**90**(2):145-148

[42] Rosencher N, Kerkkamp HE, Macheras G, Munuera LM, Menichella G, Barton DM, et al. Orthopedic surgery transfusion hemoglobin European overview (OSTHEO) study: Blood management in elective knee and hip arthroplasty in Europe. Transfusion. 2003;**43**:459-469

[43] Vuille-Lessard É, Boudreault D, Girard F, Ruel M, Chagnon M, Hardy J-F. Red blood cell transfusion practice in elective orthopedic surgery: A multicenter cohort study. Transfusion. 2010;**50**:2117-2124

[44] Cushner F, Agnelli G, Fitzgerald G, Warwick D. Complications and functional outcomes after total hip arthroplasty and total knee arthroplasty: Results from the Global Orthopaedic Registry (GLORY). American Journal of Orthopedics (Belle Mead NJ). 2010 Sep;**39**(9 Suppl):22-28

[45] Flordal PA, Neander G. Blood loss in total hip replacement. Archives of Orthopaedic and Trauma Surgery. 1991;**111**:34-38

[46] Toy PTCY, Kaplan EB, McVay PA, Lee SJ, Strauss RG, Stehling LD. Blood loss and replacement in total hip arthroplasty: A multicenter study. Transfusion. 1992;**32**:63-67

[47] Grosflam JM, Wright EA, Cleary PD, Katz JN. Predictors of blood loss during total hip replacement surgery. Arthritis & Rheumatology. 1995 Sep 1;**8**(3):167-173

[48] Hrnack SA, Skeen N, Xu T, Rosenstein AD. Correlation of body mass index and blood loss during total knee and total hip arthroplasty. The American Journal of Orthopedics. 2012;**41**:467-471

[49] Carling MS, Jeppsson A, Eriksson BI, Brisby H. Transfusions and blood loss in total hip and knee arthroplasty: A prospective observational study. Journal of Orthopaedic Surgery and Research. 2015 Mar 28;**10**(1):48

[50] Bowditch MG, Villar RN. Do obese patients bleed more? A prospective study of blood loss at total hip replacement. Annals of the Royal College of Surgeons of England. 1999;**81**:198-200

[51] Browne JA, Adib F, Brown TE, Novicoff WM. Transfusion rates are increasing following total hip arthroplasty: Risk factors and outcomes. The Journal of Arthroplasty. 2013;**28** (8 Suppl):34-37

[52] Hasley PB, Lave JR, Hanusa BH, Arena VC, Ramsey G, Kapoor WN, Fine MJ. Variation in the use of red blood cell transfusions. A study of four common medical and surgical conditions. Medical Care. 1995;**33**:1145-1160

[53] The Sanguis Study Group. Use of blood products for elective surgery in 43 European hospitals. Transfusion Medicine. 1994;**4**:251-268

[54] Bierbaum BE, Hill C, Callaghan JJ, et al. An analysis of blood management in patients having a total hip or knee arthroplasty. The Journal of Bone and Joint Surgery. American Volume. 1999;**81**(1):2-10

[55] Del Trujillo MM, Carrero A, Munoz M. The utility of the perioperative autologous transfusion system OrthoPAT in total hip replacement surgery: A prospective study. Archives of Orthopaedic and Trauma Surgery. 2008;**128**:1031-1038

[56] Smith LK, Williams DH, Langkamer VG. Post-operative blood salvage with autologous retransfusion in primary total hip replacement. Journal of Bone and Joint Surgery. British Volume (London). 2007;**89**:1092-1097

[57] Moonen AF, Knoors NT, van Os JJ, et al. Retransfusion of filtered shed blood in primary total hip and knee arthroplasty: A prospective randomized clinical trial. Transfusion. 2007;**47**:379-384

[58] MacFarlane BJ, Marx L, Anquist K, Pineo G, Chenger J, Cassol E. Analysis of a protocol for an autologous blood transfusion program for total joint replacement surgery. Canadian Journal of Surgery. 1988;**31**:126-129

[59] Axelrod FB, Pepkowitz SH, Goldfinger D. Establishment of a schedule of optimal preoperative collection of autologous blood. Transfusion. 1989;**29**:677-680

[60] Woolson ST, Marsh JS, Tanner JB. Transfusion of previously deposited autologous blood for patients undergoing hip replacement surgery. Journal of Bone and Joint Surgery. 1987;**69**:325-328

[61] Eckardt JJ, Gossett TC, Amstutz HC. Autologous transfusion and total hip arthroplasty. Clinical Orthopaedics and Related Research. 1978;(132):39-45

[62] Hart A, Khalil JA, Carli A, Huk O, Zukor D, Antoniou J. Blood transfusion in primary total hip and knee arthroplasty. Incidence, risk factors, and thirty-day complication rates. JBJS. 2014;**96**(23):1945-1951

[63] Goodnough LT, Shuck JM. Risks, options, and informed consent for blood transfusion in elective surgery. American Journal of Surgery. 1990;**159**(6):602

[64] Keating EM, Meding JB. Perioperative blood management practices in elective orthopaedic surgery. The Journal of the American Academy of Orthopaedic Surgeons. 2002;**10**:393-400

[65] Bower WF, Jin L, Underwood MJ, et al. Peri-operative blood transfusion increases length of hospital stay and number of post-operative complications in non-cardiac surgical patients. Hong Kong Medical Journal. 2010;**16**(2):116

[66] Pierson JL, Hannon TJ, Earles DR. A blood-conservation algorithm to reduce blood transfusions after total hip and knee arthroplasty. The Journal of Bone and Joint Surgery. American Volume. 2004;**86**(7):1512-1518

[67] Krebs V, Hozack WJ, Callaghan JJ, et al. Eliminating transfusion in primary joint arthroplasty—An achievable goal. The Journal of Arthroplasty. 2014;**29**(8):1511

[68] Sukeik M, Alshryda S, Haddad FS, et al. Systematic review and meta-analysis of the use of tranexamic acid in total hip replacement. Journal of Bone and Joint Surgery. British Volume (London). 2011;**93**(1):39-46

[69] Poeran J, Rasul R, Suzuki S, Danninger T, et al. Tranexamic acid use and postoperative outcomes in patients undergoing total hip or knee arthroplasty in the United States: Retrospective analysis of effectiveness and safety. BMJ. 2014;**349**:g4829

[70] Brown GD, Swanson FA, Nercessian OA. Neurologic injuries after total hip arthroplasty. The American Journal of Orthopedics. 2008;**37**(4):191-197

[71] Schmalzried TP, Noordin S, Amstutz HC. Update on nerve palsy associated with total hip replacement. Clinical Orthopaedics and Related Research. 1997 Nov;**344**:188-206

[72] Schmalzried TP, Amstutz HC, Dorey FJ. Nerve palsy associated with total hip replacement. Risk factors and prognosis. The Journal of Bone and Joint Surgery. American Volume. 1991;**73**:1074-1080

[73] Edwards BN, Tullos HS, Noble PC. Contributory factors and etiology of sciatic nerve palsy in total hip arthroplasty. Clinical Orthopaedics and Related Research. 1987:136-141

[74] Barrack RL. Neurovascular injury: Avoiding catastrophe. The Journal of Arthroplasty. 2004 Jun;**19**(4 Suppl 1):104-107

[75] Klein GS, Sharkey PF, et al. Late sciatic nerve palsy caused by Haematoma after primary total hip arthroplasty. The Journal of Arthroplasty. 2004;**19**(6):760-792

[76] Kinov P, editor. Arthroplasty – Update. The Shard, London: IntechOpen Limited; ISBN: 978-953-51-0995-2. 618 pp. [Chapters published February 20, 2013 under CC BY 3.0 license DOI: 10.5772/56149 Edited Volume]

[77] Montogmery AS, Birch R, Malone A. Sciatic neurostalagia caused by total hip arthroplasty, cured by late neurolysis. Journal of Bone and Joint Surgery. 2005;**87**(3):410-411

[78] Mounsasmy V, Cui Q, Brown TE, et al. Acute sciatic neuritis following total hip arthroplasty: A case report. Archives of Orthopaedic and Trauma Surgery. 2008;**128**(1):25-28

[79] Milhako WM, Phillips MJ, Krackow KA. Acute sciatic and femoral neuritis following total hip arthroplasty. A case report. Journal of Bone and Joint Surgery American. 2001;**83**(4):589-592

[80] Park C, Ikram A, Abdul-Jabar HB, Radford W. Sciatic nerve neuritis of no cause in primary total hip replacement. A case series. Journal of Clinical Orthopaedics and Trauma. DOI: 10.1016/j.jcot.2017.08.010 [Published online ahead of print]

[81] May O, Girard J, Hurtevent JF, et al. Delayed transient sciatic nerve palsy after primary cementless hip arthroplasty: A report of two cases. Journal of Bone and Joint Surgery. 2008;**90**(5):674-676

[82] Katsimihas M, Hutchinson J, Heath P. Et al, (2002) Delayed sciatic nerve palsy after total hip arthroplasty, The Journal of Arthroplasty, **17**(3):379-381

[83] Dargel J et al. Dislocation following total hip replacement. Deutsches Ärzteblatt International. 2014;**111**(51-52):884-890. PMC

[84] Sanchez-Sotelo J, Berry DJ. Epidemiology of instability after total hip replacement. The Orthopedic Clinics of North America. 2001 Oct;**32**(4):543-552, vii

[85] Woo RY, Morrey BF. Dislocations after total hip arthroplasty. The Journal of Bone and Joint Surgery. American Volume. 1982 Dec;**64**(9):1295-1306

[86] Lewinnek GE, Lewis JL, Tarr R, Compere CL, Zimmerman JR. Dislocations after total hip-replacement arthroplasties. Journal of Bone and Joint Surgery. 1978;**60**:217-220

[87] Abdel MP, von Roth P, Jennings MT, Hanssen AD, Pagnano MW. What safe zone? The vast majority of dislocated THAs are within the Lewinnek safe zone for Acetabular component position. Clinical Orthopaedics and Related Research. 2016;**474**(2):386-391

[88] Crowninshield RD, Maloney WJ, Wentz DH, Humphrey SM, Blanchard CR. Biomechanics of large femoral heads: What they do and don't do. Clinical Orthopaedics and Related Research. 2004;**429**:102-107

[89] D'Angelo F, Murena L, Zatti G, Cherubino P. The unstable total hip replacement. Indian Journal of Orthopaedics. 2008;**42**(3):252-259

[90] Ko LM, Hozack WJ. The dual mobility cup: What problems does it solve? Bone Joint J. 2016 Jan 1;**98**(1 Suppl. A):60-63

[91] Desai AS, Dramis A, Board TN. Leg length discrepancy after total hip arthroplasty: A review of literature. Current Reviews in Musculoskeletal Medicine. 2013;**6**(4):336-341. PMC

[92] Ranawat CS, Rodriguez JA. Functional leg-length inequality following total hip arthroplasty. The Journal of Arthroplasty. 1997;**12**:359-364. DOI: 10.1016/S0883-5403(97)90190-X

[93] Sathappan SS, Ginat D, Patel V, Walsh M, Jaffe WL, Di Cesare PE. Effect of anaesthesia type on limb length discrepancy after total hip arthroplasty. The Journal of Arthroplasty. 2008;**23**:203-209. DOI: 10.1016/j.arth.2007.01.022

[94] Jasty M, Webster W, Harris W. Management of limb length inequality during total hip replacement. Clinical Orthopaedics and Related Research. 1996 Dec 1;**333**:165-171

[95] Woolson ST, James MH, Sawyer A. Results of leg length equalization for patients undergoing primary total hip replacement. The Journal of Arthroplasty. 1999;**14**:159-164

[96] Knight JL, Atwater RD. Preoperative planning for total hip arthroplasty: Quantitating it's utility and precision. The Journal of Arthroplasty. 1992;**7**:403-409

[97] Charnley J. Low Friction Arthroplasty of the Hip: Theory and Practice. New York: Springer; 1979

[98] Rubash HE, Parvataneni HK. The pants too short, the leg too long: Leg length inequality after total hip arthroplasty. Orthopaedics. 2007;**30**:764-765

[99] Maloney WJ, Keeney JA. Leg length discrepancy after total hip arthroplasty. The Journal of Arthroplasty. 2004;**19**:108-110

[100] Parvizi J, Sharkey PF, Bissett BA, Rothman RH, Hozack WJ. Surgical treatment of limb length discrepancy following total hip arthroplasty. The Journal of Bone and Joint Surgery. American Volume. 2003;**85**:2310-2317

[101] Schwarzkopf R, Oni JK, Marwin SE. Total hip arthroplasty periprosthetic femoral fractures: A review of classification and current treatment. Bulletin/Hospital for Joint Diseases. 2013;**71**:68-78

[102] Berry DJ. Epidemiology: Hip and knee. The Orthopedic Clinics of North America. 1999 Apr;**30**(2):183-190

[103] Sarvilinna R, Huhtala HS, Sovelius RT, et al. Factors predisposing to periprosthetic fracture after hip arthroplasty: A case (n = 31)-control study. Acta Orthopaedica Scandinavica. 2004 Feb;**75**(1):16-20

[104] Lindahl H, Malchau H, Herberts P, Garellick G. Periprosthetic femoral fractures classification and demographics of 1049 periprosthetic femoral fractures from the Swedish National Hip Arthroplasty register. The Journal of Arthroplasty. 2005 Oct;**20**(7):857-865

[105] Gaski GE, Scully SP. In brief: Classifications in brief: Vancouver classification of postoperative periprosthetic femur fractures. Clinical Orthopaedics and Related Research. 2011;**469**:1507

[106] Yasen AT, Haddad FS. Periprosthetic fractures: Bespoke solutions. The Bone & Joint Journal. 2014 Nov 1;**96**(11 Suppl. A):48-55

[107] Chitre A, Wynn Jones H, Shah N, Clayson A. Complications of total hip arthroplasty: Periprosthetic fractures of the acetabulum. Current Reviews in Musculoskeletal Medicine. 2013;**6**(4):357-363

[108] Thomas BJ. Heterotopic bone formation after total hip arthroplasty. The Orthopedic Clinics of North America. 1992;**23**:347-358

[109] Ahrengart L. Periarticular heterotopic ossification after total hip arthroplasty. Risk factors and consequences. Clinical Orthopaedics and Related Research. 1991;**263**(2):49-58

[110] Naraghi FF, De Coster TA, Moneim MS, et al. Heterotopic ossification. Orthopedics. 1996;**19**:145-151

[111] Thomas BJ, Amstutz HC. Prevention of heterotopic bone formation: Clinical experience with diphosphonates. The Hip. 1987:59-69

[112] Nilsson OS, Persson PE. Heterotopic bone formation after joint replacement. Current Opinion in Rheumatology. 1999;**11**(2):127-131

[113] Board TN, Karva A, Board RE et al. The prophylaxis and treatment of heterotopic ossification following lower limb arthroplasty. Journal of Bone and Joint Surgery. British Volume (London) 2007 Apr;**89**(4):434-440

[114] Jain R. Heterotopic ossification after acetabular fractures: Prevention and management. Journal of Orthopaedic Complications. 2016;**1**(1):20-22

[115] Dahl HK. Klinske Observasjoner. In: Symposium on Arthrose. Blindern, Norway: MSD; 1975. pp. 37-46

[116] Brissot R, Lassalle A, Vincendeau S, et al. Treatment of heterotopic ossification by extracorporeal shock wave: 26 patients. Annales de Réadaptation et de Médecine Physique. 2005;**48**(8):581-589

[117] Healy WL, Lot TC, De Simone AA, et al. Single-dose irradiation for the prevention of heterotopic ossification after total hip arthroplasty. Journal of Bone & Joint Surgery: American. 1995;**77**:590-595

[118] Vogl TJ, Wolff JD, Balzer J, et al. Preoperative arterial embolization in heterotopic ossification: A case report. European Radiology. 2001;**11**(6):962-964

[119] Wick M, Muller EJ, Hahn MP, et al. Surgical excision of heterotopic bone after hip surgery followed by oral indomethacin application: Is there a clinical benefit for the patient? Archives of Orthopaedic and Trauma Surgery. 1999;**119**(3-4):151-155

[120] Wahl B, Grasshoff H, Meinecke I, et al. Clinical and radiological results of surgical removal of periarticular ossifications after hip prosthesis implantation. Unfallchirurg. 2002;**105**(6):523-526

[121] Dattani R. Femoral osteolysis following total hip replacement. Postgraduate Medical Journal. 2007;**83**(979):312-316

[122] Rubash HE, Sinha RK, Shanbhag AS, et al. Pathogenesis of bone loss after total hip arthroplasty. The Orthopedic Clinics of North America. 1998;**29**:173-186

[123] Abu-Amer Y, Darwech I, Clohisy JC. Aseptic loosening of total joint replacements: Mechanisms underlying osteolysis and potential therapies. Arthritis Research & Therapy. 2007 Jun;**9**(1):S6

[124] Shemesh SS, Moucha CS, Keswani A, Maher NA, Chen D, Bronson MJ. Trochanteric bursitis following primary total hip arthroplasty: Incidence, predictors, and treatment. The Journal of Arthroplasty. 2018 Apr;**33**(4):1205-1209

[125] Levy YD, Munir S, Donohoo S, Walter WL. Review on squeaking hips. World Journal of Orthopedics. 2015;**6**(10):812-820

[126] Traina F, De Fine M, Bordini B, Toni A. Risk factors for ceramic liner fracture after total hip arthroplasty. Hip International. 2012;**22**:607-614

Permissions

All chapters in this book were first published in THRAO, by InTech Open; hereby published with permission under the Creative Commons Attribution License or equivalent. Every chapter published in this book has been scrutinized by our experts. Their significance has been extensively debated. The topics covered herein carry significant findings which will fuel the growth of the discipline. They may even be implemented as practical applications or may be referred to as a beginning point for another development.

The contributors of this book come from diverse backgrounds, making this book a truly international effort. This book will bring forth new frontiers with its revolutionizing research information and detailed analysis of the nascent developments around the world.

We would like to thank all the contributing authors for lending their expertise to make the book truly unique. They have played a crucial role in the development of this book. Without their invaluable contributions this book wouldn't have been possible. They have made vital efforts to compile up to date information on the varied aspects of this subject to make this book a valuable addition to the collection of many professionals and students.

This book was conceptualized with the vision of imparting up-to-date information and advanced data in this field. To ensure the same, a matchless editorial board was set up. Every individual on the board went through rigorous rounds of assessment to prove their worth. After which they invested a large part of their time researching and compiling the most relevant data for our readers.

The editorial board has been involved in producing this book since its inception. They have spent rigorous hours researching and exploring the diverse topics which have resulted in the successful publishing of this book. They have passed on their knowledge of decades through this book. To expedite this challenging task, the publisher supported the team at every step. A small team of assistant editors was also appointed to further simplify the editing procedure and attain best results for the readers.

Apart from the editorial board, the designing team has also invested a significant amount of their time in understanding the subject and creating the most relevant covers. They scrutinized every image to scout for the most suitable representation of the subject and create an appropriate cover for the book.

The publishing team has been an ardent support to the editorial, designing and production team. Their endless efforts to recruit the best for this project, has resulted in the accomplishment of this book. They are a veteran in the field of academics and their pool of knowledge is as vast as their experience in printing. Their expertise and guidance has proved useful at every step. Their uncompromising quality standards have made this book an exceptional effort. Their encouragement from time to time has been an inspiration for everyone.

The publisher and the editorial board hope that this book will prove to be a valuable piece of knowledge for researchers, students, practitioners and scholars across the globe.

List of Contributors

Hiran Wimal Amarasekera
Neville Fernando Teaching Hospital and South Asian Institute of Medicine, Colombo, Sri Lanka
Warwick Orthopaedics, University of Warwick, Coventry, United Kingdom

Mark Curtin and Eoghan Pomeroy
Department of Trauma and Orthopaedics, Beaumont Hospital, Dublin, Ireland

James Broderick
Department of Trauma and Orthopaedics, Galway University Hospital, Galway, Ireland

Jan Vagner
Rehabilitation Department, Středomoravská nemocniční a.s, Přerov Hospital, Czech Republic

Ingrid Palaščáková Špringrová
ACT centrum s.r.o., Postgraduate Education Centre, establishment accredited by the Ministry of Health of the Czech Republic, Praha, Czech Republic

Pavel Přikryl
Department of Orthopaedics and Traumatology, Středomoravská nemocniční a.s, Přerov Hospital, Czech Republic

Šárka Tomková
Faculty of Health in Bánska Bystrica, St Elizabeth College of Health and Social Work in Bratislava, Slovak Medical University in Bratislava, Slovakia

Rafi Moheb
Department of Orthopaedics, Kroměříž Hospital, Czech Republic

Özgür Korkmaz and Melih Malkoç
Department of Orthopedic and Traumatology, School of Medicine, Istanbul Medipol University,Turkey

Munis Ashraf
KG Hospital, Coimbatore, India

Maximilian F. Kasparek and Friedrich Boettner
Adult Reconstruction and Joint Replacement Division, Hospital for Special Surgery, NewYork, NY, USA

Aamir H. Shaikh
North Middlesex University Hospital, London, United Kingdom

Yutaka Inaba, Hiroyuki Ike, Masatoshi Oba and Tomoyuki Saito
Department of Orthopaedic Surgery, Yokohama City University, Yokohama, Japan

Nishant Kumar Singh
Department of Biomedical Engineering, National Institute of Technology, Raipur,India

Sanjay Rai
Biomechanics Lab, School of Biomedical Engineering, Indian Institute of Technology,Banaras Hindu University, Varanasi, India

Amit Rastogi
Department of Orthopedics, Institute of Medical Sciences, Banaras Hindu University,Varanasi, India

Bharati Rajdev and Subash Sivasubramaniam
Sandwell and West Birmingham Hospitals NHS Trust, Birmingham, United Kingdom

Masoud Nasiri Sarvi
Faculty of Engineering, Department of Mechanical Engineering, University of Manitoba,Canada
AI Incorporated, Toronto, Canada

Ulrich Bechler, Bernhard Springer and Friedrich Boettner
Adult Reconstruction and Joint Replacement Division, Hospital for Special Surgery,New York, NY, USA

Guldeniz Argun
Departmant of Anesthesiology and Reanimation, Ankara, Turkey

Chang Park and Irfan Merchant
Royal Berkshire NHS Foundation Trust, Reading, UK

Index

www.ingramcontent.com/pod-product-compliance
Lightning Source LLC
LaVergne TN
LVHW081022210926
848485LV00004B/927